Nutritional Destruction of Black People

(Nutricide)

Llaila O. Afrika

Other books by the Author:

Holistic Self Diagnosis

Health Dictionaries

Pher Ankh

Pills for Every ill That Can Kill

Gullah African American History

Controlling, Understanding, and Raising Black Children

The Power and Science of Melanin

Llaila has a line of specialty disease Remedy Supplements. To order Supplements, Telephone Health Consultations, Health, and Science classes, Lectures, DVD's, and CD's contact:

Llaila Afrika
P.O box 501274
Indianapolis, Indiana 46250
Email: llailaafrika@juno.com
Online classes: llailaafrika.com
Official Website: llailaafrika.com
Telephone Number: 317-216-8088

Holistic Therapies and Education Center

P.O Box 501274

Indianapolis, Indiana 46250

Copyright 2015

ISBN: 9780997658804

Disclaimer

Production:

Melanie D. Stevenson

Cover Design:

Marlon W. Stevenson Jr.

Melanie D. Stevenson

Illustrations:

Llaila O. Afrika

Table of Contents

Forward

This book is a brief look at the current condition of Black people's health. The health of all Black peoples (Diaspora included) is controlled by Caucasians multinational corporations. Black people are forced to use Caucasian phantasy (theory) based medical technology and diagnosis. Black health practitioners accept and believe in Caucasians medical superstitions called theories. Unfortunately, Black people do not understand the far-reaching disease effect of allopathic poisonous medicine and assumptions about Black people's biochemical personalities. Black people are food illiterate and do not have adequate knowledge of how to develop wellness or maintain health. A healthy body is the only vehicle that will make us realize our full holistic potential.

Most Black people believe that if you honestly report Caucasian history and behavior, you hate whites, or are being negative. It is absurd to hate someone for having a disease such as diabetes, cancer, Narcissistic Avaricious Disorder or White Supremacy Psychosis.

It has always irritated me to use Caucasian references when I write, it is as if a Black person cannot have an idea unless it is under written, co-sign, validated by Caucasian research, literature or a degree. This Caucasian information control creates a "Scientific Plantation" and "Information Colonialism." I used some Caucasian references within the text for those Black people that are on the Caucasian's "Information Plantation" and "Myth Plantation". The only books that I recommend as references are books written by Black people, the Ancient Papyrus text books and those listed at the end of this book. Aside from this, Caucasian literature police references are theory based, have Caucasian norm values and Caucasian culture's bias ideas about health. I must follow the Caucasians "Information Plantation" rule of disqualifying everything written in this book, so that the Caucasian can not censor(control)the book and then have me incarcerated for practicing medicine without a Caucasian medical license. Therefore, this next sentence is written. "No statement in this book should be construed as a claim for a cure, treatment or prevention of any disease or should take the place of a licensed or accredited medical practitioner."

It is important that you should know that the Black community has always had traditional natural Healers. These Healers use many different techniques, methods and systems. I find that it is a mistake to compare them as each one of them are using their talent to help. The vast majority of Healers are attempting to help Black people get healthy. I greatly honor the countless ancestors who passed this tradition on. I greatly respect the Black

1

Healers, Herb stores and or Health Food stores that keep traditional natural remedy medicine alive.

To be a Black person is a blessing from God. To be a holistically healthy Black person is wonderful. The only other choice is disease. There is nothing more restrictive than a disease. It is best to be strict and restrictive with your diet than to let a disease like arthritis, fibroid tumors, high blood pressure, herpes, hypertension, kidney failure(dialysis), prostate disease, brain damage (Alzheimer etc.), PMS (Premenstrual Syndrome) or diabetes cause your life to be restricted. There is plenty of health information but very little books on the subject of African centered medicine. I see many Black people in bookstores, health food stores, at lectures, watching White health shows, searching Websites, and at Caucasian health conferences trying to make African centered sense out of the information. They usually become miseducated or dyseducated and frustrated and misinformed.

In this book, I have simplified and concentrated information to provide the reader with knowledge that will help them become African centered in their journey to health. The fight for Black people's holistic existence can be won with an understanding of the Caucasians (see Crave the Cave). Black people are biochemically different from Caucasians. Black people are from one of the oldest ancient civilizations and must be aware that the juvenile Caucasian civilization can not guide them to better health. Caucasian's are a race of "Culture Cannibals" that rape other cultures for science such as Acupuncture, herbal medicine, natural births etc. There is nothing that colored cultures can gain from Caucasians except square dancing. All things gain from Caucasians has side effects such as medicine, treaties, x-rays, nuclear energy, vaccines, GMO foods etc. Black people should search within to create a health system with no side effects

It may take some getting used to, but Black people are a race blessed by the Sun. Black people must be proactive about a non-GMO organic foods diet or else the Caucasians' corporations will destroy the foods with chemicals and destroy planet earth. The devastation of the soil with synthetic toxic chemicals robs the soil of nutrients which destroys more people, animals, insects and plants than nuclear bombs. I beg you, *do not let the Caucasian corporations' junk foods, pharmaceuticals or phantasies(theories) about diseases and health make you a prisoner in your own body*. Black peoples' culture, social life, marriages, relationships, children, economy, health, families, continent and communities are under siege by elite corporate Caucasians, Japanese and China's corporate pirates. Black people are in a junk food, polluted public water, air, clothing and soil combat zone. The fight is for the survival of the children, the Motherland and planet earth. We are in a military situation. The food industry is controlled with military logic. The Caucasians' corporations own the government, courts, science research,

2

spying agencies (NSA, IRS, Google, Facebook, Sprint, Wal-Mart, etc.) economy, police, schools, medias, internet, supreme court, lands, seas and entertainment mediums. The Caucasians are prone to violence and will attack without being provoked. They are military people and use military tactics to seize the advantage in order to dominate and control others or destroy others. Black people cannot use social science such as protest marching and singing entertainment, fighting within the system and voting, money, etc. in a military science situation. There is no such thing as peaceful coexistence or compromise with Caucasian invaders and their military. It is either victory or defeat. Black people are the only race capable of defeating the Caucasian. However, the consumption of junk foods, drugs and alcohol decreases the ability to create victory and accept victory.

Repeat this affirmation daily so that you can change Caucasian corporation's junk foods and Caucasian medicines' surgery and drugs treatments to a natural non-GMO organic foods diet and natural disease remedies. *"I will no longer be part of the nutritional ignorance of my race."* This affirmation, along with herbs that cleanse the organs, blood and colon will help us. A raw non-GMO organic unprocessed foods diet and other African centered healing systems will help change the health. We have got to get the white man (junk food corporations) out of our stomach. Remember nutritional destruction is very deadly because it is a combination of menticide (extermination of the African mind), genocide (extermination of the body by violence, chemicalized junk foods, GMO foods, vaccinations or drugs) and spiriticide (extermination of the African centered spirit). I wrote this book because I *had* to write this book. When I would sit down to relax. My spirit would not be allowed to rest until I tell this holistic truth to you. Holistic health is my language; it is how life communicates to me and how I communicate to life. It is my voice in this life.

Third Eye

This is a photograph of the inside of the human brain. The cells of the brain are magnified to the size equivalent to the size of a car. The electromagnetic galaxy-like cloud in the center is the Eye of Horus (Third Eye). It is inside the brain in a fluid filled space called the Third Ventricle. The Eye of Horus is alive and actively floats above the Pineal Gland. It is cyclic and influenced by your real and imagine thoughts, your biochemical personality, natural and social environment, emotions, diet, radiation, drugs, music, colors and personal relationship.

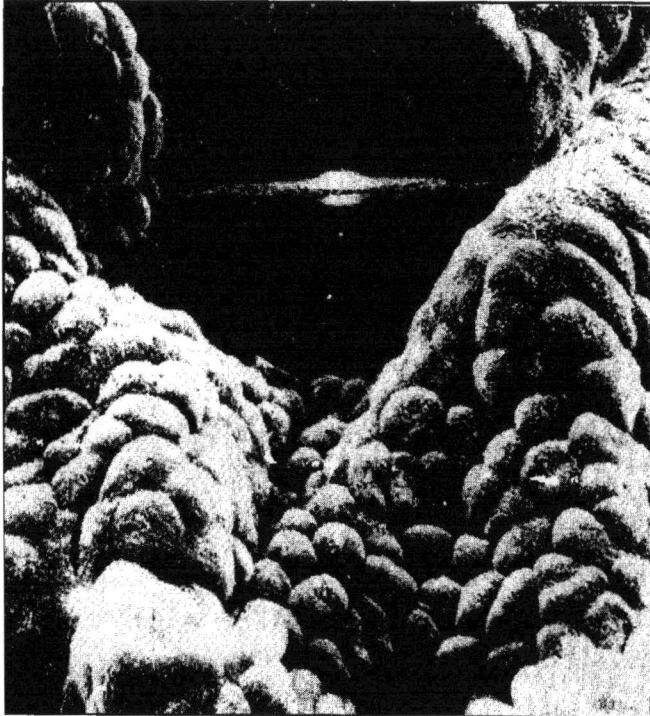

Chapter One

"If a person (*Caucasian*) would send another (Black people) into bondage (*slavery*), he would, it appears to me, be bad enough to send him to hell, if he could."

Harriet Tubman

Crave the Cave

Black people cannot fight for fresh organic fruits and vegetables in their neighborhoods without an understanding of the White corporate own food industries. The ability to organize a winning strategy for better school lunches, snacks, alternative natural medicine, herbal and supplement medicine, care for the elderly and prenatal care requires knowledge of how and why the Caucasian culture's corporations function. The foundation for their corporations is their culture and their culture started in the caves.

The Caucasians have a traceable cave history. Their social life, emotions and behaviors have been written about by and traced by the Greeks. Their cave social histories and negative relationship with Black people are not clearly stated by them. Historically, the Caucasians negative relationship with Black people was influenced by their negative association with the color black. They lived in the blackness of their caves that sometimes had the dim light of candles and fires. The black color subconsciously reminds them of the cave life that they do not face and try to deny. The color black in their culture is believed to be evil and a failure of nature (dyscrasis=bad mix). Before they had contact with Black people they believed black was evil and bad based upon their cave life, philosophy, superstitions and medicine. The ancient Caucasians medical Humors (four fluids) System gave color names for four bodily fluids. The four fluid Humors (temperaments) were 1. Blood (red hemoglobin) = Air, 2. Phlegm (clear liquid) = Water, 3. Yellow Bile (part of bilirubin) = Fire and 4. Black Bile (sickness, an evil in the body) = Earth. These four Humors were believed to be the vital metabolic fluids in the blood and each had Elements (Air, Water, Fire and Earth). They believed that the second part of digestion in the liver produces the four Humors and the waste of bile, urine and sweat.

The four Humors are based upon superstitions, theories, the influence of cave life, myths and Gods. The four Humors are not culturally neutral; they are derived from the culture of ancient cave civilization. The Humors concept has a traceable social progression beginning with the blackness of cave social environment. In the cave social environment, the color red was associated with the red blood from injuries, eating bloody animals, menstruation blood rituals and cave bloody wars. The concept of the element Air in cave philosophy was associated with animal stench of fumes, offensive smelling animal and human manure and stale urine, foul smelling watery phlegm liquid fluids, diseased smells of the snot of colds/flu, sweat odors, tears and diseased spit, the Fire concept came from the burning of wood and the burning of candles made of rancid animal fats, the color brown and black soil smells of rotten waste embedded in the soil of the Earth element and foul human ammonia and sulfur (smell of their moist hair) body stench smells was embedded in the soil of the dirt floors, walls and ceilings. The cavies (cave people) had many gods associated with Elements, especially in Greek mythology Gaia goddess of Earth, Apollo god of life's blood (4 Humors), Zeus and Hades gods of evil underworlds, Hygeia goddess of hygiene provided curses for Black evil diseases etc. Their many gods used miracles, divination, curses, evil fluids, plants, menstruation blood, insects, human and animals sacrifices to do spells and wicked deeds. This provided a deep emotional attachment to colors especially the black color of African people's skin.

In the four Humor (fluids) System the color black was considered a curse of nature and the curse of diseases by the Gods. When the pink colored skin of Caucasians gets injured the skin turns purplish black, they get black eyes from blows and dead necrotic injured or diseased tissue turns black. These physical things are stored in their cave minds. The cave influence on the Caucasian psychic DNA reminds their subconscious that the color black is evil and Black people are ungodly and inferior. In contemporary times, at the end of the backside of the toothpaste tube there is a small square color bar code that indicates the purity of the contents of the paste or gel. The black color bar indicates an inferior un-natural, synthetic, toxic chemical mixture of impure paste; the blue color bar is a toothpaste with drugs and some natural ingredients; red is unnatural and natural ingredients and green indicates natural ingredients and can contain the poison Triclosan a pesticide, fungicide, herbicide that causes cancer, lung and nerve damage which is ban from use by the FDA and only allowed in toothpaste/gel. Caucasians are unaware of their negative attitude towards the color black and label a crashed airplane's computer box that contains data of the cause of the crash is called the black box despite the fact that the box is orange. It is embedded subconsciously in the Caucasian's genes (DNA psychic) that the color black indicates evil, death, bad luck or a curse of the gods. Black people are considered too cursed to be good or evolved and too much of an animal to escape their inferior human nature. The cavies (cave people) essential relationship to Black peoples remains the belief that the black color is a mistake of the gods. White people are unaware that the sight of Black people's black skin stimulates White people's self-hatred. White people hate themselves because they come from caves. Therefore, they subconsciously get rid of their self hatred by criminalizing, lynching or shooting Black people, practicing White Racism, oppression, putting Black people in jail, over charging Black people for loans and interest rates, using racial slurs, having sex with and marrying Black people to feel superior, having dysfunctional Black people on reality shows to satisfy their addiction to their self hatred. The Caucasians exercise their negative beliefs on Black people and their White self-hatred. They store negative beliefs and self hatred in their institutions. Institutions are not alive, people are alive and run institutions. Institutions are an abstract name for groups (tribes) of people acting as an institution (type of tribe). In other words, Caucasian people mistrust Caucasian people (institutions=tribes) because they mistrust and hate themselves.

In the Caucasian social systems and institutions there is built in corruption and mistrust. They mistrust themselves and mistrust of their governments, political groups, scientist research findings, news reportage, manufacturers, companies and industries. The companies and industries maintain misguiding propaganda and diseases that create problems and social paranoia. In modern times, Caucasians do not trust other Caucasians to follow agreed upon rituals (laws, rules, contracts, policies, trade agreements etc.). They have formed standards for drug and food, automobile, appliance, book, medical devices, medical safety procedures, fabrics, clothing, water, housing, machinery, boats, toilet paper, bridges, buildings, roads, toys, sanitation, furniture, vehicles, meat, shoe, and toothpick. Because they mistrust each other they have inspectors to make sure that other Caucasians follow the quality, safety, hygiene and health standards (rituals, rules) of production. Despite inspectors, treaties, laws, standards, rules, security systems, cameras, drones, computer profiling systems, voice and facial recognition, industrial spies, DNA test, fingerprints and various types of rule (rituals) enforcements the Caucasian have not and do not follow their own rules (rituals/ceremonies). These systems of rules (rituals) give the illusion that their crimes against themselves can be eliminated and their systems are self purifying. History is the evidence that White people will not correctly behave (follow rituals). White people do not behave when they are making sure other White people behave. They have rituals (laws, rules) that are used to avoid rituals (rules, laws). They constantly upgrade the corruption of rituals. In their histories cave leaders had corrupt spies and policing enforcement tribes (gangs = armed forces, police force) that disobeyed and corrupted the rituals for corruption. The level of mistrust, corruption, deceit and deception is beyond correcting. It is internally built into their culture. Whenever the Caucasians make a ritual (law, rule) they also make a ritual that allows them to break the ritual called a loophole or amendment. They use their courts, judges or investigation committees to find a way to corrupt their rituals (laws). The indigenous colored races such as Native American Indians told Black people that before they believe the words the White man writes on paper see their many, many treaties (legal agreements) that they have broken with the Native Americans. White people do not behave. They do not obey their own laws (rituals) and do not respect or behave correctly with others race's rituals and human rights of sovereignty. Misbehavior is related to the

8

cave past and built in their social systems and institutions (the institutions of marriage, education, finance, justice, banking, courts, corporations etc.).

In the Caucasian cave past people had no allegiance to countries, rituals and ceremonies. The cave society's social atmosphere put people at constant health safety risk because of diseases, cannibalism, attacks by adult and/or child gangs, attacks by animals and/or insects, unstable weather and food supply shortages. Mentally ill (crazy) children and adults wandered around cave settlements murdering other insane people and murdered sane people, people were constantly exterminating each other with diseases, had fights until death and there were murders in personal relationships and physical and emotional brutality; people were murdered as sacrifices to the gods or murdered to combat a superstition. People could die from injuries, could be sold as a slave, deaths were caused from the drinking of polluted water, sexually transmitted diseases, child birth, eating rotten meat and vegetables and eating diseased people and animals etc. Cavies used spells and superstitions for protection from the weather, bath water, disease, the mentally illnesses, the dead, each other, ghost, the gods, animal attacks, night spirits, defeats in battles, etc.

The cavies believed their allegiance to their mates, families, clans and tribes was temporary. They could not remain faithful or truthful in those relationships. The clans and tribes did not trust each other. This caused a need to use slaves and create human puppets (so called citizens) for a government (clan). The citizens are psychologically seasoned (trained) similar to pet dogs that are trained to protect the owner (clan oligarchy=government). Their pet dogs are substitute Black slaves that they subconsciously miss. An example of mistrust is ethnic groups (tribes, clans) behavior towards each other, in one area of a country the ethnic group tribe called Germans (Danes, Dutch, etc.) would be fighting the Arabs while in another area of the same country the Arabs and Germans would be united to fight the Danes. The ethnic groups such as the British, Germans, French, Portuguese, Chinese, Asians and Spanish continued to have intertribal conflicts and clan gang warfare within their societies. Therefore, there was mistrust, suspicion, corruption, deceit and hatred between ethnic groups within a tribe and ethnic groups such as the French, British, Portuguese, Chinese and Germans. This caused Caucasian oligarchy (small groups that controls people) gangs to mistrust the loyalty of their Caucasian soldiers and sailors. The soldiers and sailors distrusted the loyalty of their clans and tribes to protect their family and land. This resulted in Caucasians tribal oligarchies using Black slave sailors (historically British sailors were 60% Black) and soldiers in their military. The White oligarchies did not fully trust their Black military slaves because at any time the slaves might revolt. Therefore, White tribal oligarchies were forced to unite to protect themselves from themselves.

9

The only thing that kept them united was the social engineering, bonding brain washing of their populations with patriotism (citizenship) to oligarchies (countries control by a small group). The bonding of the people required the use of common rituals and ceremonies (Halloween etc.). Cavies spoke over 200 different languages and Black slaves spoke over 2,000 languages which made language a barrier and unity impossible. African countries have over 100,000 languages. For example, one country such as Nigeria has over 400 languages. The many languages caused people with common languages to bond together against other people with a different language. The hot iron branding of Black slaves on the palms of hands or body parts, cutting off the vaginal lips and the cutting off toes, tongues or ears helped Black people to have a common mutilation bond that unified them against the Whites. The relationship of Black people with White people was always a relationship with corrupt Caucasian clans of criminals. Black people existed in a constant atmosphere of mistrust of Caucasians. When the Black slave soldier or sailor revolted, it intensified the Caucasian mistrust of Blacks. Black people's countries were controlled directly or indirectly by Whites which maintain and sustain White Domination, White Supremacy and White Racism. Therefore, Black people have an unspoken mistrust of White people. Black people had no route that lead to trusting White people. This caused slavery traumatized Black people to constantly maintain an emotional and psychological state of self-defense for protection from cave traumatized Caucasians. This racial unhealthy relationship has many facets. It is doubtful that the untreated slave traumatized disorder of Blacks and the untreated cave traumatized disorder of Whites will ever result in a healthy relationship between the races. If the races could be treated it would be by the use of White psychology's phantasy of Oedipus Complex's divisions of the mind into an animal mind, suppressed animal desires subconscious, consciousness, id, ego, and superego and the Right Hemisphere and Left Hemisphere of the brain Myth. White psychology's therapies are based upon myths and phantasy. They are connected to the emotionality and mentality of cave civilization. The little amount of the social history of cave civilization that is known is not enough to explain what is not understood about Caucasians White supremacy psychosis. Unfortunately, the Caucasians have the vocabulary of intelligent people, but do not have the social, cultural or intellectual history that could produce their claim of intelligence. The Caucasian's words of intelligence and vocabulary is stolen from the ancient Greeks and an Africans. Their vocabulary expands more and more and the meanings of their words explains less and less.

In the past many Caucasian writers have reported on the natural social behavior of Caucasians. And, there is a multitude of documentation of their natural behavior and emotions in cave type literature painted on walls of caves, cave calendars, writing on bones, tools, graves, and fossil remains. The

Caucasian cave remains are treated as if they are not languages. All art and science is a form of cultural languages. Art and sciences are not culturally neutral. Aside from this there are the volumes of the Greek's literature such as the philosopher Plato (428 -347 BC) in his book "The Republic" in seven and eight volumes contains the "Allegory of the Cave" which is an analysis of cave life. In the "Allegory of the Cave" it is revealed that centuries of Caucasians living in caves has effectively caused the Caucasians to have a distorted perception and understanding of reality. The cave society of Caucasian is the foundation and template that they use to create their present and future society. In other words, the cave provides the emotional and intellectual structure for them to have societies and lifestyles. This is explained in their theory based science as "nurture" (social and environmental influences) and "nature" (DNA genetic influence). Nature has left a type of social DNA signature and a self imposed emotional apartheid and emotional schizophrenia (belief of superiority while knowing they are inferior) upon them. The trauma of cave life is buried subliminally and subconsciously in their spirit, emotions, mentality and behaviors. In ancient Greece, Aristotle's (384 -322 BC) student Theophratus (371-287 BC) wrote in 319 BC the play titled "The Characters". In it is a description of the type of emotions, morals, behaviors and mindset of cave traumatized Caucasians. He stated the Caucasian belief that "life is ruled by fortune (superstitions, power over people and material success) not wisdom (morality)". In the play titled "The Characters" written by Theophratus he used different characters to reveal aspects of the Caucasian's emotional and mental personality. In it he used different characters to represent psychological condition of the Caucasian's personalities traits. One of the characters was called "Ironic", this person pretends to talk about having a good personality and good behavior while making mockery of goodness with cruel words and thug behaviors; there is a character called the "Flatterer" which is their personality trait of being an insincere person acting nice and giving excessive praise to others in order to exploit them; the character of "Garrulous" trait is of Caucasians to inferiorize others with excessive rambling words in order to be superior, the "Boor" type personality trait uses inappropriate words to steal from people so that they can charge them for trying to find what was stolen; "Unreasonable" type trait of a rude ill-mannered Caucasian that has distrust of people that are trustful, "Officious" trait of having a high opinion of themselves and giving unrequested talk of freedom and justice while taking away another person or race's freedom and justice; "Complaisant" is their personality trait that means the lack of intelligence and understanding of truth and uses untruthfulness while letting others search for truthfulness in White peoples untruth; "Stupid" their personality trait of acting agreeable, unable to understand themselves or others, lack the ability to use just and gracious to help while they deny others their rights; "Reckless" doing exploitative unstructured defiant acts to others with no concern about the harm it does to others; "Avaricious" appetite that cannot be satisfied with more objects/money, this causes them to constantly ignore others human rights and sovereignty while increasing behaviors to take other's sovereignty, land and resources, they can only be satisfied by taking more of other people's sovereignty land and resources; "Patron Rascal" trait that causes the use of cruel dishonest annoying ways to commit crimes that are illegal and immoral; "Evil Speaker" their motives is to be deceitful and always belittle others intelligence with no intention of talking mannerly; "Late Learner" personality aspect that causes them to be slow to understand, their desire to be intelligent exceeds their ability to be intelligent; "Oligarchy" a type of tribalism that unifies a small minority group that exploits the majority of the people; "Coward" a behavior that causes them to socially engineer others to be heroic and fight battles, invasions and wars that protects their wealth and rights not to fight battles, "Arrogant" personalities that assumes their intelligence is above the ignorant listeners; "Boastful" always brags about themselves as a higher civilized person in all matters, "Mean" their goal is to defeat the loser with deceit and deception, then destroy the loser's culture and history, they constantly character assassinate the losers personality, harass and embarrass the loser for fun and enjoyment; "Petty Ambitions" their trait that causes them to take important things from others, and stay successful by taking things of no importance or of no consequence or value to their success; "Unpleasant" a trait which creates the need to cause others discomfort and pain by being offensive self-righteously superior; "Pompous" pretends to know or discover all knowledge; "Offensive" likes to cause hurt to others, exploited them, displeased them while claiming to be giving pleasure to others; "Distrust" others and feels that other people's morality, intelligence and abilities cannot be trusted, "Grumbler" excessive obsessive compulsive ranting, whining and complaining about other people's being inferior while claiming themselves to be superior; "Superstitious" beliefs without rational or emotion proof, they believe that nature and reality is a mistake, they have no rational process to connect their ideas to each other and use myth or fantasy ideas to prove their beliefs, "Tactless" bluntly offends others and lacks sensitivity of others culture; "Thankless" does not appreciate others contributions; "Backbiter/Backstabber" when others are not present they commit slanderous negative attacks on others reputation; "Rough" speaks of irregularities of other others character and assume they are perfect; "Vicious" grossly immoral and depraved; "Surly" behavior of having a discourteous, rude, sullen bad temper attitude with others and expecting others to accept their attitude , "Gossip(Newsmonger)" uses a constant flow of rumors, fake stories, unfound facts and idle misplaced ideas about others , "Shameless" lack of respect, they have no feelings of disgrace for their unacceptable behavior while taking other peoples sovereignty, land and resources. They emotionally, psychologically and physically exterminate people, "Penurious" miserly, stingy with wealth (billionaires) while others are starving, homeless, unemployed and poverty stricken; "Gross" hoards wealth and resources while simultaneously creating more poverty for others etc. Other critiques of the Caucasian's character logic are Overbury's characters in Sir Thomas Overbury's poem "A Wife (1615)", Titus Maccius Plautus (254-184 BC) play about the flawed behavior and personalities of White heroes and great White people, the "Characters of Virtues and Vices" (1608, by Joseph Hall, Bishop of Exeter) and "Barbarian" a play by William Anderson.

Any specific Caucasian personality trait can be active or stimulated separately, or in simultaneous combination or clusters. Any of the traits can be stimulated emotionally, intellectually, subconsciously, indirectly and or directly. The reaction to a trait stimulation can not be satisfied by any specific emotion or behavior. The trait that is dominate (strong) or sub dominate (weak) at one moment can shift to another stimulus response trait within the same moment (find an outlet of anger etc.). This short term and long term memory switching is caused by the emotional value (crazy response) the Caucasians apply to a behavior. Unstable and mixed negative responses (weird, crazy) to normal actions and reactions of Black people. This is a trait that stems from the poor emotional intelligence (craziness) of the mental illness (being crazy) of cave trauma. The problem with any White rationale (word order) thought process psychology (based upon their fairytale myth) is it has mental blind spots. This causes the inability to be mentally healthy (sane).

A critique of the character traits of the Caucasians are in the Greek play titled "The Characters" and a July 4,1852 speech of the ex-slave Frederick Douglas (1818-1895). A collection of the words he used in his speech to describe Caucasians are; emotionally and intellectually unjust, unreasonable and oppressive, plotters of mischief, act hideous and revolting, false to the past and false to the present, have blasphemy in thought, have swelling vanity, do crimes which would disgrace a nation of savages, they are opposed to laws of God and of man, they hate all change but silver, gold and copper change, have no principles of right action nor bowels of compassion, to them humanity is a base pretense, they are imposters, have personalities with customs of hurtful character, shameless disregard of the forms of administering law, they are involved in the most awful responsibility of which the mind can conceive, convert the very name of religion into an engine of tyranny and barbarous cruelty, notoriously hate all men whose skins are not colored(white), they have doubtful application of the principles of justice, practice inhuman mockery and sacrilegious irony, mercy to them is a crime,

13

do evil work with social impunity, breed insolence, rob religion of its significance making it utterly worthless etc. When he was a slave he observed them in their private lives, religious practices, business dealings, sexual and family behaviors, slave treatments, rape of children and while free he worked for them in business, served in their government and gain undisputed insightfulness.

White peoples emotional and physical behaviors cause many White conscious humanistic individuals and groups to try to make the majority of White people behave correctly. Conscious white groups use social movements, politics , protest and strikes against the corrupt minority rulers of the White banking industry, (oligarchies), they protest against low wages, protest against the oil drilling, pipelines and oil fracking companies, protest against putting people off welfare, polluted public water, microfibers and prescription drugs in public water, debtor's prison, creating homeless people, they death penalty, police violence, prison companies, invasions of countries, predatory loans, cost of drugs and hospitals, protest against war, GMO foods, student debt, rape on college campuses and in military, child abuse, etc. The constant attempts by a few conscious Whites to make other Whites behave will fail because White people as a group ignore White Supremacy Psychosis, Post Traumatic Cave Disorder, and Narcissistic (love of self= White Supremacy) Avaricious (always wants more) Disorder. They need treatment for their addiction to their emotional illnesses and treatment for their emotional illnesses. The cultural roots of their lifestyle have to be clearly defined without social science and psychology type of words. This could help them to see their combinations of mental and emotional illnesses.

All human social behavior is confined to two types of activities which are; 1. Rituals, and 2. Ceremonies. The Caucasians use different names for rituals such as rules, tradition, sex mating, treaties, agreements (shared rituals), romance, manners, economics, physical fights, courtesy, laws, principles, grammar (word order), laboratory test, games, order, mathematic formulas, music, crimes, etc. Ceremonies are given various names such as a court of law trial, athletic competitive games, weddings, parades (marching), capital torture punishment executions, news programs and newspapers (history ceremonies), education classroom academic ceremonies, war, funerals, internet social media, etc. When you have a ritual, and add other people or food, dance, music, specific clothing, candles, bells it becomes a ceremony.

Caucasians are controlled by the "Rule of Mobs". Mob control has many different names such as surveys, polls, statistics, the idea of an average person fantasy, consensus opinions, think tanks, banks, Wall Street corporations, democratic voting (majority of people have oppression over the minority), movie ratings, board of directors (clans), staff (clans), juries, councils, committees (clans), licensing boards (clans), riots, lynching's, talk show panels, etc. These types of mob rule are used to get the people to follow the opinion of a select few. It is oligarchy disguised as the belief of the majority while it is in effect the minority of the few people that put together the process (ritual) for doing the statistics, survey, polls, consensus, riot, lynching etc. (see books Microbiology, Mob Rule by Adrian Woolfson, The Myth of Mob Rule by Lisa Miller and Mob Rules by Louis Ferrante).

There are negative affects of being an abandoned cave child. Many Children did not know their birth parents, siblings or relatives. The children were used as money, soldiers, slaves prostitutes and this has caused an emotional injury to the child. The injury is carried into adulthood. The child's conception could have been from sexual intercourse between father and daughter, mother and son, sister and brother, an orgy or a product of rape. These abandon children had a social life that permanently traumatize them. In cave life, a child is prevented from reacting to their fears. The child has no choice but to suppress and inferiorize their awareness of fears. The continuous suppression of fears dysfunctionalizes their emotional network of nerves causing them to escape that fear emotion with violence, anger, rape, self-hatred and abandonment of reality into craziness. Aside from this, incest biochemically causes a high degree of mental illness and emotional birth defects. Currently in the USA, 1 out of 5 White marriages are between cousins because of the imprint of their ancient cave life. This contributes to Caucasian social acceptable emotional illness called normal behavior. Cave children were disciplined with physical violence, hair pulling, beatings with sticks or stoned (beaten by throwing rocks at them), herded by dogs, slept with dogs and developed a special unending bond to dogs. The children hunted rodents, pigs and insects to eat, drank the breast milk of dogs, lambs, pigs or a breastfeeding female, drank blood, ate stillbirth dead children, ate placentas, raped each other, were used in human sacrifice rituals, played with each other and animals, masturbated, and had fights with each other.

Children formed gangs to protect themselves from other dysfunctional wild children. The Children gangs were a way for a single abandon or group of abandon children to protect themselves from adults and other children gangs. Many runaway children formed gangs and child cave communities. They formed raiding parties that roamed in the wild and attacked adult cavies and other children gangs. Many herds of abandoned wild children roamed day and night terrorizing individuals and settlements. Currently emotionally abandoned children form internet social media gangs that raid other child chat rooms, bully, torture and do character assassinations on other children. This sometimes leads to suicides or physical violence, emotional abuse, rape and or terrorist activities. The activities of cave gangs are in the modern books and movies such as the "Lord of the Flies" by William Golding.

15

Caucasians can easily relate to the abandoned child themes in stories such as the abandon children called Superman, Cadillac, Chrysler, Pinocchio, Snow White (a slut that had sexual relationships with 7 men), Cinderella, Hansel and Gretel, Jesus, The Old Lady (slut and single mother) that Lived in a Shoe (father abandon the children), Little Red Riding Hood (father abandon her and her mother abused her) etc. They enjoy stories about cave rodents such as mice (Mickey Mouse, Mighty Mouse etc.), bats (batman), the rodent in the rat family called a rabbit such as Bugs Bunny, Easter Bunny, Ever Ready rabbit, Playboy Bunny rabbit, and spiders (Spiderman), dogs (Rin Tin Tin, Lassie) etc.

The social DNA for the current Caucasian societies is the caves. The Caucasians recipes and diets started in the caves such as eating rare, and or raw bloody meat, cooking foods that can be eaten raw such as spinach, celery, onions, potatoes, kale, cabbage, fresh wheat berries, apples, orange (pasteurized=cooked), tomatoes, poor food combining, seasoning food, fried foods, etc. Their dietary, family and sexual behaviors origin is from the caves. The Greek fairytale Oedipus myth reveals cave sex. The boy Oedipus wanted to have sex with his mother so he murdered his father, then his mother married him and had sex with him and had children. The myth exposes Caucasians sexual relationship behaviors.

Caucasians had heterosexual and homosexual relationships. In Greek culture, men would have a "best man" which was their homosexual lover. The term "Platonic" friendship was used for the same sex homosexual marriage, it was named after Plato's homosexual marriage. The Greeks would select sex mates at orgies held in gymnasiums. The gymnasiums were used for socializing, political meetings, business meetings, pornographic plays, philosophical discussions, exercising, sports and all the activities included sex. Homosexual mates were selected by a pat on the buttocks. Male homosexual prostitutes were called parasites or a "hore (whore)". The "whore" performed sexual acts for pay similar to a hore hound dog that performed tricks and acts for their master (owner) for the payoff of food, masturbation, oral and physical sex with their master.

There were no formal cave marriages. Sexual relations were sporadic and temporary types of rape or shared acts of sexual intercourse (orgy). Incest was normal and used to breed additional "people herds", slaves, herds of breeding women or wives. Polygamous or group type multiple marriages of an entire cave village were formed by incest and harem sexual intercourse. These were open polygamous marriage in which the individual freely had sex with others. Women were kept in harem gangs to be used as slave labor for hunting, agriculture work, prostitutes, or military units. Harem gangs fought each other for possession of caves, food or men for breeding. The women harem groups had women slaves that protected their caves. The heterosexual and homosexual women were used as money, breast milk providers for men, women and children, childcare services, indentured slaves or rented out to others.

Charles Darwin (1809-1882) used economic science theories(superstitions) to develop his superstitious belief called the Theory of Evolution. Darwin believed the White race started in the cave past as a race of primitive humanoid type animals. Darwin's superstitious myth called The Theory of Evolution claimed that a slimy reptile like creature that lived in a cave under water crawled out of the sea. And, this creature crawled to a land cave and eventually became a white skin furless ape. The furless ape climbed up into a tree and fell out of the tree grunted and started walking and eventually became the modern white man. The primitive reptile like Caucasian existence were Darwin's subconscious words for the Caucasian cave civilization. Darwin stated that the modern White man (Caucasians) still has the thought and emotional reptile like cave brain DNA genes. Darwin and Freud substituted symbolism and superstitious words for the cave past. They like most Caucasians are in denial about their cave social past. Denial is part of Trauma Disorders. The traumatized disease causes blindness to the obvious. A traumatized and mentally ill people develop blind spots in their ability to send and receive emotional, moral, psychological, and relationship ideas. The blind spot is similar to the natural physical visual blind spot(scotoma) in which the optic nerve inside each eye blocks the retina nerve from detecting an image (natural blindness) and limits the eyes visual range of sight. The most difficult thing for emotionally ill cave traumatized Caucasians to do is to see and accept the obvious. It is obvious that Caucasians came from a cave society. It is admitted by Caucasian historians and symbolically and theoretically admitted by Freud and Darwin. Freud only did psychoanalysis and research on Caucasians. Therefore, his theories and conclusions about psychology are exclusively derived from the White mind. Incidentally Darwin's economic basis for evolution superstition is not correct, the ancient Africans and ancient Greeks taught and classified economics as a philosophy (social science) not as a form of economic mathematics. Economics is the practice of using propaganda to make people emotionally desire a product (sneakers, diamonds, cars, clothes, perfume, etc.) and then creating an emotional value for the product. For example, people want to emotionally satisfy their desires. Their desires were created by advertisements/commercials. And they want to own the advertised product to satisfy their emotional desire to have something of emotional value. Economics is the emotional manipulation of people to satisfy their emotional desire to be unique (different from others) and have an emotional valuable (important) life. It is a form of fantasy used to escape their cave life in order to believe that material satisfaction gives emotional satisfaction of desire and value. Only a cave culture that existed in funky dirt caves would give emotional value to yellow dirt (gold), silver dirt or transparent dirt rocks (diamonds).

The cavies have an emotional need to escape. They emotionally deny their cave beginnings by escaping into others' countries with invasions that they call exploration. They call their invasion of Africa, the Americas and America's islands (Caribbean, etc.) exploration instead of violent invasions, extermination and enslaving of peoples, colonizing and stealing of natural resources. Their invasion of China is called the Opium War, invasion of South Africa the Boer War. They did invasions of Korea and Vietnam. The oligarchy that economically controlled the northern American colonies plan the invasion of the southern colonies to capture the control of the southern oligarchy's production and wealth was called the Civil War. The Caucasian clans and tribe's invasions, murdering and stealing of colored peoples (red, brown, yellow and Black race) human resources and natural resources and lands were not called invasions they were called explorations or wars.

The cavies in the invasion armies of clans and tribes had no allegiance to their country. Their allegiance is to their ethnic groups of clans and tribes. They created the borders in other people's countries and created countries. This is the oligarchies method of dividing up the land and dividing peoples so that the people can not fight back as a united group. The Brussels Conference (1890) and the Congo (Berlin) West African Conference (1884-1885) allowed White countries of thieves to divided land between themselves. They eventually divided Africa into countries. France, Britain and Germany got occupation and control over the most African countries, Belgium controlled the Congo and Niger River basin and killed over 50% of the Black people. Cecil Rhodes murdered over 2,000 Zimbabweans (Rhodesians) each week in southern Africa. Later in history, Sargent Major Mahatma Gandhi in the British Army murdered Black people in the Boer War. He never apologized for the murders and all his life thought Black people were inferior and could never enter heaven because they were chosen by God to be forever untouchable/Dalit in the lowest caste. Dalit are the 160 million Black people in India. Dalit is a word that means niggers. It was the Ottoman Empire (1453) that invaded Constantinople (built in 7 B.C., known as Istanbul) that blocked the Caucasians from having complete control of India, North Africa and the Red Sea. The Portuguese had to avoid invading south west Asia because of the Mongol Empire (Genghis Kahn). This allowed the Arabs and eventually France, Britain and Portugal to control the Trans-Pacific Slave Trade and sell African slaves to China and India.

The cavies currently invade and explore planets, under sea and outer space, improve genetically modified animals, plants and insects, nuclear radiated foods, artificial foods rather than explore their cave civilizations and

18

improve their cave life understanding. The Post Traumatic Cave Trauma Disorder and their Narcissistic Avaricious Disorder is an emotional and mental illness. Denial of their juvenile delinquent civilization, self-hatred and the cave social life is a disease too diseased to see a reality. They use their fantasy psychology, symbols, myths and superstitions with abstract numbers (called science theories) to see reality.

The fantasy superiority complex of White Supremacy is part of their Narcissistic Avaricious Disorder and is their cave reality. White people as a group are cultural infants that think that they can walk without crawling. The majority of White people desire to escape their exploited social life by escaping into the ruling oligarchy minority. They in effect want to recreate the social disease that is destroying them. Cavies desire to escape their emotional contradiction by creating a mental illness state with the consumption of synthetic chemicals to get stimulated or high or drunk. They use recreational synthetic chemical drugs to create a mental illness condition which they call being high, drunk, or feeling good. The typical drugs are the concentrated chemicals of nicotine, caffeine, synthetic chemicals from burnt tobacco and marijuana plant leaves, refined sugar, alcohol, stimulants, psychoactive drugs, methamphetamine, morphine, opium, cocaine and other types of narcotics. These synthetic drugs alter the mind, mood, emotions, physical biochemistry and state of consciousness which means they make you mentally and emotionally ill (crazy) or so called give you a high or good feeling. This diseased mental illness feeling is the state of emotions and mentality that they had in caves called Cave Traumatic Stress Disorder. Diseased feelings and sickness was their state of being normal. The cave life of the oppression of reality would make a normal person crazy and denies the development of the ability to behave properly. Expecting the mentally ill Caucasians to behave normal is in itself a mental illness. The denial and oppression of cave civilization and culture adds to their Cave Trauma mental illness. In a constant traumatized state, it is difficult to select behaviors. The mind is filled with thoughts of "I could do this" and "I should do that". It is doubtful that proper selection of thoughts and behaviors could be made and if made they could not be performed by a mind drunk in a cave reality.

Behaviors are developed from a people's culture, parents, physical environment, social conditions and innate DNA. An examination of a people's behavior is connected to their past. Anthropology and Archeology are sciences that use their culture as a filter for the examination of a race of people's past. These sciences indicate that the cave past of 40,000 years ago is considered pre-history because there are not formally written book records of the cave people during that era except cave wall and ceiling paintings, symbols on graves, hunting devices, utensils and markings on tools. The paintings are not decorations any more than African Egyptian hieroglyphics are decorations. The cave paintings are a type of written language. The writings use bison, horses, hunting scenes, calendars, Aurochs, deer, finger flutings, spotted horses, decorated cows, women, birds and people swimming to communicate ideas. Cave writings are of the Stone Age (2 million to 30,000 years ago) can be found in the Americans, Spain, Germany, France, England, Australia, Chauvet Cave in France (30,000 BCE), Coliboaia Cave in Romaina, etc. Caucasian cave life is depicted in the movie "Brute Force" by D.W. Griffiths, a 1914 silent film, and in cartoons such as Flintstones. The Caucasians do not reveal the social conditions of the Neanderthals or the Paleolithic period, or the two Caucasians species of Australopithecines multiple branches. However, the writings of the Greeks and Romans reveal the behaviors and mentality of those Caucasians coming out of the caves.

In social science traces (derivatives) of a people's current behavior is connected to their past behavior. And, the symbols such as letters, numbers, designs, art figurines, geometrics, graves, hunting tools, clothing, foods, weapons, decorations and cooking utensils connect to a social past, superstitions, social ideas and social behaviors. The books "A Book of the Beginnings" by Gerald Massey and "Pher Ankh" by Llaila Afrika provide methods for recovering and reconstituting a people's origin by using derivatives of symbols, language and behaviors.

Black folks should be aware of Caucasian cave mentality and social history. Instead, Black folks focus on critiques and analysis of colonial Caucasians and slave history. Over 99% of Black history books (includes Egyptian History) are written by Caucasians for Caucasians while less than 1/100 of 1% of the subject of White history are written by Blacks for Blacks. Without reportage of a Black perspective on the cave social origin of White Civilization, Black peoples fight for freedom will be similar to a blind man with a gun shooting at unseen shadows of people. An old African proverb can help reveal a truthful understanding of White people, if you want to know the truth about the hunting of Lions for the Deer's do not ask the Lion ask the Deer. Unfortunately, Black people ask White psychology and White history's perspective (Lion) and White psychology (Lion) about the hunting of Deer instead of African-Centered Black scientist and historians (the Deer's). Cave social history reveals that White Domination of other peoples human and natural resources is supported by their belief of White Supremacy which is defended by White Racism. Oddly enough, Black folks have untreated Post Traumatic Colonial/Slavery Disorder while Whites have Post Traumatic Cave Disorder. Untreated disorders will stop a healthy relationship between the two races. The cultural centers (cosmology) of the races are in conflict. And, they have different social values and suffer from the side effects of centuries without conflict resolution between the races. For example, White civilization advances and improves itself with gadgets, robots, promises of the future, theories, gene editing's, Nano surgery and robotic surgery, computers, artificial intelligence, GMO, drugs, money, war, space exploration and new material goods. Black civilization advances itself by improvements in the lives of children, the elderly, the family and the male/female relationships. This is two different cosmologies (cultural centers) and value systems. Only freedom from Cave Trauma and Slavery Trauma can produce the level of intelligence needed to resolve the problems of the white and Black races.

White Domination, White Supremacy and White Racism are extensions of the social DNA of Caucasian cave civilization. The military, jails, school systems, games, wars, government, slavery, entertainment, colonialism, drug and food industry are extensions of the cave civilization. These social activities cannot escape the DNA roots of cave civilization. Caucasians carry the social DNA traits of their original cave social system. Within their society are the social tools used to dominate and control Black folks with misdirection, deception, corruption and bait and switch tactics of military logic. Consequently, White Domination, Supremacy, Racism and military logic are new names for the old cave behavior characteristic of Avaricious, Mean, Offensive, Vicious, Shameless, Superstitious, Surly, Backbiter, Pompous, Offensive, Petty Ambitions, Arrogant, Coward, Boastful, Patron Rascal, Reckless, Officious, Boor, Garrulous, Flatterer, Ironic, Grumbler etc. It is typical of cavies to use computers, wars, education, institutions, sex, artificial Caucasian intelligence, drones, gadgets and genetically modified organism, antibiotics, pesticides, gene editing, herbicides and processed food as weapons to dominate others. The White Domination, White Supremacy and White Racism problems cannot be solved using Caucasian cultural rituals and ceremonies called psychology, laws, science, treaties, agreements (rituals) and religion (ceremonies).

The problem is the thinking used to solve the problem creates the problem. Thinking that something outside yourself such as a savior, a prophet, gadget, miracle, science, multicultural concepts, nature, etc. can save you from yourself instead of confronting the diseased cave social behavior and mentality that causes problems. Thinking that improvements of an automobile's motor, car's safety features, future science advancements, head and tail lights of cars, tires, gasoline or electric fuel makes driving safer instead of improvement in driving skills such as alertness, reaction time, driving free of prescription drugs, talking on phones, text messages and free of marijuana and alcohol consumption makes driving safer. It is typical of cavies linear thinking to improve gadgets (material objects) or weapons of war instead of improving the social and economic conditions which lead to stopping wars.

The social, physical, emotional, dietary and economic violence against Blacks cannot be changed by the tactic of singing and marching forms of protest entertainment (ceremony). Black folks have made the tactic of singing and marching (strut dance), voting, carry protest signs, giving speeches, being jailed for protesting, and getting White permits to protest the way to get freedom. Protest has become a way of life instead of a tactic to use. The protest entertainment (ceremony) type marches with songs and speeches do not cure the cave mentality and will not create sovereignty and the human right of freedom. Aside from this, Black slaves were brought to Americas and Caribbean to serve White folks as cotton, cane and crop pickers, work in mines and work as fishermen, carpenters, cowboys, tailors, doctors, deep sea divers, linguist, pornographic entertainers, midwives, medical experiment subjects, musicians, soldiers, book keepers, sailors, teachers, sports entertainers (i.e. boxers), music and dancing entertainers. And, today Black folks still resort to entertainment of White folks and themselves with the singing and marching entertainment as a form of protest and civil unrest disobedience entertainment ceremonies. In any case, currently Black folks entertain themselves with singing and marching protest (ceremonies). It is obvious that Black lives matter to businesses especially the private prison industries, Chinese restaurants, wig stores, special education, junk food stores, illegal drugs, bleaching crème and hair relaxer industries which are controlled by the oligarchy Chinese and East Indians capitalist. White owners of businesses depend upon Black lives for profits such as professional sports entertainments (soccer, boxing, basketball, football, etc.), predatory loan, payday loan, pawn shops, men's depilatory (shaving heads bald), furniture and appliance rental companies, alcohol beverage industries, used car industries, school dropout industries, criminal justice and bail bond industries, etc.

It is the method of thinking that creates the problem instead of creating a solution. For example, when a child has problems in school the teacher usually gets a solution by consulting the parents to get the child's behavioral history and to understand how the parent may be contributing to or creating the problem. Consulting parents helps to arrive at a solution to the student's problems. When White Domination, Supremacy and Racism causes the problem then consult (examine) the social parent of Caucasian culture the cave civilization. Instead of looking at cave society, Black folks examine oppression, the school system, voting, profiling, politics, institutional racism, White privilege, slavery, colonialism, the police force, poverty, unemployment and drugs. They are part of the problem but not the creation of the problem. Oddly enough, there are many Black and White people addicted to watching White people misbehave. The White People Watchers are similar to Bird Watchers that observe the bird's colors, mating, fights, flight movements and feeding and do nothing about it. White People Watchers get excited about gossiping (news programs) about the Caucasian's misbehaviors and watching

22

misbehaving individuals, governments, organizations, politicians, businesses, police and militaries. They give each other White People Watchers awards (Pulitzers, Izzy awards etc.), get degrees in the analysis of misbehavior, do independent media reports, make movies, write books, make documentaries films that investigate White misbehavior. White people seem totally surprise that other White people misbehave. The White People Watchers constantly talk about current misbehavior as if it is new misbehavior. White People Watchers believe that they are exposing truths that will eventually cleanse White people's culture of corruption and somehow cleanse their lives of cave DNA behavior.

White Supremacy belief is used to identify a few types of selected White behaviors. White Supremacy could not and cannot invent itself. White Supremacy is an attribute derived and invented from culture. It is a mental illness belief that a race's white skin automatically makes their race intelligent and their culture superior to all colored races particularly the Black race. Beliefs have their origin in culture. Culture uses rituals and ceremonies called rules, taboos, traditions, laws, proper and improper behaviors, art, science, religions, cosmology, dress, folktales, fairy tales, songs, games and language to bond people together (civilizes them). Culture uses ritual and ceremony socialization processes to create citizens. People that share the same ethics (rituals and ceremonies) are called an ethnic group (i.e. Bantu, Ashanti, French, and German). The source of Ethnic groups behaviors are in their recorded history. The source of African people's world view (cosmology), lifestyles, sovereignty and traditions of Maat = truth, justice, balance, harmony and reciprocity can be found in ancient hieroglyphic writings, text books (papyrus) and pyramid text. Incidentally, indigenous sovereign Black Africans (Black diaspora) are made to think of themselves as citizens of a former White colony or a citizen of the White country of their birth. They do not claim a worldwide indigenous native's citizenship of Africa with sovereign human rights privilege nor are they recognized by Whites as indigenous sovereign natives of Africa. Black people claim a White citizen's civil rights (rituals)of a Caucasian country. They are trained to be citizens (follow the White rituals) under White Domination instead of citizens of the planet earth and Africa. The source of the present day White domination, White Supremacy and White Racism can be found in cave literature (so called drawings), Greek writings and modern day writings on the subject of the subconscious and evolution. The White Supremacy belief is an extension of Caucasian's cave culture.

The impact of cave culture upon present day Caucasians is consistently denied, ignored and believed to be non-existent. The impact of cave life causes the disease of Post Traumatic Cave Disorder. The terrifying cave life experience distorts emotions, moods and states of consciousness resulting in severe anxiety, intellectual treason, self-hatred, uncontrollable emotions, thoughts, beliefs and behaviors, real and unreal subconscious flashbacks, avoidance of facing reality, negative feelings about others (colored races), numbness to others feelings about White supremacy, difficulty in maintaining healthy relationships (with the Black race), aggressive violence (lynching, profiling, shooting of Blacks), self-destructive addictions (drugs, sex, gambling, White racism, wars, etc.) and denial of the cave trauma (Whites believe they are normal). Caucasians deny themselves a psychosocial examination of the cave life that created their culture. Caucasians suffer from "Pathological Incredulity" which means that the mention of their primitive uncivilized behaviors is too incredible to believe. Therefore, they do not believe or accept the Black person's statement about Caucasian's juvenile primitive behaviors. The Caucasians dismiss the statements about White people's violent nature as Black anger or Blacks dismisses statements of crude cave primitive behavior as too incredible to believe. "Pathological Incredulity" causes Blacks to dismiss reality. However, an examination of cave culture behavior of White Supremacy can reveal their reality. The meaning of "Pathological Incredulity" is Pathological = sick and Incredulity = ideas that seem too abnormal and too incredible to believe.

White Domination, White Supremacy and White Racism are modern terms that identify the behavioral traits of cavies. They are not self-created behaviors but behaviors that crawled out the caves with the Caucasian. The modifications in present day Caucasians civilization behaviors are very small and reflect their past. They cannot escape their social DNA past with new names such as "White privilege", "Accidents of Peculiarities of the Subconscious". The "subconscious" trait is metaphorically defined in Plato's ancient Greek play titled "Analogy of the Divided Line" which is in his books titled the Republic.

The classification of body fluids (4 humors) was an outgrowth of the cavies classifying evil spirits, and lesser spirits that controlled and influenced the weather, darkness, rocks, birth, the dead, smoke, animals, plants, fire, ghost, sex, sounds, dreams, the wind, the Gods, war, bowel movements, pain, the placenta, insects and disease. This was followed by the classification of people called the "Great Chain of Being". At the top of the chain was the superior White man followed by the good and bad inferior White women, then Asian, dead people and lastly the inferior Black people that were assumed to be ape-like humans. According to the cave idea of "Great Chain of Being" hierarchical rule was natural, fixed and cannot be changed. The problems with the White race and Black race cannot be resolved without therapeutic intervention. It is stated in Natural History by Jared Diamond that "No two peoples on Earth were less equipped to understand each other".

Asking the Caucasian scientist and historians to explain cave life is similar to asking a drunk (chemically alcohol intoxicated) to explain the biological, emotional and intellectual effect of being drunk. Obviously, it's best to ask a non-intoxicated person to explain the drunken condition. White people do not know what they do not know about the cave life. Every word they use to explain their cave life subtracts from their intelligence and adds to their ignorance. White supremacy belief protects them from the consequences of their ignorance. Using social deconstruction of their current civilization, behavior analysis, ancient Greek and Roman writers that observed cavies, cave writings, games, customs, superstitions, myths, war tactics, food supplies, fossil manure and their myth (Oedipus) and theories (left and Right Brain Theory) of psychology can help to expose their past and present lifestyles. They deny their current behaviors is from cave primitiveness. Denial is part of Caucasians Cave Trauma Disorder. Consequently, they do not talk about or examine the psychological impact of their cave beginnings. White people as a group do not know their cave history and do not want to know the cave history. They are missing an understanding of themselves. They must accept that a tree (culture) grows from its roots (cave civilization).

The remnants of cave social functions are in White people's modern life. For example, the oligarchy owners of the computer industry (tribes of corporate elite) have a herd of peasant computer laborers (slaves) that must give away their un-copyrighted intellectual property (ideas) to the cave chief. All intelligence belongs to the chief. The chief acquired his position by being able to steal from others (a good thief), a good hunter, terrorist, invader and warrior. This violence gave the chief power over cave settlements. His position attracted clans and tribes of cave people to his cave for a livelihood, protection and a source of food. The chief acquired land, human and natural resources, livestock, food stock and people stock. The exploitative corrupt means of getting stock was never more important than the end result of power. In other words, the end results justify (wealth) the means(slavery). The method used to get the results is not important only results are important. Products (commodities) equal to money which means power which means control over people. Money is a form of people (stored labor) and represents the people that money can and does control. The more money you have the more people you can control (own). People are a commodity to be used, misused and abused. Protection was provided by the chief's ability to attract warriors, raiders and invaders. This social structure varied from one chief in a single cave to another chief with cave villages (settlements).

Warfare with other cave settlements was influenced by the food supply of the cave settlement, weather, topography and superstitions. Cave warfare attacks were usually during the daytime because at night they could easily mistake their cave friends for the enemy. There were comparatively few battles in early summer or early winter. More attacks were in spring and early autumn because they had food stored inside of their caves and cave attackers needed food eat. Cereal crops and animal feeds were stored inside caves. Unfortunately, cereals stored inside caves were easily flammable which made fire a weapon to use to burn cereals, people, animals, fur and leather clothing, grass, straw and wood huts inside caves. Cave settlers were in constant fear of vandalism, arson and raids for stealing food, animal stock, dogs and cats. Ironically, men leaving their cave to fight battles left their families unprotected. This caused many families to be stolen, murdered, and boys, girls, men and women were raped. The attackers of caves would mentally terrorize returning warriors to their cave settlements by leaving the bodies of the dead people with eyebrows beaten down into the eye, and fingers, penis, noses, ears and breast completely cut off, scalps removed, teeth beaten out of the mouth, amputated heads on sticks and or tied to the necks of the dead, amputated feet stuffed in the mouth of the dead, half eaten legs, buttocks and/or arms roasting in a fire, bleeding babies stuck on sticks, spears in the vagina or the anus, mangled corpse, etc. Paranoia and fear was influenced by these traumatizing sights. And, you cannot un-see the mutilated bodies of victims. This was a visual terrifying traumatizing method to make cavies fear their enemies and stop them from wandering too far from their cave settlement areas. Many cavies were forced to sleep without campfires this made them inconspicuous to attackers. This also exposed them to the cold night temperatures and animals and insects that attack at night. Cave settlers were constantly in fear of the night and darkness spirits and the slightest sound of night spirits. This caused sleep deprivation and constant colds. At night, they would not leave their sleeping pits. When sleeping in the pits they curled up like dogs. In the sleeping pits, they would urinate and have bowel movements in their clothes to avoid night attacks from their own cave residents, snakes, predatory animals and wandering cave gangs that were always inside the cave.

The Caucasian personality and behavior is of a Psychopathological Racial Personality, Narcissistic Avaricious Disorder with White Supremacy Psychosis and self-hatred. They bring these diseases subliminally to every aspect of their society such as art, finance, education, work places, movies, computerized games and learning programs, color, sports, personal relationships and are totally unaware that they have the cave trauma disease. In contemporary times, mannequins that model clothes or jewelry in stores have amputated heads, fingers, hands, arms, or feet, only torsos, scalped heads, and are eyeless and toothless. In stores there are people are on display counters. It was part of the cave experience to constantly see such sights. The sights of mutilated mannequin's bodies subconsciously relive the cave life experience and reinforce that traumatic misbehaving cave life reality. They have never been treated for cave trauma diseases and are in denial about their cave personality. They crave cave sexual behavior and enjoy watching others have sex because in the cave sexual activities were in full view of others. They must have a constant murder, stealing, violence attacks and wars and betrayals in their movies, television shows and computer games. They "Crave the Cave" so they watch other's sexual activities (pornography) to satisfy their craving for the cave. Currently the cave craving is satisfied by watching "political correct" pornography in parental guidance rated movies, television shows, computer games, and listening to sex jokes. The pornographic partially nude dressed cheerleaders at sports events use sexual intercourse movements, and use batons to do pole dance type sexual movements and hold two fluffy testicles "pom-pom balls" and shake the fluffy testicles as if they are moving during sexual intercourse. This is subconscious sexually erotic stimulation. The public display of pretend sexual activities reinforces their cave trauma disease addiction and socially keeps them connected to their cave addiction.

The environment does not create people. People's behavior can be influenced by the environment. The caves did not create White people. White people adjusted their innate inborn DNA behavior to the caves. No environment is uncivilizable (made tame and livable) from the Arctic cold to deserts because people adapt to survive and civilize the environments. A civilization can begin in a specific environment and wander into other areas. A civilization cannot be conquered or colonized or made primitive by an environment. No part of the world is uniquely privileged to be civilized by people and no people are uniquely made for an environment. Cave people bring their cave DNA behavior to all environments. White people cannot be civilized by an environment or another race. People were not created by an environment and cave thinking cannot be uncreated by an environment. The impact of the caves cannot be uncreated. The cave people's food hunting and gathering lifestyle existed at least 30,000 years. Around 5,000 BC, the Neolithic or first Agricultural Revolution began. This forced cave tribes into cereal farms and into other cave tribes areas and into other animal farm territory. Cavies had cave war refugees, in-migrations and intermingled with other cave settlements. Cave areas were often subdivided into sections for the poor, rich, family clans, food storage, toilet, animal, sleeping, cooking and recreation areas. Some very small groups of cavies became conscious and or vegetarians and peaceful (conscious) while the majority remained violent war mongrels, meat eaters with Narcissistic Avaricious White Supremacy Psychosis and social alcoholics. In their past rotten contaminated food was soak in alcohol before eating to prevent diseases this eventually caused their entire race to become socially acceptable alcoholics. This gave rise to the custom of saying "Toast" before drinking because hard toast bread was soaked in alcohol before it was   drank so they would say toast and then drink the alcohol and bread mixture. Aside from this over 90% had rotten teeth or were toothless because the teeth had rotten out of their mouth. They could not chew bread. Eventually toothless groups of conscious cavies abandon the savage cavies and formed settlements. They usually lived in environments where other cavies found the weather and food supply too hostile for existence. The hostile war mongrel cavies dominate the Caucasian social, political, military, economic, agricultural, academic, religious and social landscape.

The Cave people's (Neanderthal and Cro-Magnon) social structure had three levels:
1. Trogloxenes (troglo= cave, xenes= temporary)- they used caves as temporary shelters, night time sleep to hide from prey and wandering gangs of thugs. They spent most of their time outside of the caves. Usually used several temporary cave shelters for following animal herds and plant harvesting seasons.
2. Troglophiles (troglo= cave, philes=lover of caves)- They used caves for shelters, rituals, ceremonies, storage of food, animal and human livestock.
3. Troglobytes (troglo= cave, bytes = to live)- they spent 90% of their life in caves on ground level and underground caves. Some caves had tunnels connecting them to other caves. They had poor eye sight and very pale white skin.

Remnants of the cave social structure is called the "lower class" = Troglobytes, "middle class" = Troglophiles and "upper class" = Trogloxenes. The cavies' superstitions are beliefs, science myth beliefs that use scientific words, numbers and mathematical symbols which they call "theories". Theories, postulates, hypotheses, and axiom are beliefs supported by beliefs which cannot be true and require no proof which means they are superstitions in abstract form. Cavies have many superstitions such as Theory of Relativity, Evolution Theory, Auxiliary Theory, Electron Orbital Theory, Left and Right Brain Theory, Genetic Disease Theory, Wave Function Theory, Weight Gain Theory, Germ Theory, Contagious Disease Theory, Structural Information Theory, Black Hole Theory, Hygiene Hypothesis Theory, Probability Theory, Causal Inference Theory, Speed of Light Theory, Pessimistic Induction Theory, Standard Model Theory, Stimulus Theory, Gestalt Theory, Inference Theory, Object- Salient Perception Theory, Sumatic Mutation Theory, Quantum Theory, String Theory, Dark Matter Theory,

M(Matrix)- Theory, Brain Plasticity Theory, Intelligence Quotient Theory, Antibody Response Theory, Free Market Theory, Essentialism Theory, Group Theory, Standard(particle) Model Physics Theory, Grand Unified Theory, Conservation of Energy Theory, The Theory of Anything, Cause and Effect Theory, Supply and Demand Theory, Information Theory, Intrinsic Geometry Theory, Entropy Theory, etc. All theories are extensions of a culture. Their theories develop into living myths. They should be avoided when looking at reality. There are two processes used in mathematics which are addition and subtraction. No matter how sophisticated or advance a science claims to be they can only use a form of addition (tracing forward) and subtraction (tracing backward). Reverse Engineering, Behavioral Deconstruction and Derivatives are types of adding or subtracting (tracing backward and forward) one behavior, idea, belief or myth to arrive at the original behavior, idea or myth. These methods were used to trace the ancient past of the Caucasians superstitions that they call theories, rituals, ceremonies and emotional and mental state of consciousness. The Caucasians use science words and mathematics to decorate their superstitions and science myths so that you cannot see that they are beliefs supported by beliefs = superstitions. In other words, any explanation of belief is a belief itself. They use a belief to explain a belief and worship their belief myths and demand that others honor and respect their superstitious beliefs (theories). They believe and then see. They do not see to believe. Their history can also be traced by their dictionaries origin of words and then looking up the god or myth and social history of the people that used those words. This tracing backward will eventually lead you to the caves.

Cavies have a superstitious fear of small animal bacteria and small insects such as mosquitos. Contemporary Caucasians use cave type shelters and building that have a cave atmosphere such as monasteries, jails, eat in dark rooms such as in restaurants, dark night clubs and pubs, watch movies in the dark, paint their bodies at sports games etc. This originally was a superstitious practice to protect themselves from evil loser spirits or to call for spirits to protect them, entice the sex spirit and have ceremonies to kill evil spirits (enemy team effigy doll) and burn the doll in the fires of hell. This is called barn fire rallies for burning a sporting event's opponent doll of effigy. They use amputated body parts (heads, feet, hands, fingers, arms etc.) to model underwear, hats, clothes and jewelry. They use sex rape and sex orgies activities and drink alcohol before, during and after sporting events to celebrate victories and use fire dancing by running around fires in a circle etc. In the past, they would hunt and capture, rape, hang and burn Black people to celebrate White Supremacy. The Caucasian custom(ritual) of pouring liquid black rubber or black oils on Black people and then sprinkling feathers on them was a ceremony used to symbolize the feather wings of the Black Imp evil angel spirit that fell from the grace of the gods. After feathering a Black person, they would burn the black person to return their Imp spirit back to hell. When they did not tar and feather the Black person they would hang the Black person and burn the Black person while alive or burn them while the Black person was choking on the rope. The rope and pieces of the skin and oils from the dead Black person were sold and or kept as souvenirs. The social tradition of saying "God Bless you" after someone sneezes is used because white people once believed a sneeze could causes the spirit to fall out the noise resulting in death. If you sneeze and live then God has blessed you. They still refer to alcohol liquor as a "spirit" that possess your body causing it to be uncontrollable in movements (drunk behavior) and the spirit could not restrain sex desires. They call mucus dripping out the nose a "cold" caused by the cold wind of moon. Caucasians keep dogs in their house, sleep with dogs and kiss dogs because these social activities come from their cave past. White people keep dogs as pets to practice owning slaves on a subconscious and emotional level. The Caucasians do not want to know where their ancient rituals, ceremonies and superstitions come from because if they admitted that they knew it will validate their primitiveness. Their denial of cave social history distorts their reality and condemns their future. They emotionally deny the presence of ancestral DNA genes in their thoughts and behaviors.

In Cave life, the wearing of the different colors and smells of animal fur and skin were a sign of status. Currently they wear the mink rat's fur as an indication of prestige. Animal skin is worn in clothing and used for seats, furniture, shoes, hats and this sustains the cave social life. Different colors and smells of animal fur and skins symbolize victory of killing an opponent, control over another race's women, and a trophy from successful hunting. Currently their military and police wear mock plastic animal skin colors on their jackets or shirts to symbolize status and or victory in combat battles.

Men and women use a types of military sexual mating conquest rituals and call it romance, dating or the battle of the sexes. Caucasians men and women have social drinks of alcohol and get socially drunk (feeling good=mentally ill) and listen to love songs. The song's words are suggestive of sex which is a form of seductive rape stimulation. Women are used as sex objects or commodities at sports events. The women stand seductively and dance or walk around partially nude in bikinis at boxing and martial arts matches and sports entertainment events. This stimulates   various types of rape and confirms ideas that sex is a reward for victory. Heterosexual and Homosexual Rape was a part of cave battles victories, mating and life. There are three types of rape:

1. Petty Rape: Women are emotionally blackmailed by men or a woman to use sex as a payment for car or household repairs, payment for bills, to get or keep jobs, pay their rent, or car note or credit card.
2. Seductive Rape: Men date women that must wear partial nude clothes, skin tight pants or yoga spandex pants, consume drugs, alcohol and or marijuana to loosen their morals, do sex related dancing, listen to sex related songs, watch politically correct pornography in movies or computer games and or watch X-rated pornography.
3. Violent Rape: physically over power or use weapons (guns, knives) or date rape drugs to force women to have sex against their will.

The cavies trained children with the same methods used to train dogs, horses and other animals. Disobedient children were beaten into submission to adult authority. Obedient children were rewarded with treats, food, hugs, petted, sex, toys, sugary snacks, etc. Some children were products of rape or stolen, adopted or made into sex slaves. Children were often herded together for training, schools and daycare. Public schools use a type of intellectual herding of children called a standard school education and standardized test play and games (intellectual herding). Children in herds function with mob rule (peer groups). Mobs or peer groups influence serve as their primary parent, nurturer, source of knowledge, pleasure, guidance and source of fear if rejected by their mob. Rule of the Mob guidance is still used by Caucasians. The cave children's caretakers were elderly, handicap individuals, drunkards, the diseased and or mentally ill, had dysfunctional behaviors, or useless non-breeding menopausal women or child abusers and rapists.

Mental illness (schizophrenia, neurosis, anxiety, depression, suicidal behaviors, etc.) amongst cavies was an epidemic. The mentally ill or people that stutter, children with birth defects, people that were cross eyed, bow legged, lisp (misarticulation sounds of words), retarded, thumb suckers, crippled or blind children were seen as possessed with demons or evil spirits. The treatment was torture, beatings, bloodletting, castration, sexual abuse, sacrifices to the gods, rape, and murder. They were also used as bait to catch animals, used as animal feed and or eaten.

The cavies that lived outside the protection of cave settlements lived in huts under cliffs or in the woods or types of tree houses perched in tress. Inside the caves and thrown on the dirt floors were the stench of manure covered leaves and grass used as toilet paper, there was crawling and flying bugs, fleas, frogs, snakes, flies, scraps of rotten food on the floors, manure from bats, rats, roaches, dogs and cats, menstruation blood, human and animal urine, vomit and spit soaked into the floors. There were constant sounds of animals, insects, people fighting and arguments, dogs barking, babies and adults crying, farts, laughing, sneezing, coughing, hollers from pain, moans, groans, sexual related sounds, screams from torture etc. Aside from the constant irritating noise (sound pollution) the smoke from the cooking of meats and the smell of candles made of rancid animal fat, combine with the foul stench of the people was accepted as normal air (air pollution).

The herded people and herded animals (elk, deer, horses, pigs, etc.) were moved seasonally in order to follow the harvest of ripe plants. The herded cavies were usually captured during battles, raids or stolen. They were used for labor, breeding, money, soldiers and for food during times of famine. Cavies had constant head and pubic lice (crabs), matted moist hair from sweating that trapped the stench of Sulphur and ammonia fumes from their pores causing a dog-like hair smell, dandruff, athletes foot, rotten tooth cavities, bad breathe, used urine as a deodorant, skin sores, bumps that oozed out pus, body rashes, warts, moles, sexually transmitted diseases, did not take baths because of fear of the water spirits, women had vagina stench, people had manure caked on their behinds, had constant attacks of diarrhea and flatulence (farting), yeast infections and athletes foot. They had sperm drinking rituals called oral sex. They had anal sex ritual games called pen the tail (tongue) on the donkey's ass hole (usually used dogs, sheep etc.). These activities increased diseases. Their cave culture and gods said they were normal.

Cave groups had circulating mobility and radiating mobility. Keep in mind that different cave settlements had different languages. Some cave settlements were composed of blood related individuals (clans) or tribes. Some had different types of incestuous female and male bonding (marriages). Some of the leaders had sexual rights with all females and males. The cave men followed a pecking order to avoid sexual conflicts with other males. Cave settlements were in competition with other settlements over territories, food, slaves, herds of people and water. Incidentally, during America's slavery era Black slave's pictures were on all paper money because slaves were money. In the modern era people's faces are on money because the leader of the people (wealthy oligarchies, rich, corporate elite) represents the highest form of money. People are money. Without people commodities, natural resources and land means nothing. In cave society, it was clear that the more people you had in the cave settlements the more wealth you had. Therefore, the good hunters and warriors had people under their leadership because a good hunter could provide food, land and protection to people. And, a good warrior could invade and steal more food. Therefore, people settled around good hunters and or warriors.

The high amount of warfare and territorial battles caused many injuries, handicaps, destroyed families and caused deaths. Women during the Caucasian cave era was equal in physical built. Many of the female warriors because of the physical stress of constant battles did not menstruate and were infertile. Many escape women formed herds. The women ran away from settlements because of the many gang rapes. Women refugees from settlements joined together and formed new settlements. The women gangs would randomly have attacked groups of men and villages. The female warriors gang stole the food supply of others and stole food crop fields. They raided small villages and stole other cave villages' children to use for their military and use for slave labor. The raids and battles for human resources (slaves) and natural resources (wood, animals and plant crops) caused many injuries, handicaps and murders. Diseases were a constant outbreak and caused deaths. Childbirth problems caused many deaths. The female's health deteriorated from many births, miscarriages and multiple breast feedings of adults and children which caused many deaths and anemia. Females had sex and masturbated while pregnant and menstruation as part of their normal life. The elderly women and men that were physically unable to hunt or fight in battles were usually abandoned, murdered, eaten, or used as bait to capture animals.

The cave life is indirectly depicted in movies such as the "Planet of the Apes". The apes are symbols of evolved cave people. The cave life usually is indirectly explained using such characters as apes. Cave life is represented by the subconscious myth of the woman's womb (cave) as a symbol of the cave. And, tombs (caves) are used symbolically as the burial places or birthplaces of cave leaders or spirit prophets. The prophets usually come from their origin (cave) with social rules and order.

Many of the war games of Caucasians originated from cave games. The war games were used as a type of social engineering that reinforced and conditioned (domesticated) the cave people to behavior in manners that sustained the cave settlement. In games the three types of strategies are;
1.) Confrontation- used to find the combat position and man power strength of an enemy or the mental and or physical condition of your opponent.
2.) Battles- used to achieve an advantage that gains a superior position over the opponent
3.) War- used to transfer power (natural and or human resources). The games use "misdirection and deception" which is the military state of mind.

"Misdirection" means to pretend or fake going in one direction while actually going in another. For example, "Emancipation" of slaves was a misdirection and believed to be freedom of slaves. Emancipation's definition is "transfer of ownership". The ownership of slaves was transferred from an individual owner to the state, government, group and or corporation as the owner of the slaves. The slaves remain a slave. The USA government paid the slave master for each slave he freed. In other words, the USA government bought the slaves from the slave owner and became the new owner of slaves. The other war mentality is "deception" sometimes referred to as lies, propaganda and corruption. Deceit is when a corrupt government promises to help all the citizens while only helping a few rich people become richer. The corrupt government should be viewed as the owners of a gambling casino house. It is known in gambling you cannot bet against the house and win. In other words, citizens bet with their incomes and civil rights against the house (government) to gain more income and civil rights while the government (owns the gambling house) takes away more of the citizen's income with corporate tax breaks, trade agreements, agriculture (food) and natural resource subsidies. And they take away rights to privacy with by spying on citizens. The gambling casino (government) buildings are monuments (of the wealth of corporate elite) built by the losers (citizens). There are many versions of "misdirection and deception" war mentality. Wars are fought with a war mentality. Guns, missiles, Drone airplane bombing of the enemy and politics and economics are an extension of the war mentality.

Each time a war game (soccer, chess, computer games, basketball, football, tennis, etc.) is played the spectators, gamers and athletes' war mentality is reinforced. The games reaffirm a selfish desire and belief that "if you are not for me, you are against me". The games reinforce the selfish idea that you must win at all cost. Victory is not shared-there is a victor and a victim. The teams and individual's tactics, maneuvers, weakness and strengths are not equally shared with the opponent. Sexual marriages are a type of war or battle of the sexes. The women dress to kill (capture a mate) and put battle paint on their faces (make-up) and are emotionally forced to want to breed while the men are predators that hunt for women for sexual intercourse. Sex is used by White men as a symbol of power (victory over an opponent) not a symbol of togetherness, emotional unity and sharing. If each member in a war game were sharing tactics and the responsibility of following the rules (rituals) of the games then there would be no need for referees, officials and penalties. The success of the Caucasian cave corrupts and traumatized individual in games or relationships is based upon disrespecting and ignoring the rights (sovereignty) of the other person (the opponent). This behavior is an extension of the cave civilization.

The war (cave) mentality is reinforced in written language. Ideas, thesis, narratives and paragraphs are written pro against con (pros and cons) battles. The village of written words (paragraphs) must support the cave chief (main idea). The peasant village of words such as verbs and adverbs, adjectives and nouns, must work for the main theme or idea. The main idea of a narrative supported by sentences is equal to cave chief (main idea) of the village (sentences). Caucasian use of words is an extension of cave culture. The culture gives to people beliefs, beliefs create emotions, a person's reactions to emotions are called feelings, and a feeling of long duration is a mood. Caucasian feelings are an extension of cave culture. Feelings of anger, fear, power, stealing, exploiting and mistrust of other people (enemies) are created by the cave culture and its use of words. Language (word order) is an extension of culture.

Historically ancient Africans had no words for jail, orphanage, nursing homes (warehouses) for the elderly because there were no jails, orphanages and nursing homes. Nursing homes for the elderly are places to wait for death. Caucasians language has words such as rape, jail, incest, masturbation, pedophilia (sex with children), necrophilia (sex with the dead), sex with animals (zoo-philia) and homosexuality, because these things existed in their culture and continue to exist.

The Caucasians believe that modern technology and new theories (superstitions) will improve their emotions, mentality and social life. However, there has always been modern technology. For example, at one time in ancient history the invention of the wheel, hammer, shovel, writing, fire stick (matches), toilet, candle and arithmetic were a modern technology. With all the technologies, the Caucasians continue to misbehave like their cavies' ancestors by exploiting the poor, needy, and elderly, exterminating people, invading countries and terrorizing, destroying clean air, water, soil and stealing others human and natural resources. It is easy to satisfy the needy by eliminating slave wages, ending predatory loans and mortgages, providing free education, health care and shelters for all. The greedy can never be satisfied (Narcissistic Avaricious Disorder). The greedy stealing of other peoples and natural resources is not isolated to material objects and commodities (oil, gold, water, pork bellies/bacon, minerals, etc.). The greedy corporations are committed to emotional, intellectual and spiritual stealing. For example, when Caucasian's corporations lie about the safety of water, history, African science and history, tobacco, cars or babies toys they have "stolen the truth" and replaced it with a lie.

Caucasians juvenile delinquent culture is constantly in search of new technology and new theories (superstitions) to save them from themselves. The technologies did not create them and cannot uncreate

35

their heritage of cave life DNA genes. In ancient times, they were after the magic fountain of youth or elixir. Currently, they are after the magic drug, magic technology, magic surgeries, magic computer intelligence or disease fighting gene and magic theory to save them from themselves. Superstitions keep them bonded to cave civilization. Superstitions are the voice of culture. Caucasian superstitions are subliminally embedded in their religions such as water turning into wine, burning bushes that are not on fire, perfect people born in immaculate conceptions without sex between men and women, rebirth (resurrection) in a cave, etc. Their religions have failed to change their behavior. Caucasian religions for over 2,000 years have failed to make them behave. This should be enough evidence to convince Black people that they cannot make Caucasians behave. However, Post Traumatic Slavery Disorder keeps Black people addicted to trying to change Caucasian culture.

The juvenile Caucasian civilization has blurred the real with the unreal. For example, they have written scripts and rehearsals for reality television shows that are presented to the audience as unrehearsed spontaneous depictions of dysfunctional black women and black couples. They mix Computer Generated Images (CGI) of people and places with real places and objects. They have CGI fantasy sports events and use CGI images of living athletes. There are black judges granting equal "justice" in reality court of law (rituals) television shows. In reality, Caucasian courts use jail term sentence for revenge punishment of people. Their jails are not used for rehabilitation of people but to punish. The Caucasians would rather recycle trash than recycle rehabilitated Black prisoners. The Caucasian courts of law (rituals) sentence, convict and arrest black people at a higher rate than white people (no justice). However, Black judge's reality shows pretend they dispense equal justice. They have Black host of television game shows giving away money and gifts "equally" to Blacks and Whites when in reality Blacks are the last to receive "equality". This presents a make-believe reality and blurs consciousness with a mixture of the unreal combined with the real. This blurred reality enters the viewer's intelligence. This has outsourced black people's intelligence to computers. The viewers watch computer generated scripts, computer generated news broadcast people that read computer generated news articles. The computerized world is another extension of the Caucasians cultures cave superstitions disguised as intelligence. Computer science uses mathematics theories (superstitions) to generate information. People are no longer censoring information because the computer censors it for them. The computer generates Black people's profiles for businesses to hire Black people. Corporations market their products and send words and images that entice Black people to buy products from White owned corporations. The corporations are an extension of Caucasian culture that maintains the ideology of the cave.

The corporations make IPhone, laptops, IPad with computer monitor screens that stimulate the visual and auditory centers of the brain. This increased stimulation of the visual and auditory centers increase the connections in the neuronet synaptic density. There is more wiring type connections (synapse) in those centers that has wiring that interconnect to the emotions. This causes the person to let information into the brain uncensored. And, this changes the brain as a physical organ. This brain change causes a focus on the "here" and "now", short term memory and fight or flight responses. Fight or flight was the constant state of mind of the cavies. In other words, the computer causes a cave mentality. It reduces the field of vision and the head does not move to the left or right, but stays looking straight forward, like cavies that kept their eyes looking straight forward to the cave entrance on guard for cave bandits and cave gangs of thugs trying to enter the cave. Aside from this, the computer eventually causes digital dementia (senility) and delays cognitive intellectual maturity "retardation". The person's intelligence is no longer used. Intelligence has been outsourced to the computer. The computer has become the leader of the cave settlements of people with IPhone, IPad and computer operators (IT, artists, musicians, social media, etc.). It is a cave gang leader with a gang of people with loss Cognitive Episodic Memory (long term), loss Reflexive Brain activity which causes a decrease of cognitive (intellectual) concentration by viewing screen pop-ups. This will eventually increase nerve deterioration leading to senility and eye macular (transparent skin) degeneration cause by LED lights of the computer. The brain has physically changed and is a new brain and not the old normal brain of 1970. The old brain is depicted in textbooks and used as the basis of psychology theories.

The computers decrease the ability of the brain to filter and censor morality. They decrease the brain's physiological development of the interconnections of the prefrontal brain's neuronet synaptic density. The brain has changed because of the computer reliance and usage. The brain's prefrontal cortex associated with censorship of thoughts and emotions is used less and less and the visual and auditory senses enter the brain uncensored and are used more. These auditory and visual senses are trained by computers to follow step by step procedures (socially called a ritual) and how to use step by step rituals to avoid a ritual. They call disobedience to an encrypted computer procedure (ritual) hacking. In other words, Caucasians are using the computer to be delinquent and misbehave. This misbehavior is a continuation of the cave outside the cave.

The cave mentality continues with little girl's pedophile sexual arousal fashion shows and beauty contests. The girls dress like adult females, wear make-up and sing adult songs that have sexual connotations and are suggestive of sex. This causes pedophile sexual stimulation and reinforces females to have fear of rape thoughts. Fear was a constant in Cave life. People were fearful of rape inside and outside the cave and fearful of physical violence with others as well as insects and animals inside the cave and fearful of attacks outside the cave by insects, animals and roaming gangs. The car chase scenes and fight scenes, scary rides at amusement parks, science fiction human-like creatures from outer space or animals or insects or diseases attacking Caucasians on Earth, boxing, wrestling and horror movies stimulate fear. Fear emotionally re-creates the constant fear of living in a cave societies and satisfies the craving for the cave.

Fear cause by cave living stimulates the bipolar (negative and positive thoughts) pathological (disease) defense reaction. This prolongs sympathetic flight or fight nervous system stimulation which results in catabolic overdrive. This weakens immunity, drains emotions and decreases the use of right and wrong behavioral response. It retards the ability to mature and locks a person into a juvenile state (stunts emotional growth). In other words, their emotional disease keeps white people in a perpetual Juvenile Culture Delinquent State and sustains the emotional and mental illness called Post Traumatic Cave Disorder.

White people's food combing started during cave life. During cave life food was scarce, so they ate what they found which caused wrong food combining. Consequently, they found wild onions, bugs and rats and ate all them together, then ate many different types of insects, then found wild grapes and potatoes and ate both of them together, then found wild flint wheat berries and crab apples and ate them together. In contemporary times, they crave the wrong way to combine food such as fruit (raisins) with starchy wheat berries (cereals), onions and tomatoes (fruit) with wheat starch (flat wheat bread) called pizza because they crave the cave. In the past, the cavies ate illogical food combination for survival (Theory of Survival of the Fit) which is the alternative to their Theory of Reductionism (combine food properly for a healthy life). Cavies lack the intellectual stamina to figure out that eating is for achieving wellness instead they eat for stimulation of taste. They use the questionable emotional values of their food theory beliefs. In a traumatized condition of Cave Trauma Disorder, it is difficult to select proper eating combinations. And, if they could exercise proper food combining they lack the intellectual ability to do proper food combinations. The emotion of fear of starvation guided their past and current wrong food combination

38

such as sweet fruit with starchy carbohydrates, milk with fruits, and starch with meat. Cavies current food combination are connected to their past, so using social Reverse Engineering (tracing backwards), Behavioral Deconstruction (tracing backwards to see how behavior is constructed) and Derivatives (tracing backwards) to find the origin of a word or behavior will lead to the caves primitive life style. By eating improperly cavies reaffirm their emotionality, mentality and behavior of cave life. They can only crave the past (existence) because their future does not exist.

The cavies search and research for any and everything such as bacteria, virus, outer space, drugs, planets, oil derivatives and ancient colored cultures lifestyle to find their place in the world. Their problem is no other race befriended them or desired to bond with them. They assume that if they knew why they exist they would find the key to life. They ask themselves why do White people exist, where did White people come from and are White people really the perfect race. If White people could know their reason for existence they would know it. Their explanation for existence is religion mixed with superstitions and theories. They actually believe a boiling hot massive piece of dirt blew up and sprinkled out the plants, the sun and the Earth. They believe the explosion made a loud big bang sound. However, there was no one alive to hear the sound, so it made a silence. It could have been a big splash of hot water. Sea water boils and the results is a white dirt called sea salt (sodium chloride). In other words, the Big Splash of boiling hot water sprinkled out the dirt called the planets, stars and Earth. Big Bang or Big Splash are both a fantasy unproven fact which means a superstition that uses scientific terms. The Caucasians emotionally cannot accept the ancient wisdom of Africans because that would make them accept being a juvenile civilization and culturally immature. Ancient Africans stated you cannot get something for nothing. There must have been something already existing to create a Big Bang or Big Splash. Ancient African civilization was trying to tell the juvenile Caucasian civilization that you cannot know the beginning of the elements that compose water such as hydrogen and oxygen. You can only calculate the age of water (fossil frozen water) or layer of dirt but not the elements that compose water or dirt. You cannot know the age of an element and you cannot know the age or birth of God. All ancient colored civilizations told the cavies not to hurt Mother Earth or Mother Earth's waters, air, soil or violate or exploit living things because you hurt, violate and exploit yourself. The few conscious Caucasians started social movements in order to be in harmony with nature and create a better life for all. These conscious white people (social activist,

Whistle blowers = expose illegal activities (rituals) of government) are punished by the oligarchy and called spies or put in jail.

The only safe place to practice cave culture and for the Caucasian to live is inside the caves. Because the world's colored peoples, and Black Africans and the few conscious Caucasians cannot make the majority and oligarchy minority of Caucasians behave. There always exist in a Caucasian social construct a few people that see and behave and act on a harmonious reality that a majority cannot and will not follow. For example, in a total population of people there will always be a small percentage of teachers, vegetarians, writers, drug addicts, professional athletes, artist, bankers, entertainers, genius, politicians, soldiers, sailors, beggars, prostitutes, etc. In the Caucasian socialized population, there will always be a few Caucasian people that can behave amongst the misbehaving majority.

The Caucasian mindset creates the false image for black people that Caucasians were in the cave and every white man dressed in suites, wore white shirts and neck ties, shoes, had haircuts, wore deodorant and their women dressed in gowns, polish their nails, used make-up, wore high heel (stilts) shoes, use salon hair styles, had clean shaven legs, armpits and arms and both men and women spoke in proper English, listen to classical symphony music and read Shakespeare's plays and played bridge or chess. Black people are made to accept that Caucasians were always totally civilized, intellectually superior and in charge of the planet earth. The effect of Caucasian brainwashing is written in the book "The Emperor's New Clothes" by Hans Christian Anderson (1805-1875) which is an adaption of Aesop Fables (620 -564 BC) a book written by a Black man that contains wisdom past down from ancient African civilization. In the fable, the Emperor is told by a tailor that his new clothes are perfect. However, the clothes are invisible and the emperor is naked. His citizens must believe that the emperor is not naked and is wearing perfect clothes. If they tell the emperor his new clothes are invisible they will be murdered. Therefore, all the citizens said the naked emperor's clothes are visible and perfect. The Caucasians must tell themselves they are perfect because if they do not, then White Supremacy (Emperor's new clothes) will not exist. Without the psychotic fantasy of White Supremacy, they will exist as naked fools and would have to be put back in their caves. The false belief that Caucasians are not primitive people (cavies) is socially engineered into Black people's mind. Any spoken or written words by a Black person about the Caucasians primitive juvenile civilization causes Slavery Traumatized Black people to get angry or to label the Black person as a racist for the reporting Caucasian character traits. These Black people think that the historical truth is too incredible to believe, so they dismiss the truthful facts. These brainwashed Black people suffer from Pathological Incredulity Disorder. They say to themselves it is too incredible to believe and do not accept or believe the facts. Their emotions override their intelligence. It irritates their addiction to White people and bothers their co-dependency addiction to White people. White people have successfully programmed Black people to believe that Caucasians have no currently existing social primitive behaviors. When cave traumatized White people tell their fantasy truth about the caves they lie. Then they lie about the lie until their truth is a lie and their lie is a truth. Caucasian DNA contains their genetic innate behavior, and their DNA physical, mental, social, emotional and spiritual records. And, the emotional injuries, emotional wounds, emotional scars and their emotional stunted retarded growth is contained within their DNA. They have a past of being herded on people farms called cave settlements.

Cave people were raised in types of people farms similar to animals. In the people farms (today called urban cities) the conditions are created so that people will destroy their spiritual, emotional, physical and social lives. When living in people farms (over populated urban cities) you are only free to choose the wrong thing. The fear of being robbed causes people in people farms to lock themselves up in gated housing community jails (pay police to watch them), buy spying devices such as camera monitors, alarms, sensors, detection devices, locks for doors and windows that are digitally operated. Anything the people own that is digital allows them to be spied upon and the digital information is owned by the government and can be sabotaged by a hacker. The hacker can be an individual thief or the government's surveillance spies. They out sourced spying to private own companies and private militaries that have spies that work for the government. The privately own companies use citizen workers to spy on citizens. They are the governments collection of citizen thieves that steal other citizen's private thoughts. This allows the government to punish you for thought crimes (your imaginations ideas can be a crime). The crowded urban lifestyle pushes people together and violates personal space (social distance between people). Farmed people (urban dwellers) are seeking a life free of the never-ending cycle of work, eat, pay bills, sleep, work, pay bills, sleep etc. They use sex, masturbation, reality television shows, game shows, sports, gambling, pornography, martial arts, night clubs or pubs, social media, gun violence, prescription and non-prescription drugs to get relief from the routine of spending their lives working to provide money (pay bills) for the oligarchy. And they die in wars to protect the oligarchy. They use drugs to escape their social condition. The drugs cause a temporary and permanent change in the moods, state of consciousness, biochemistry and emotions. This is the

41

technical language for a drug induced mental illness which means drugs make temporarily people crazy. The drugs create a fantasy world to escape into called being high and feeling good. Drugs can cause physical illnesses to escalate. Drugs are used to escape and hide from physical illnesses and the emotional pain of a constant cycle of work, eat, pay bills, sleep, work, eat, pay bills, sleep, work, eat, pay bills, sleep, etc. This is the repetitious cycle of the life of people herds owned by the oligarchy.

Drug addiction related crimes can lead to a jail terms and provide free labor for the corporations. Legal prescription and non-prescription Drug Addiction creates permanent customers for the health (sick) industries hospitals, clinics, surgeons and drug pharmacy business. The farmed (urban) people escape from their herded animal programmed life with social medias, internet games and internet surfing until it becomes an addiction. Each time the people herds living on people farms try to escape they are re-captured by their profiles that are created every time they use their computers or any digital device. The computerized big data profiles create a type of social engineered fence around their emotional, mental and physical cave settlement. Animal herds and people herds on people farms is part of the DNA cavie past life. The cave chiefs are the new word for corporations which is the new word for oligarchy. The cavies (urban lifestyle) are like pets that buy their own feed and keep their social engineered caves and cages clean and pay for the cage (home owners) or rent the cage and buy MRI, CAT scan pictures of their path to death.

Cave and Slavery Traumatized people are vulnerable to all sorts of emotional accidents and injuries that can cause physical diseases. Emotionally traumatized people can create a continuous cycle where by their emotionally injured family and emotionally injured group (race, culture, gang, oligarchy) causes a self-inflicted emotional wound. The journey of an emotion is interconnected by synapse (similar to interstate highways) in a type of neuronet spider web connected to other spider webs of emotions that influence each other even when they are not intending any emotional harm. A negative emotional injury is frequently harmful to another emotion while it can be a pleasurable emotion to another distant emotion. This means that no single emotion is in control of the emotional neuronets journey's path of the brain.

Traumatized people's emotions can become hypersensitive to unreal or real emotional attacks. Emotions can become very sensitive to actions that are suggestive of an insult, or a perceived emotional interference with rights or seem to be put-downs, and/or felt as pain. Consequently, traumatized people have an emotional radar that monitors another person's emotional signals. They interpret emotions so that they can mobilize their defenses and mount a counter attack against explicit or implicit or subliminal real or unreal emotional behavior or physical action of others. Traumatized people tend to attach negative emotional meanings to insignificant actions and exaggerate their actual importance. The results are traumatized people tend to feel hurt, upset, revengeful and or angry with others. They are supersensitive to rejection, humiliation, failure, resentment, success, betrayal and or criticisms causing them to be susceptible to a vast array of neuronet connections to pain sensations. Emotional pain can cause stress, distress, disease and pain more intense that physical pain. A traumatized person can relive the emotional pain with any stimulation of their sense of smell, taste, touch, sound, color or seeing someone else in a similar situation. In other words, the cave trauma or slave trauma follows them with no expiration date except eternity. The cave trauma follows the Caucasian in their diet, science, sports, sexuality, art and social activities with Black people. The cave trauma distorts their dreams and distorts their future. They are forever craving the cave because they have a subconscious addiction to the caves. Addiction causes a person to emotionally override their intelligence in order to satisfy the addiction. White Supremacy Addiction gives them emotional comfort in their misbehavior with the Black race. Their misbehavior is part of their social systems and the cave culture. Cave culture is addicting and addictions do not go away with some type of therapy that is not related to or developed by the addictive caves.

Ancient Black people that were the most successful with controlling the white cave people and making them behave were the Black people of the Kuba kingdom. They were motivated to control the cavies by the ancient African popular saying which was "When the first white man (makes settlements) lives in the land (African) the Black nations would die". This phrase kept the Africans cautious about the cavies. Historically Black people were mindful that it was something terribly wrong with the Caucasians (Cave Trauma Disorder). Therefore, ancient Africans totally rejected engaging in a social relationship with the whites. However, a succession of violent attacks and invasions by the Assyrians, Persians, Greeks, Romans, Arabs and the Turks from 1475 to 1675 (200 years) and the fall of Egypt forced the Kuba kingdom to deal with the cavies. The European violent invading cave tribes of Germans, Danes, France, England, Spain, Italy, Portugal had surrounded the African countries and controlled the coastal areas of Africa which forced Black people to come in contact with them and engage in warfare. The Whites offered choices of "Trade or Raid" trade with them or be invaded by them or "Sell a slave or Be a slave".

The Kuba kingdom (began before11 AD) set up a Commissioner of White People. Whites coming to Kuba had to check in and check out with the Commissioner of White People, they were given a temporary day pass. The cave Caucasians had to complete their trading and leave by sun down. They were not allowed to hold any social or religious position, could not own land or live in the kingdom, could not marry a Black person, all their trade transactions were taxed, transportation caravans were taxed and disobedience of Kuba laws were punishable by death (for more information see "Destruction of Black Civilization" by Chancellor Williams).

The Kuba Black Africans that converted to Islam invited their white Muslim brothers into the country. The white Muslims intermarried with the Black Muslim women, made villages, established trade outpost (increases their armed military forts) to protect their trades, commodities and money. They eventually increase their army's weapons and used their white armies to invade and capture African land and murdered and enslaved Black people. This caused the destruction and fracture of African culture and the down fall (destruction) of Kuba. The cave whites lied to the Kuban's and said their large armies were in Kuba to protect their forts that stored goods. However, the militaries used their modern weapons to destroy Kuba. The White cavies large army outpost sole purpose was to invade and capture Kuba land.

The great Kuba kingdom was composed of many ethnic groups that merged and created new languages, new rituals and ceremonies that had attributes of each ethnic group. Some ethnic groups lived in Kuba before the newly merged ethnic groups such as the ancient indigenous Kete and Cava tribes. The Kete and Cava lived in the Kuba area since the world began. The unity of the African ethnic groups and organizing factors were based upon the principles of Maat which is Truth, Justice, Harmony, Balance, Reciprocity, Propriety and Rightness. They had the Sky God which was the Sun God that symbolized the "One God" concept. This one God and Maat glued the groups together. The Black people universally believed that the cavies were violent barbarians, pagans, superstitious and had many gods. The cavies' male gods were violent and murdered people with floods and punished people with the fires of hell. Their male gods made the cavies a unified invasion military group. The Kuba people could not find a way to help the cavies. The Kuba's Maat principles were against the cavies' superstitions, rituals (rules) for violence and their male gods. African spiritual systems have female and male gods and their god does not do evil to people. This African spirituality and Maat caused a cultural clash within the White cavies' mind. The cavies had an emotional need to classify Black people as primitives. They thought Black people are beyond being cave civilized. This emotionally justifies the White Supremacy Psychosis. Today the white people subconsciously or consciously think Black people have an inferiority genetic problem. White people see themselves as a superior race without emotional and mental problems (Cave Trauma Disorder, Narcissistic Avaricious Disorder, White Supremacy Psychosis). They have not developed and will not develop a treatment for their problems. They crave the mental illness state of the mind that they had before they lived in the caves.

Nutricide

Food used to destroy Black people is a type of genocide. White people's corporate own junk food business's deliberately and systemically alter foods in order to cause physical, emotional, and mental dis-eases, genetic mutations and/or death for profit. The impact of junk foods low in of nutrients causes problems with pregnant women resulting in problems in their children. The infant death is higher than 33 nations. Baby's mortality rate is better in Singapore, Japan and Sweden. The March of Dimes Birth Report Card rates the USA the worse grade. USA has 500,000 deaths a year. Human Experimental Toxicology indicates increase vaccinations increases the death rate. The Mapping Health US birth and maternity care indicates that it is cheapest in Turkey and China and is free in Denmark. The CIA's Fact book puts the USA baby's death rate as the same as Iran. The statistics always indicate the worse outcome for Black children in the USA and in all other countries including Africa. Northwestern University Feinberg School of Medicine 12-year study indicates white children are 30 times more likely to abuse drugs than Black children. The study indicates that Black people as a racial group are less likely to abuse drugs, 1 in 3 Blacks are put in jail for drug use and drug related crimes while 1 in 17 whites are jailed. It is the effect of White Supremacy that causes drug abuse amongst Black people as well as the high arrest rate of Black children.

Black children that eat junk foods are deprived of vital nutrients. Nutrient deprivation cause attention span disorders (senility), learning problems, behavioral disorders and hyperactivity. It is typical to find a Zinc deficiency in boys and Iron deficiency in girls. Iron deficiencies in boys are ignored. Black boys in Philadelphia Public Schools were having conduct problems, disruptive behaviors, restlessness, irritability and learning problems. They were found to have an iron deficiency. Iron is the nutrient needed by the left hemisphere of the brain. It is the part of the brain used for school work, cognitive skills and manages reason and logic. This is the region needed to do well on standardized tests. When a Black girls or boys have an Iron deficiency they perceive information differently and do not respond well.

Black children who eat Caucasian junk food and cooked foods aside from having an Iron deficiency also have a deficiency in a vitamin called Thiamine. Thiamine deficiency causes the Black child to be sensitive to criticism and have poor impulse control, can become aggressive and hostile, anger easily, develop depression, and have headaches and or sleep disturbances, (Institute for Bio-social Research, Tacoma, WA). The Black child's emotions, mind and behavior is destroyed by MSG (Monosodium glutamate) found in fried foods, fats, and Chinese foods. MSG can cause heart problems, headaches, itching, nausea, reproductive problems in men and women, high blood pressure, kidney and Liver diseases, allergic reactions, DNA mutations, problems in pregnancy, lactation problems, brain and nerve damage, infertility, bone damage, etc. MSG has other names such autolyzed yeast, calcium caseinate, hydrolyzed protein, gelatin, hydrolyzed corn, gluten, hydrolyzed soy, monopotassium, pea protein, yeast extract, textured protein, plant protein glutamic acid etc. It is present and not listed as an ingredient in bouillon, malt, carrageenan, citric acid, maltodextrin, enzymes, flavors, seasonings, soy sauce, whey protein, soy protein concentrate, infant formula, baby foods, Kosher food, low fat and no fat milk, protein bars, drinks, wines, waxes applied to fresh fruits and vegetables, vaccinations, nasal spray, IV fluids, drugs, barley malt, herbicides, fungicides, pesticides and added to fertilizers used in agriculture. Added to this, the artificial sweetener Aspartame, can cause brain tumors, seizures, violent outburst, menstruation problems, constipation, tiredness and genetic mutations (clones).

The white corporate controlled public schools (educational plantations) books promote junk food, cooked food and a high concentrated sweetener (white sugar etc.) diet. The American Academy for Pediatrics reports that the average child spends more hours on social media, texting, playing computer games, and watching television than they spend in school. The child eats a sweet snack for every two hours of being on the computer or television viewing. The average Black child is on the computer and watches more television and eats more sweets than White children. Children, especially Black children, oppressed, or in poverty eat more junk food, fast food, sodas and snack foods than poor White children. The majority of Black children and 22% of White children do not eat breakfast. They usually eat snack junk foods (Citizens Pubecy Center in Oakland, CA). Junk foods are nutrient deficient and have addictive chemicals which includes hormones, poisonous table salt = sodium (salt) chloride (bleach), sugars, cancer causing coal tar dyes and perfumes (makes them smell good). They do not have natural B complex vitamins, B_6, Niacin, Folic Acid, Riboflavin, Iron, Potassium, Chromium, Vitamin C, Beta-Carotene, Phenylalanine, Lysine, Glutamic acid and the nutrients the brain needs to function. The White corporate junk food business is deliberately processing out nutrients and not giving the child the vitamins, minerals, trace elements, fiber and amino acids that they need. This is done deliberately because milling or processing grains such as brown rice, corn, whole wheat flour and sugar cane grass increases its shelf life, which increases profits. Shelf life is the ability of foods to stay on the store's shelf without spoiling. Processed foods have become a type of synthetic dirt or manure in the stomach and colon which clogs organs, arteries and veins.

The junk foods include synthetic eggs and rice made of plastic and potato starch, which is the same as eating a plastic bag. Synthetic meat composed of toxic glues, meat scrapes, plastic and potato starch. Ideally the child should eat non-GMO organic grains (amarantha, spelt, millet, whole wheat, brown rice, yellow grits, etc.) that have vitamins, minerals, proteins and fiber, and have a short shelf life. The short shelf life is against the profit margin of the long shelf life junk foods. Selling non-GMO organic natural foods would decrease business profits. The GMO crops must use specific synthetic fertilizers. Consequently, the junk food diet of the Black child makes them a diseased sacrifice for business profits. (A book such as *Psycho-Nutrition* by Carlton Fredericks can be a resource).

Children's brain suffers allergic reactions from stress, nerve damage, pain, GMOs, junk foods, and concentrated sweeteners. They cause learning and behavioral problems. There are various types of plants processed and refined to produce white sugar such as beets, corn and cane sugar. Any one of these processed sugars can cause brain pain. When the brain feels nerve damage (so called pain) it changes the ability to think and changes the moods and state of consciousness. The brain cannot feel physical pain it reacts to nerve signals of pain with mood changes, problems with emotions and thoughts. The food corporations only have to report an ingredient such as sugar and not the synthetic chemicals used to make the sugar or any ingredient. For example, sodium chloride (table salt) contains close to 32 synthetic chemical ingredients that are used by the wholesale manufacturer of the salt. However, the retail company that bought from the wholesaler only has to put on the retail label that the ingredient is salt. The corporate owned White junk food companies and international trade agreements put harmful synthetic chemicals into foods that destroy the human body. Black children are mentally, nutritionally, and physically abused by international food trade agreements and government institutions. The National Institute of Health's Genetic Factors indicates that food companies use chemicals to alter the brain and drugs to genetically modify and control the behavior of nutritionally deprived Black children. Added to this supplement and herbal remedies are made as candies. Candies that use all types of chemically laced sugars from plants, cancer causing Triclosan (FDA ban from use in agriculture, but used in toothpaste or gel), coal tar type sugars, artificial sugars and animal's collagen, and cartilage and petroleum jelly that is used to make gelatin gummies (C.A. Frazer, M.D. explores allergic reactions in children in Parent's Guide to Allergy in Children).

The 1988 Surgeon General's Report on Nutrition and Health reported that diet influences and causes 60% of diseases. The diseases destroy the body's ability to function and to protect itself. White junk food companies are in business to stay in business. Their foods deplete the children of energy and lead them to a life of diseases that will put them on special education drugs, prisoner's drugs and junk foods and in a cemetery.

Disease and death are a byproduct of poor nutrition. Food has become Caucasian corporations weapon to control people and destroy Black people's wellness. Black peoples high amount of food illiteracy and CGI artificial intelligence and social media zombies that causes them to make the wrong food choices. Allowing Black people to have financial access to non-GMO organic natural foods is not the government's design or purpose. This information is published in "The Food Gap, Poverty and Malnutrition in the United States" (Washington DC. Government Printing Office 1969) and in N. Kotz's Book, *Let Them Eat Promises: The Politics of Hunger in America.*

It is a total illusion to rely upon the White corporate junk foods or allopathic disease causing drug medicines to save Black people. The drugs are made in the form of candy such as chewable gummies. This makes the child addicted to sugar and addicted to the drug. This is a double addiction that locks the child into a spiral of diseases from diabetes to cancer. White people's nutritionist, doctors, dieticians, and health practitioners eat as much junk food as the general public and use corporate created faulty and fake scientific research and text books. This makes them unreliable for nutritional guidance. If one of their theory based science gangs decides to be humanistic or allow Black people to use their culture's herb medicine or African centered hygienic health treatment system or non- GMO organic natural foods diet, then one of the other disciplines (science gangs) will attack them. They attack each other in order to keep the Black caucus alive long enough to drain more economic profit. They identify the disease early so that they have a long time to sell drugs to the Black person. They also take pictures early (MRI, CAT scans, x-ray) and cause Black people to pay for pictures on their journey to death. The old saying was kill a donkey, buy another; kill a slave, breed another. Black people breed children and train them to eat death causing junk food.

The White people do not have an intelligent brain that supervises White Supremacy or divide and conquer techniques or selfish individualism or violent wolf pack attacks upon Black peoples. They use emotional manipulation and the cave instinct for survival. Historically, the basic emotional unit of their society is the emotionally dysfunctional family. The White civilizations family structure is divided. Basically, their normal cave dysfunctional family is a loose collection of individuals that will betray and deceive each other. They have deceit and deception emotional addiction and enjoy their dysfunctional addiction. In their distant past, they would deceitfully sell bricks that were cracked to each other. They would hide the cracks in the bricks with wax (deception) and sell them as good bricks. Eventually a house built with cracked bricks would fall apart. They have a saying left over from their deceitful behavior and we sign letters with the word "sincere." Sincere means the cracked bricks are not sealed with wax.

The deceit and divided characteristics of their cave civilizations family, spirit, emotions, minds and countries is still present in their social DNA.

Cave civilizations dysfunctional cave families and mixtures of cave families called clans were blood related and fought each other. Then after a battle against a common enemy they would fight amongst each other. Individuals in their families would betray, deceive and abuse each other violently and sexually. White people's cave dysfunctional broken homes would unite, and then break up their unity. Then the cycle of dysfunctional families, clans and tribes would continue. This led to dysfunctional kingdoms and governments. This cycle of dysfunctional governments was repeated in America when dysfunctional European families separated from homeland governments were sent to America by feudal kings. The oligarchy kings were seeking businesses profit. Oligarchy kings used the homeless, criminals, thieves, prostitutes, beggars, mentally ill, orphans, indentured wage salves, and some were blood relatives of the kings for their business profits. The newly arrive oligarchy thieves used European social waste that they brain washed into believing that they were citizens and patriots to steal the land and natural and human resources, murder native Americans and Carib Indians. They used the profits from stealing the native Indians gold, coal, wood, tin, iron and labor of African slaves to finance the so-called American revolution. The revolution was the act declaring themselves free to steal the European own land, slaves and businesses of the feudal kings. After stealing the property, they set up a corporate own government called the USA. They had the people (so-called citizens and patriots) fight and murder their blood relatives which was the same behavior of cave life. Later in history, the corporations fought over stealing the ownership of the human resources (slaves), and natural resources of Africa. They again had their brain washed citizens fight other brainwashed citizens (their relatives) over possession of land in Africa. They called the stealing of America's land and resources the American Revolution. The thieves loosely united again and fought their own blood relatives and clans over control of the American colonies economy which was the War of Northern Economic Aggression against the South (so called Civil War). It is inherent in Caucasian civilization to be dysfunctional, divided and prone to violence. They have families that behave like an animal pride and family members that will lie and steal from each other. This dysfunctional family structure builds their nations and corporations (see Crave the Cave "The Characters" play)

The cultural ingredients for White dysfunctional families is within the cave civilization. This civilization began the illogical food combining habits of eating a meat and starch centered diet. This diet and the disease the diet causes has been forced upon Black people. Any race that has the ungodly misfortune to have to associate with White Supremacy diseased cave people will become divided and conquered, inferiorized, use group sex, masturbation, use stimulants (caffeine, nicotine, sugar, alcohol, cocaine, etc.) use violence upon its members, use homosexuality, have dysfunctional families, junk food diets, have corporate created inflation, depression, and recession economy, use drugs, practice revenge call justice, human torture in isolation in jail, have abortions and won't know their history (White people do not know their cave history). Black people that follow White culture have reproductive failures, rotten teeth, suicides, rape each other, have White Gods and Saviors, follow theory based science, and commit wild wolf pack attacks upon each other (gang warfare).

The chemicalized junk foods are addicting and biochemically help to support addiction to White people's behaviors. Biochemically the brain nourished by junk food has a predisposition for addiction, which means it can become easily addicted to other things.

Black people suffer due to the nutritional level set by white theory based science. White women and girls' diets are the most nutritionally deficient. For example, Black people have the highest level of malnutrition, stress, degenerative diseases, birth defects, venereal dis-eases and even the most headaches. John Hopkins University's research reports that the poor have 60% more headaches. Added to all white corporate own research is the dis-eases caused by White supremacy. White medical science totally ignores White Supremacy's disease effect when evaluating Black people's diseases. They would rather blame Black people's diseases on a virus or bacteria instead of White Supremacy.

Junk food is used to destroy Black people's health while at the same time that same constipating synthetic chemicalized GMO junk food makes an abundance of profit for white food corporations. The dis-eases caused by junk food makes profits for the Sick Industries which are hospitals, doctors and drug companies (disease industry). Incidentally, aspirin and laxatives are the two largest selling chemicals of drug companies. The cooked junk food causes the headaches (aspirin use) and constipation (laxative use). Black people are indoctrinated (so-called educated) to believe that they are born to be sick and born in sin. Indoctrination teaches you what to think while education teaches you how to think. Black people are indoctrinated until they believe that they are going to get sick no matter what they eat or do not eat. Black people think that they must die from disease and often say, "You gonna die from something, so why should I eat health foods."

There are many white corporate own countries, (United States of America, Canada, England, Italy, Sweden, Portugal, France, etc.), that have populations that are walking sick outpatient people that go to hospitals that feed them fast food stores, and have junk food machines and drug stores that sell junk foods. Many times, the hospitals are very large buildings because they know their disease market of sick people is permanent and always increasing fixture. They sell drugs for dis-eases at gas stations, grocery stores and amusement parks and everyone buys them including doctors, nurses and morticians (undertakers). Black people are carefully taught in movies and by television, games, commercials sport events, to be junk food addicts and functional alcoholics. They are merely permanent hospital outpatients with some type of walking dis-ease believed to be caused by a bacteria or virus instead of the White junk food, White Supremacy and drug medicine businesses. Because of the manmade synthetic junk foods, Black people are food illiterate and walk around with a fear that their own body will fail to be healthy or that their body will fall apart or self-destruct from a mysterious germ that has attacked them. It is the disease-causing actions of junk food and drugs that have attacked all Black people. Furthermore, "certified Negroes" reject health food and will say that they are not dietary extremists like the Black health food and vegetarian dieters. Consequently, they eat in "moderation" which means their diet is a mixture of junk food and health food. "Moderation" is used as an excuse to stay addicted to junk food, junk culture and junk religions.

Junk culture is a mixture of White people's cave culture in a superior position and African culture in an inferior position. These "certified Negroes" accept all non-black cultures that so not accept them. And they can be seen wearing European tuxedos and African Kente cloth bow ties, high heels and straightened relaxed hair with an African gown; celebrating Christmas, Halloween, Thanksgiving, Valentine's Day, or St. Patrick's Day or other White people holidays. They pledge allegiance to White people's cultural perversions of ancient African spiritual systems that white people call religions (Judaism, Christians and Muslims) with books written by and for Caucasians such as the *Torah, The King James Version of the Bible and the European Arabic Koran*. These religions refer to Black spirituality as sinful and inferiorize African culture. In any case, junk food, junk culture and junk religions addicts may call themselves multicultural or "moderates." However, the deadly effect of all junk foods and drugs is death.

There are many alibis (excuses) used by junk food addicts. For example, the addicted Black people say that all White people are not racist or that some White people are nice. There are also "nice" alcoholics, drug addicts, thieves, rapists, cancer patients, diabetics, etc. Being "nice" does not stop white folks from having the disease of White Supremacy just as being nice does not stop diabetes. "Nice" White people accept the benefits of their white skin (White Privilege) and do not actively or militarily stop other whites from being White Supremacist or White Racist. Nice and or conscious white people are guilty of White Supremacy by passive participation and association. They live in a white culture (white racist) house and accept the

51

economic benefits and social advantages from supporting the white culture (White Supremacy). If they were truly "nice" they would move out of the White Supremacy mind set or try to destroy White Supremacy without any Black person telling them to do so. "Nice white folks" is another excuse Black people use to stay addicted to White people's junk food, junk culture and junk religions.

The White people distort and lie about their own history and Africa's history. This helps to force their human relationship dysfunctions and dietary ignorance upon Black people. In their history writings, they state that Black people were never taught in schools (so called "rite of passage" a German term invented for school) or read about health and nutrition. The historical lies about Black food science or the wealth all white countries stole from Africa supports their myth of White Supremacy. In fact, Black people never view themselves as a holistic part of world history or a part of the science of nutrition. In any case, omitting nutrition and food as a part of history causes the reader to assume that all people basically ate the same as white cave civilizations people and use allopathic drug medicine.

There are words that hide the White crimes of using junk food and drug medicine to destroy Black people. White people use the words "Western Science," "Modern Man (the white man)," "The Western Countries (white countries)," "manmade (made by whites)," "Modern Medicine (white medicine)," "Scientific (white) Proof," "Statistics (white assumptions)," "Education (white degrees)," "Professional (white) License," "Certified (white approval)," etc., all of which means White peoples civilization must be followed. It is not "Modern Man" that has polluted the earth, it is the White people. It is not "Western Medicine," it is White peoples drug medicine. It is not an "Education," it is a White people approved "Indoctrination." It is not junk food, synthetic fertilizers, poisonous drugs; it is White people's corporation that own junk foods, synthetic fertilizers and poisonous drugs. It is not "a war on terror"; it is White people that cause a world of terrorist, war and violence. They get money to pretend to solve the problem that they have created and in so doing create new problems (collateral damage).

Black people everywhere must eat non-GMO organic foods to be healthy. White people are the ones producing these natural foods for other White people to eat. In the process of producing the foods they slowly pollute the food. A White person on an organic natural food diet is still a White Supremacist. It is the White corporate own natural foods industry that believes that they will always be in control of food and the planet earth and Black people will always be consumers of white products and never producers. In the past, the White people have had control over health food movements and perverted them. For example, the White doctor, Dr. Kellogg and his brother were pioneers in the health food industry. They started the use of fibrous and nutritionally rich whole corn flakes. Today, Kellogg's corn flakes are a GMO junk food. There are more nutrients and fiber in the cardboard box than contents the flakes than are in the corn flakes. Dr. Kellogg performed many surgical removals of parts of the colon to adapt it to junk food. Another pioneer in the health food movement was Dr. Graham. He started the use of nutritionally rich and fibrous cracked whole-wheat crackers. Today, his "graham" crackers are GMO bleached white wheat and white sugar with a little cellulose wood fiber = junk food. One of the remnants of white people's early health food movements is the meal time salad. Today the salads are reduced to a junk food with synthetic cooked oil (a type of oily drugs) salad dressing and ascetic acid(vinegar), cooked meats, cheese and cubes of white bread usually made from recycled day old stale bread. The White people's health food movements usually come to a complete ruin. White people eat health foods in order to run from diseases. In African culture, health food was part of the Maat and wellness.

White people's health food corporations usually ruin itself because it has to add addicting synthetic chemicals to the foods because the pharmaceutical, health (sick) care and agriculture industries are part of their health food industry. Those industries have to maintain profits and the addition of synthetic addicting chemicals stabilizes their market share. Those industries pay scientist to discredit the value of health and pay them to generate fake research that supports junk food. The high prices for non- GMO organic foods force Black people to eat junk foods and get sick and then take drugs that make them sick and then take drugs to fight the side effect sickness caused by the drugs. Usually the high prices of health foods keep Black people out of those stores.

The health food store or drug store and both are own by the same multinational corporation. The natural foods industry is still an unnatural racist industry. White people manufacture supplements and herbs for themselves without respect for Black people's specific biochemical personalities. Black people are becoming sick and White people are becoming healthy with a White Supremacist cave civilization mind. Black people's former slave masters ate non-GMO organic foods and still hated the Black race. White corporations are totally capable of destroying Black people on many levels. It must be historically noted that it was White Arabs on non-GMO organic health foods that operated the Northern and Trans Pacific slave trade. The Arabs, East Indians and Chinese maintained the most vicious evil form of chattel enslavement for over 1,000 years. The Orientals and Indians usually bought 4 Black women slaves to each 1 male slave. They used them for breeding. The Europeans usually bought 4 male slaves to 1 female slave. Males did the labor-intensive work. After the Arabs and oriental enslavers, the White people (England, France, Spain, Portugal, Dutch, Germans, Russia) called Eastern Europeans and Western Europeans (includes China and India) participated in the slave trade. They were on cooked non-GMO organic foods diet when they stole the African slave trade from other white people. This slave trade forcefully brought Black peoples to North and South America, Caribbean, India and China. Slavery and colonialism contributed to the mass murder of at least 200 million Africans.

White psychologist label any White person that has killed 5 or more people a mass murderer. The mass murderer is scientifically proven to be emotionally and mentally ill. Then they look into the history of the mass murderer and identify the behavior that created the killer's insane mind. If Black people use white psychology's evaluation standards then by definition the White race is one of a mass murderers (killed over 200 million Africans) with a Psychopathic Racial Personality added to Cave Trauma's emotion and mental illness. Examine White history and it will reveal the cave behavior that shaped their insanity. Ironically, any Black person that truthfully labels and identifies the White race as a race of mass murderers, liars, thieves and prone to violence with at biochemically imbalance, and emotionally, and mentally illness that Black person is called a racist. White people have murdered the natives of north and south America, Caribbean and Black peoples on the continent of Africa. They claim themselves to be peaceful and use policing (control) of the world with bombs, drones and soldiers to invade, terrorized and take over countries. Their takeover of countries includes the extermination of innocent children and women. They send junk food care packages and their drug medicine to the drone bombed peoples. This creates life time customers for their synthetic chemicalized GMO agriculture foods, drug medicine while they instill the hate of Black people's to other races. Black people with a "slave's mentality" will use negative words to attack and character assassinate any Black person that speaks truthfully about the violent nature of cave trauma whites.

Slave Trauma Black people tend to have Pathological Incredulity Disorder. They automatically assume the White behavior is normal and it is incredible that someone would say White people are prone to violence and have Cave Trauma. Black people that read the truth or listen to truth about the many lies that white people tell about their discovery of America or their lies about being the greatest white country are attacked by white people. When those same Black people are presented with validate facts about white people's non-stop violence and cave behavior most black people will automatically say it is an incredible lie. During slavery, these Slave Trauma Blacks believed that when the master was sick they were sick and would say "master we are sick we got a cold".

Caucasians on health foods murdered, raped, enslaved and destroyed Africa's human and land resources. Again, physically fit White people are still white supremacist. A book such as *How the White Man's Diet Affects Natives of Africa* by Albert Schweitzer can give some insight. Using White health standards and junk food is destructive to Black people before birth and after birth. In Black culture a natural delivery, is drug free and allows the umbilical cord to stop pulsating before being cut. The baby's delivery is in the squatting position. Relatives, extended family and a midwife are present, and Afrocentric rituals and ceremonies are used. The natural birth allows the contractions to stimulate the baby's muscles which moves lymph fluid and activates immunity, stimulates the cerebral spinal fluid and helps send nourishing blood, oxygen, and nutrients to the child's brain. Drug induced contractions nutritionally rob the brain, causes an acidic sympathetic response in the child which, weakens the immune system, pollutes the liver, pancreas, thyroid and leaves dead brain cells in the brain. A Cesarean Section (C-Section) interrupts the synchronized cyclic hormonal rhythm between the mother and child. This interruption causes bonding and lung diseases, behavioral problems, slows the growth and or retards growth. Instead of nutritionally solving this problem White doctor's drug medicine add to the problem with their interruption and interference with the Bonding and Emotional Rites of Passage of birthing.

There are psychological aspects to White people's interference with African culture births. For example, White people indoctrinates Black people to believe that a baby has a birthday. This logic is used to inferiorize women and de-Africanize Black people. In African culture the mother (Isis) has a birthday as she gives birth to the child. The child cannot birth itself. The child has a day of "emergency" as it emerges from the mother's uterus(womb). The Greeks called the uterus a womb because they believed the woman's penis was cut off by the gods to punish her for creating sin. In any case, the only true emergency occurs as the baby emerges from the uterus at birth. It is a part of White peoples diseased cultural individualism to think "I had my own birth" or "all for me" or "me for me." It helps to affirm their White Supremacy psychosis which is the belief that white people are the center of the world's knowledge and civilizations. They believe that their theory base science use of drugs is the solution for all diseases for all people. They proceed to solve the medical problems that they created (with their junk foods, GMO chemically polluted foods) by creating a synthetic chemical (drug) problem.

White theory medicine defines any problem the child has after their drug and surgery medical interference with natural birth as a biochemical problem of the baby. They use drugs to torture the Black child's entire body combined with the torture of the C-Section surgical operation. What awaits the child as a consequence of a C-Section are drugs for asthma, bronchitis, behavior problems, colds, learning problems, and synthetic hormones. Books by R.S. Mendelsohn MD, titled *Confessions of a Medical Heretic and Male-Practice*, document the Nutricide crimes.

White medical theory based science medicine problems started prenatally and during the birth process are never corrected. The white junk food diet compounds the problems. White medical science proceeds to classify problems that they created as the Black child's genetic brain illness that causes violence, and learning problems. Ritalin or similar type drugs are given in addition to Genetic altering drugs. Ritalin is a narcotic that is in the same category as cocaine. It retards growth, increases blood pressure, attacks melanin, weakens immunity, digestion, reproductive and excretory systems weakness, causes uncontrollable emotional out breaks, menstruation difficulties, causes learning problems and damages the brain and nerves. The use of drugs such as Ritalin has not been documented to increase intelligence or performance. The drugs make the African child a dope robot, prone to addiction, alters the normal biochemistry and gives the child a predisposition for relationship problems.

Ritalin is a chemical solution for the educational systems failure to educate and White peoples' cultural bias educational system's that is design to make Black servants to white Supremacy. This social engineering and indoctrination into white culture is called an education. The mental, emotional, cultural and physical chemistry between the Black child and the White educational system failure to educate is the problem, not the Black child. Aside from this the drugs that are given to Black children by the public schools are actually based on money. It is profit motivation that causes the schools to drug Black children. The schools, hospitals, theory based medical science, and junk food companies run a cash and carry business. They receive cash money for every child that swallow's drugs. Schools get more money from the federal government if they can qualify Black children for certain behavioral problems. The federal government offers more money to schools that have children with mental or behavioral problems. The federal money given to schools to treat children with special problems is used for salaries (extra pay), supplies, books and other items that the school needs and the drug is last on the list of pay outs. The corporate own schools desiring the money can conveniently find that 40% of the children have behavioral and or mental problems or brain damage. The drugs are given to Black children despite the unscientific diagnosis for their use. They give Black children such narcotics as Ritalin or other behavioral drugs such as Toframil, Cylert, or Dexedrine. Black children are basically drugged because of the nutrition less junk food problems of the mother that were created prenatally and after birth the child eats junk foods, sugary foods and drinks acidic cow's milk (mother's milk is alkaline).

Drugging the child covers up the School systems failure to educate, psychologist failure to counsel and parent's lack of parenting skills. The Black parent tries to be the village to educate the child. However, a parent is not a village. The parent compensates for not being the village by giving the child expensive clothes, Iphones, computers, computer games, or X-rated shows and movies to watch and allows social medias to parent the child. This further dysfunctionalizes the Ritalin sugar addicted child and creates a co-dependent child addicted to white culture.

A co-dependent child is a non-drug-addicted schoolmate of an Ritalin addicted child. Non-addicted school children are forced to socialize with the addicts. This causes the Ritalin addicts classmates to develop distorted emotions, feelings, thoughts and behaviors in order to survive the addict and socialize with the addict. Co-dependency creates a dysfunctional personality. This once mentally healthy co-dependent classmate of the addict changes their personality in order to get along with the addict. When the non-addicted child does not do things the addict desires it may cause a fight. The non-addicted child learns to take physical and emotional abuse, and they have to pretend to be friendly. The non-addicted child learns to curse and be violent to defend themselves. The co-dependent playmate of the addict changes into a personality that can complement, maintain and feed off the dis-eased Ritalin addict. The non-addicted child only feels normal when they are abused. The addict's entire classroom of children becomes affected and infected with forms of co-dependency mental illnesses. Co-dependents grow up to have dysfunctional relationships and dysfunctional children in order to feel normal.

A dysfunctional Black person is by definition a "seasonin" Black slave that is an economic benefit to Whites. Whites earn money (capital, profits) from all types of dysfunctional Black children and adults. Dysfunctional Black people buy material goods to be comfortable in their mental illness, oppression and wage slavery. White Supremacy can only be successful if and only if Whites create and maintain dysfunctional Black people.

Once a disease (Dysfunctionality, AIDS, Cancer, Hyperactivity, Crime, Co-dependency, White Supremacy, etc.) becomes an industry it never dies. The disease industry maintains and protects itself by coming out every year with a new model (drug, research findings, disease). This means new signs and symptoms for disease, new research findings, new names for White Supremacy (white privileges), new crimes (hate crimes), new treatments and drug therapies. White science constantly redefines diseases, create a new disease within the old disease so that the industry can expand its market share and profits. Dis-ease no longer functions as a disease; disease functions as a business. The drug industry uses the pink color as a symbol to raise money for research, and people run, march, donate money, and buy pink garments to donate money to the drug industries. Drug companies create diseases to sell their vaccinations or make a law that you must buy their drug vaccinations. The use of Vaccinations is based upon the Germ Theory which is the basis of the Contagious Disease Theory that supports the Immunity Theory. You cannot be immune to polluted air or polluted water. Your body will react to polluted water. If your body does not react it is called immunity. Immunus was a city in Greece that did not pay taxes and they did not react to the king's order to pay tax. Aside from this there is no physical system in the body called the immune system. Black people were in slavery, which means they should be immune to slavery. If you actually believe the theory belief of the White people then you have Post Traumatic Slavery Disorder (mentally ill = crazy). White people's vaccination belief theory means they use a belief (theory) to support a belief (theory) that is a belief (theory). The theory belief of white theory based science is the factual reason to take a vaccination. A belief is NOT a fact. This belief system of beliefs is "science fiction (fake)" science. White people believe that giving a person a disease (laboratory made synthetic vaccination drug disease) protects them from a natural disease. If you use that logic (craziness) then Black people can be given a White Supremacy vaccination. Black people have been around White Supremacy so long that they should have a naturally acquired White Supremacy vaccination protection and they have acquired the craziness of the whites called assimilation and intergration. In any case a religion is a belief and does not have to be proven because it is a belief. It is alright for white people to have a belief but it is not alright to force their belief on Black people. This is their arrogance to believe Black people must accept white beliefs as reality and fact.

The Black junk food addict arrogantly defends White junk food. "Arrogance" is a trait of White people. Arrogance occurs when a White people exaggerates their fantasized superiority over Black people in an overbearing manner and defends it with pride. White people's disease of arrogance is exhibited when Black people arrogantly assume that one Negro group is the only group that is aware and conscious. For example, Black people that are Christians, Jews, Muslims, Khemetics, Vegetarians, Health food dieters and history, political and social activist groups assume that their individual groups are the only Black group that is aware or conscious of the proper way to be a Black person, or how to eat, or be African-centered, or be spiritual, or have the path to Black people's freedom. These Black people will arrogantly state that the other Black groups are not conscious and holding back the race from progress. By the by, the assimilationist and integrationist Black person is an invention of White people so they can hide their mental illnesses of self-hatred and White Supremacy psychosis. Assimilationist and integrationist are Black people created by crazy white people. Most Black people regardless of their level of consciousness or awareness, are working to uplift the Black race. Arrogance is a type of slave or colonial mentality. Assimilation, Integration and arrogance is another tool given to Black people to destroy themselves, their culture and their children. It is Black children that need nutritional salvation from White people assimilation and integration ideological plantation.

Eating junk food causes a slow degenerative disease process. Junk food and drug induced deterioration is disguised because Black people are trained to think that constantly getting sick or being sick is normal. They are trained to think that the habitual taking of non-prescription and prescription drugs drinking alcohol and cooking oils in tobacco and marijuana is normal. It is normal for White people to be sickly but not Black people. Prescription and non-prescription drugs, medical procedures, concentrated sweeteners, alcohol, caffeine, sex stimulants, GMO foods, salt (sodium chloride), fried foods, cooked nicotine oil and cannabinol oil, and junk foods cause physical, mental, and emotional diseases.

Junk food destruction is supported by the blind religious belief in theory based science. This is a science that solves nothing and cures nothing. Theory based science is designed to create and support White Supremacy theory (psychosis). Science means to "know". Historically, it has been ancient Africans that "know" astrology, Dogon Star, Sirius, Galaxies, cycles, God, architecture, nutrition, acupuncture, human relationship, biology and chemistry. White people copy the knowers (Black people). White people do not know and have to search, research and then write fantasy superstitions theories in a science language. They write fiction and fake science and call it science. Scientifically speaking, if Black people flushed all the white theory science books down the toilet, it would be the worst thing to happen to the toilet and sewer and the best thing to happen for the Black science students. The health junk foods damage is scientifically disguised and misdiagnosed. They blame disease on a bacteria or virus and never admit that they are the emotionally and mentally disease people causing the disease. For example, the hospitals non-cyclic control of light and dark in infant nurseries can cause the degeneration of the body, decrease the cleansing of the brain and cause gland immaturity. Light manipulation and LED lights weakens the ability of the body to defend itself and predisposes the child for disease. Aside from, the separation of the newborn from the mother causes emotional damage in the child.

Junk food meat tissue grown in test tubes and meats have been irradiated and exposed to nuclear waste, synthetically fertilized, insecticide, herbicide, cloned means plants combine with bacteria, germs, human cells, insect and animal cells which makes a freak plant. The foods are processed with synthetic chemicals. The plants are grown in polluted air, soil, and

59

water, radiation waste from nuclear plants and run off waste from animal farms. It is the emotionally ill minds of the cave traumatized White Supremacist that sometime in the future one of their theories will save the world. In other words, Black people should not be afraid of the created monster Frankenstein (junk food). Dr. Frankenstein (the White mind) is the creator of the monster and it is he that must be feared.

The protection and reparation to "nature" are the spiritual right of plants, air, water, soil and the planet earth. Reparation to people for the damage of white corporate own junk foods and their poisonous drugs is beyond the comprehension of the cave trauma White people. White people are addicted to insanity (White Supremacy) and practice daily their insanity. Black people that plead to white people to behave and ask White people to voluntarily pay reparations might as well ask white people to stop having white skin. A new standard of reparation must be developed to meet the requirements demanded by Black people because the white standards for reparation are for "Whites Only."

The standard for reparations is entrenched in cave superstitions and White Supremacy psychosis. For example, theory science, theory nutrition, theory medicine and theory social sciences use the theory belief that the natural existence of life is confusion, antagonistic, a conflict, life becomes confused, and chaotic. This white linear theory logic justifies White peoples continued psychotic need to dominate Black people and steal Black people's human and natural resources. In White people's drug allopathic medicine (medical doctors) the fundamental theory belief concept is that "contrary cures opposite." This means that to be against nature cures nature from being nature. If reparation is left to the devices of White people it will follow the theory concept that contrary to reparation solves the reparation problem. White people will use "Reparation" as another tool for destroying Black people.

Black people thinking that they can get reparation from emotionally and mentally ill cave traumatized White people is in itself a crazy concept. Sane people can pay reparations to sane people. However, any demand of reparations from the emotionally and mentally ill White people is questionable. In other words, Black people would have to decide how much the White violent thief should keep of what they have stolen. This is what Black people call reparations. No thief has any rights to claim any part of what they have stolen. White people will never accept themselves as being insane thieves and prone to violence that are in need of punishment and habilitation. Reparations means that all of the White corporate own countries, and corporate own religions must pay money for killing over 200 million Africans during colonialism and slavery. Added to this, they must pay for the Black people that were lynched by rope and by drugs, police murders,

60

jail tortures, drug experiment murders, medical treatment injuries and deaths, junk foods diseases, mis-educated mental deaths, alcohol, cigarettes, lead poisoned, syphilis deaths, those killed in Caucasian wars and abortion deaths. White people must pay for the death of potential offspring of those murdered. Aside from this, the White people must give back the economic profits they got from 450 years of free slave labor and the East Indians, Chinese, and Arabs must pay for 2,000 years of free labor. White people must pay for the money and profits of the over 10 million dollars in gold and jewels given to the U.S.A. for distribution to ex-slaves by Emperor Menelik in 1865. Pay for the patents stolen from George Washington Carver and many other Black inventors. Pay for the stolen music copyrights of Fats Waller and other musicians. Pay for the stolen natural resources of Africa such as gold, diamonds, books, tin, wood, land, uranium, plutonium, trees, ivory, oil and treasures looted from ancient cities and Egyptian tombs. Again, no thief has any rights to claim what they have stolen. Therefore, white corporate own countries must give back what they have stolen, and then reparations can begin. Anything else would be an insult to the ancestors. Only a sane people can be punished or pay reparation. White people would have to be habilitated. Habilitation means they must learn to live in holistic harmony with themselves, nature and other races. After habilitation, the White people should be holistically balanced (reparations) and then rehabilitated. Reparations in White people's linear logic means punishment while with Black people it means healing and harmony (Maat). Reparations for junk foods destroying Black people are part of the reparations that the White people must confront in order to gain some form of sanity.

African Women Nutricide/Cultural Genocide

African men and women are faced with one reality and that is to rid Black culture of nutritional and cultural destruction. White people use their cave sexism against the Black people to exploit, oppress and deny them of sovereign human rights. Black people were taught sex behavior and relationship behavior by white rapist pedophile slave masters and white cave culture. Black people have become white and see sex as Cultural- less and non-spiritual activity. Sex is a behavior language of a culture. Currently, the Black woman sexuality is White in its emotional, mental and physical behavior women's sexuality is different because they have 34 nerve endings per inch of skin 17 nerve endings, women have a different hormone ratio and balance, women's fatty tissue grows vertically upward under the derma while men's fatty tissue grows horizontal to the derma and men, women's midbrain is larger than men's, the brain's language center is larger, women's breast age faster than her other skin, men's breast skin age relatively equal to other skin, women immune system is twice as large as men's etc. "Seasonin" during slavery caused the mental, emotional and European cultural enslavement of Black men and women sexuality. White type sex needs to be eliminated. Black people must start saying a prayer before having sex because sex was created by God and is a spiritual activity that puts you in contact with God. The child produce from a Godly activity of sex will be the technology the race needs to destroy White Domination, White Supremacy and White Racism. A holistic sexual balance requires new words and deeds of behavior from Black people's sexuality. The resurrection of African centered sex is risky. Risky because a new definition for the Black man and woman's sexual mental, emotional, spiritual and social past behavior has to be cleansed and redefined without white culture. Black people sexuality is learned in the process of learning and simultaneously healing sexuality. Healing Post Traumatic sex slavery activity is the responsibility our history and ancestors have placed upon us. The mistakes made in the process of healing slave sex trauma will be healed by the use of Maat. There will be some moderate emotional injuries that will heal as we are in the healing process. This redefinition has to start with trauma injured ex- slaves united with Maat on a cleansing and healing path. An emotional injury that has causes Black people to do mutilation called infibulation, dilation and curettage the cutting of the inner skin of the uterus, outside vagina lip excision, hair relaxers, circumcision (boys and girls), wearing of earrings, navel rings, nose rings, nipple rings, penis and vagina labia rings, cursing while having sex, sex spanking, using whips and chains in sex, toxic tattoo dye, bleaching cream, and high heels (stilts) makes the body a sacrifice to the White culture. In the historical past, Black people would mutilate and disfigure their bodies by stretching the lips, ears, penis skin, vagina skin with plates or heavy metal, scar the skin with knives so that white slavers would not put them in slavery. Unfortunately, white slavers captured them and sold them to circuses. Black people are a living commercial for the white culture and white standards of beauty. Black people call their African clothing customs or only wear them once a year during Kwanzaa. Black with the "we are the same as white" mentality want to merge or assimilate integrate into white culture or say do "They not see skin color" use it as a way to merge, assimilate or integrate into whiteness. They feel that having white friends or having sex with white people or marrying white people gives them the same freedom as white people or somehow protects them from being a "nigger". They are emotionally seeking protection from being a "nigger". This has not worked in the past or the present. Black man getting haircuts to rid themselves of kinky nappy curly African hair and Black women relaxing heir kinky hair so it resembles limp white hair has not and will not save them from being "niggers". The Black race is sending the subconscious messages that they want to be white and hate being Black. Black male sexism as well as female feminism heterosexual or homosexual activities requires the power to have human rights. Human rights can only be guaranteed by a group that has control over human and natural resources and land. There are no individual or relationship human rights without a group to defend and protect the rights and the ability to attack your enemies. Without a group, there are no freedoms and no sovereignty. Civil Rights means following the rituals and ceremonies of the white people. White people give the civil rights and they can take away the civil rights. Sovereign human rights are a birth right. However, in this white and Black relationship with the white cavies' Black people must claim their culture and then create a path to freedom.

The Black males and females imitate White people's relationship problems and assume they have the same Black problems. It is the same as a slave saying, "Master we are sick." White people's sexism and feminism are based on European culture. Cave Trauma and Slave Traumatized individuals are creating traumatized male and female relationships. Black people assume that they can use white people's relationship books and shows. White people's culture is intact and created the relationship theories. Black culture is fragmented and not intact. Therefore, Black people's relationship is based upon spiritual, political, military economic and social with a focus on our talents and jobs aimed at securing freedom from white people's culture. The Black relationship must be a military cell that incubates children that will defeat white people. The Black relationship is a revolutionary cell devoted to being able to practice African culture at all times and in all situations. Therefore, the relationship is about cleansing each other of slavery traumas. It should not be used to make each other more dysfunctional. The relationship should not divide other person's personality so that they can be conquered as an object of love. Typically, the Black relationship is based upon emotional illiterate vocabularies. And, the adults had parents that were not culturally focus. Each person comes to the relationship culturally homeless and emotionally damaged. In most cases, each person comes to the new relationship as left over used waste from a previous emotionally damage failed relationship. If the previous relationship was successful they would still be with the person. Love defined by White people is a mysterious feeling, an accidental falling in lust (love), a battle of the sexes and a confusing thing. White people's love behavior used by Black people creates culturally home-less feelings, confusion resulting in divorces, emotional abuse, and adultery that destroys children and destroys culture. All social customs, rituals, ceremonies, dance, music, make-up, artifacts, clothes, relationships, and current values must be disrupted, lives upset and a new Maat holistic relationship formed.

Relationship are formed without the help of the elders or communication with ancestor spirits or a complete emotional vocabulary. The relationship are dysfunctional and bonded to white culture. Bonding is best when Black people are breast fed 3 to 5 years because this develops the bipolar emotional vocabulary. Without emotional intelligence which strarts from infancy, toddler, teenager and adulthood a dysfunctionality will exist. Problems will develop when the Black man was not married to the Black woman by Maat, the family, emotional maturity and the elders' decision process. Both people in the relationship should have been raised on a non-GMO organic foods diet and trained in the academic schools on how to be an adult and trained in the schools on how to be married called a rites of passage the relationship will not create the revolution. Both people in the marriage should know how to use sexual regeneration (non-climaxing sex, non-ejaculatory). The Black man and woman have to stop erotically looking at each other's bodies or buttocks. Buttock watching comes from Greek and cave life; the buttocks shape was used to determine the sexual ability of a homosexual male. Black men should naturally look at a woman as a spiritual being instead of her buttocks and breasts. A black woman's buttocks that have a Round Shape indicates there is there is more fat the top of the gluteals, Square Shape buttocks indicates there is more fat in the low abdomen, Triangle Shape buttocks indicate there is more fat in the upper thighs and the "V" Shape buttocks indicate there is more fat at the top of the buttocks than the lower buttocks. However, if the couple uses White people's romance phantasy instead of Maat and spiritualized unity the relationship becomes another tool of White Supremacy. The relationship will be a slave plantation relationship and African culture-less.

Black relationships are not normal because they are under White cave culture siege with psychosocial battlefield conditions. The Black relationships suffers from the side effects of cave life. The Black relationships that use white psychology's culture values alienates Black people from African culture and adulthood. In a white type relationship, Black people alienate each other from their life's purpose. The Black relationship is viewed by white people as a sensual hypersex relationship. Sex is sometimes used by Black people as a way to hid from the traumatic emotional, cultural, mental and spiritual impact of slavery.

The Black woman's cultural, intellectual and emotional partnership with the Black man is believed to be controlled by the moon instead of Maat. The use of the Moon as a timing device of the galaxy can indicate changes. It is believed that the moon's sunlight reflection has an impact on menstruation. The moon's cycle is 29 and 2/3 days while a woman's cycle is 28 days. Ironically, the Black man's body has 10% more water (moon relationship) than the Black woman and the women have 10% more fat (earth attribute) than the man. So, it would follow that the man's body would respond to the moon with equal if not greater force than the woman's. It must be taken into consideration that the man's body is half female in hormonal and anatomical structure (he has nipples).

Historically, it is documented that Black women were soldiers, presidents of countries, and types of Supreme Court judges (Chief of the Council of Elders). Black men equally parented and raised children, wore dresses (gowns), make-up and mutilated their bodies with earrings. White people created and maintain the myth that Black men are irresponsible parents. The Johns Hopkins Children's Center, of Baltimore, Maryland, study (1992-1993) of married, separated and single parents indicated that over 74% of the Black fathers were active in parenting and during pregnancy. The Black man's attributes of being a "gentle-man" or having a Female Principle are depressed. The Black man's depressed Female Principle energy and emotions allows the Black woman's exploitation to go unchecked. Black people are forced to be emotionally and economically poor under White domination. All Black disease rates the highest. Diseases decrease the quantity and quality of life. Diseases in Black people are caused by White corporate own social and environmental factors. The Department of Health and Human Services Task Force on Black Health reported this information from its research.

The disease of Premenstrual Syndrome (PMS) is being used as a weapon to distort the relationship. The females body is being taken over by the imbalance of hormones and estrogen (3 hormones group as one hormone) has an effect on the parietal lobe(section) of the brain used for mood, listening, language and thought processing. PMS causes at least 5 to15 days of each month to be emotionally and intellectually hostile for men as well as women. This hostility can result in arguments, negative feelings, divorces, fights, crimes, and promiscuous sexual behavior and child-abuse. PMS goes untreated because White chauvinistically defined theory science says it is normal.

The body, emotions, and mind react to being nutritionally starved by lifestyle choices, junk foods, drugs and the poisonous chemicals in perfumes, deodorants, sanitary napkins, toilet paper, hair solutions make up (amounts to 5 pounds of poisons a year). There is an epidemic of additionally sex organ disease PMS or fibroid tumors. For example, the junk diet is low in Riboflavin which affects memory, low in Beta-Carotene which decreases cognitive skills, low in Manganese, which results in early menopause and has low pituitary and thyroid functions. Low Manganese decreases women's ability to nurture as well as bond, instinctual responses, and contributes to diabetes, high blood pressure, hypoglycemia, epileptic seizures and myasthenia gravis, while low dietary potassium is related to hypoglycemia, high blood pressure and heart problems. Low selenium is related to sudden infant crib death; low copper is related to postpartum depression and hyperactivity; low manganese is also related to irritability, muscle tremors, depression; and low vanadium is related to decreased birth weight, diabetes, and high death rates. These are just some of the nutrients lacking in Black woman's diet when she eats junk foods and takes drugs. This diet causes the Black woman to be emotional and physically weak. And, cause the inability to nutritionally in control your life and health. The state of the Black women's body is the state of the Black race. Many Black women are unable to create children (fertility problems) and the Black race is losing its ability to create freedom. Black women are not tested for nutrient deficiencies. If tested, it is by the normal standards of the White woman. These White standards for normal nutrient levels indicate a subclinical form of malnutrition in Black women, children and men. Because Black people have a higher mineral level, low in raw cholesterol and lower protein. Chlorophyll is needed to stabilize protein and is a natural deodorant. Black people's melanin skin absorbs the most sunlight that converts to Vitamin D. Black people have a higher Vitamin D level related to the Liver's metabolism of ultra-violet rays from the sun.

When Black people's high nutrient level is reduced to a low White people's nutrient state level the White theory science reads it as normal. No ethno-medical steps are taken to convert white standard into the Black health levels needed to make Black people healthy. Instead they wait until Black peoples nutrient level falls low into the normal white standard and then view it as normal. In other words, the white normal level is a sick level for Black people and makes the Black woman is twice as sick as the White woman. Therefore, the Black woman's PMS, and other dis-ease, disease reactions and recovery is twice as horrible. Added to this, junk food caused diseases to continue and multiplies a simple mild dis-ease to a chronic disease.

A non-GMO organic natural foods and raw foods diet could stop the dis-eases of premature births, birth defects, spontaneous abortions, menstruation difficulties and holistic disease bodies. (*Nutrition Against Disease*, by Roger Williams reviews these problems). Aside from foods caused dis-eases, eclampsia which is a disease of poor nutrition which strikes the poor severely. Black people are forced to be poor and undernourished under White corporate own food domination. This makes all disease rates the highest.

Eclampsia is a toxic convulsive condition of late pregnancy. Hypertension is usually a contributing factor and statistically higher in Black people. Black people suffer the most from hypertension. The Black woman with eclampsia will have swollen feet and legs, spots before the eyes, severe headaches, and dizziness which if left untreated leads to a coma and death. There is mild eclampsia and just as in any disease, there are various degrees of torture. Eclamptic behavior can be noticeable and unnoticed. The American Medical Association has offered no cure for eclampsia, or the common cold for that matter. Black women fall prey to all of the White woman's diseases by eating the junk foods and taking drugs. The White corporate control of research, drugs, disease symptoms, treatment modalities, medical schools has made Black people disease slaves in their bodies. Aside from this White Domination, White Supremacy and White Racism causes diseases. This the White corporate medical oligarchy ignores different types of symptoms. The same disease are expressed differently in men, women and children, and in different races. Aside from this the nutritional or environmental causes of dis-ease are ignored.

The White junk food diet causes hormonal imbalances in Black women. Hormone imbalances cause cholesterol to accumulate. The Cholesterol Theory has been proven wrong. Cholesterol is used in a crisis and will be high to fight the crisis. The constant high levels can cause low bile acid in the Liver's gallbladder resulting in gallstones. The gallbladder holds about two cups of concentrated bile. The acidic junk food diet stresses the alkaline ability of the pancreas and Liver. This causes exhaustion of the Liver, pineal, pituitary, thyroid, pancreas and sex glands. The exhausted Liver is not able to emulsify fat, get rid of toxins, stores energy (8-hour supply), alkaline food, generate heat to warm the internal organs, hypothermia of organs weakens them, Liver fails to make Vitamins or hormones properly, get rid of excess estrogen and makes inadequate bile which decreases the pancreas enzyme affect. When the Liver is weak, cholesterol is not emulsified and it sticks together, clogs the blood, cause nutrients to stick together and forms stones. Women are at a higher risk for stones because estrogen imbalances or stress can increase the cholesterol.

Emotional or physical stress allows waste to accumulate in the body causing arteriosclerosis, heart bypass surgery, senility, hemorrhoid veins, leg pain and tingling, varicose veins and atherosclerosis. Clogged or blocked vessels can cause coronary artery bypass surgery to replace constipated, blocked or clogged coronary vessels. Coronary bypass replaces 2 to 3 inches of a vessel while leaving the other 99% of the artery clogged with liquid manure called plaque. Long pig veins or plastic veins are surgically used to replace clogged veins, which eventually get clogged from the junk food diet.

The University of California Medical School has increased nutrition, to people which lowered the fat and cholesterol and removed 70% of the plaque from clogged vessels. The Medical Review Board cannot prove that the bypass operation medically solves the problem. After the bypass operation, the patient develops plaque in the new arteries within 5 years.

The mutilation of the Black people's body can be subtle, such as earrings, harmful synthetic chemical tattoos, circumcisions, cutting of the skin inside the uterus called dilation and curettages (D and C) or overt. During slavery, African people's tongues were cut out (removed). Tongues were removed to prevent Black people that spoke the same language from communicating a rebellion. Front teeth were knocked out with hammers so that Black people who protested slavery by starving could be forced fed. Furthermore, Caucasians would remove (amputate) feet, legs, hands, arms, lips, ears, slit noses, cut hamstring muscles and other body parts, or cut open a pregnant woman's abdomen to remove the unborn baby and then cut up the unborn child as punishment for attempting to run away, talk back, fight or in any way demand human rights. Slaves that attempted to hit a white person would be mutilated (whipped) in the face until the flesh hung from the face.

White people started scalping the heads of Black people to serve as evidence that a slave had been murdered. The scalp was then turned in for payment for catching a slave. Scalping mutilations are not an American Indian (Native) custom, but a White cave civilization custom. Native Americans used in scalping retaliation to the White scalpers. Scalping is connected to cave civilization cannibalism ceremonies. Incidentally, mild forms of cannibalism is practiced when White children eat human-shaped vitamins, gingerbread boys, or raw Livers or raw fish. This keeps White people attached to the caves and the Ice Age mentality.

Black people that still mutilate the Black woman are unwholistic as well as those who give bloodletting and animal sacrifices spiritual significance. Black woman's vaginal lips and clitoris are removed because of the influence of White cannibalistic behavior. Excisions, or removing the clitoris and infibulation, the removing of the vaginal lips' leaves the uterus exposed is done among the Dogon, Mandingoes, Tukolor, etc. This practice is performed in hospitals such as Gabriel-Toure, Hospital Bamako, Mali and is still performed in Niger, Somalia, Egypt, Yemen, Jordan, Benin, Southern Algeria, Syria, Iraq, Ethiopia, Saudi Arabia, Sudan, Senegal, Guinea, Burkina Faso (Upper Volta), Ivory Coast, etc.

Mutilation is a crude symbolic emotional need to dominate people. If the mutilation was just, (and it never is) a man would remove all the skin around the head of the penis (foreskin) to symbolize a connection to a myth, superstition or a god. Women's sex organ mutilation by men mirrors a dysfunction of the culture.

Black women where praised as the most holistically beautiful women in the entire world. Great African women such as Queen Hatsheput, Nefertari, Ty of the Egyptian 18th Dynasty, Queen Candace of Ethiopia and Queen Katabla, 16th century Queen Nzingha who defeated the Portuguese, 18th century Queen Aora Poku, leader of the Baule of the Ivory Coast, Queen Zenobia, Queen Ngokady, Pyann, Ngeede of Kuba Kingdom and the Queens who ruled Cush for 600 years.

There are numerous unsung contemporary sheros (female hero) such as Harriet Tubman or Mary Seacole (Florence Nightingale stole her knowledge), Charlotte Ray, the first African American lawyer (1872), Rebecca Lee, M.D., (1864) first African American woman doctor and Pigs Foot Mary (Lillian Harris) (1901), first Black woman to accumulate a large fortune, etc.

White people have a great fear of the Black woman's emotional, physical and spiritual superiority. Therefore, white women inferiorize Black women. White women are imitating Black women by making their limp fur like hair kinky (curly), wearing brassieres, wearing buttock pads or getting plastic or fat cells inserted in their behinds, wearing Egyptian (African) clothes to sleep in (night gowns), using cosmetics to darken skin (dark pink cheeks), eyes and lips, doing lip and buttock enlargement operations, wearing girdles to imitate Black women's muscular gluteal hip development, sun tanning, buying sex manuals to imitate Black peoples physical sex movements, trying to dance like Black women, and attempting to have the rhythmic walk caused by the muscular structure of Black women (so called switching). The Black woman is represented by ancient paintings and statues of the Black Madonna (Isis) which are found in countries such as Italy, Germany, Poland, France, Spain, Guatemala, Greece, etc. The mutilation of the Black woman's beauty with weaves, wigs, tattoos, false nails, and eyelashes, hair relaxers, bleaching cream, high heels, and drugs is profound. Physical and cultural mutilation deprives women of an essential part of holistic life such as bonding and sexual regeneration.

Sexual regeneration is the reabsorption of the elements of injaculatory fluids by the lymphatic tissue. Some of those elements and nutrients are selenium, methionine, glycogen phosphorus, zinc, lactic acid, lecithin, calcium, choline, histidine, Vitamins C and E, trace elements, melanin hormones, electromagnetic energy, etc. The elements that compose nutrients are not ejaculated out of the body of the woman or man. Instead, these elements are injaculated (recycled) and serve to stimulate the pineal gland, melanin centers of the brain, chakras (melanin centers of the body), and cells within the body. Elements make substances such as Hydrogen(H) and Oxygen(O) equal H_2O which is water, Sodium(Ns) and Oxygen(O) makes Potassium, and Potassium and Hydrogen makes Calcium etc. The brain has high amounts of the same elements as those contain in seminal fluids. Consequently, recycling the elements of seminal fluids makes them available for the Liver to make substances for the nerves, bones, muscles and the brain. Excessive ejaculation causes element deficiency. The loss of vital elements (nutrients) can contribute to the degeneration of sex organs and immunity. One ejaculation is equal the elements (nutrients) needed to run 20 miles. This nutrient drain from multiple ejaculations can contribute to sugar cravings, mood swings, outbursts of violence, unstable personalities and memory

69

storage difficulty. The sudden climatic ejaculation causes shaking, and a climax of tension. The tension release caused by the sudden drop of energy is erroneously called an orgasm.

The mucous lining of the woman's uterus absorbs the nutrients in the ejaculated seminal fluid. The ejaculation nutrients can be found present in the woman's blood an hour or more after sexual intercourse. Normal injaculated secretions absorbed by women can be found in the cerebral fluid, fluid filled ventricles of the brain, and the sympathetic and parasympathetic nervous system. A highly acidic diet (junk food, drugs, cooked food), excessive ejaculation and sexual excitation (from movies, song lyrics, curse word, dance, videos, games, music) over stimulates the reproductive hormones and organs which can weaken the prostate and decreases trace nutrients.

Regeneration requires that sexual intercourse is stopped just before orgasm is reached and the organismic feeling is kept inside the body and recycled to the pineal gland (injaculation). In sexual regeneration no sperm is ejaculated, and it is called injaculated. The orgasm sensation is visualized (pretended) to be sent to the brain and pineal gland. This is called regeneration.

White people have castrated Black peoples culture and destroyed the melanin bond between mother and child, man and woman, and man and child and are forcing "self-centered," competitive, conflict, and "non-family centered" relationships. Damaging the bonds between Black people is caused by assimilationist and integrationist Black people adopting white culture. Black people then use White psychology to form groups or to unify. White theory based psychology comes from White culture. It is a produce of White culture. It has not and cannot work to form Black unity or Black liberation. White Supremacy could not exist if it allowed the Black family or Black people to bond. Black people that practice the mutilation of the Black woman sex organs are diseased by white culture, and white psychology. They do not see or understand the side effect and social poison of White theory based psychology applied to Black people. It is not something Black people addicted to mutilation and White culture can solve. Solutions and thinking are culturally centered. Solutions for white people are on an individual therapeutic basis while solutions for Black people are cultural, family and community (group) process.

The White people use a thought (thinking) process and have the ability to memorize ideas in a step-by-step linear manner-process. White people's thinking is a linear process and adds one word to another word to make an idea. In other words, White people do not think or conceptualize and improvise thinking. White people follow thought order which they call thinking. To think you have to be creative. Creativity is a cyclic improvised emotion and thought motion. In order to be creative one has to use emotions to enter the mind. Thinking is a creative process. It is not in the body, it is of the body; it is not solely in the brain, it utilizes the brain's ventricles (holy waters), emotional centers in the brain and is rhythmic.

Black women should not be forced to mutilate (deprive) themselves or disfigure their body parts (clitoris, labia) or cut out holes in the skin, tattoo, wear wigs, false eyelashes, relax their hair, shave the hair under their arms or off the legs or vagina, dress half nude, wear make-up to appear as White beautiful. Black woman try to stay slim. Staying slim on White people's junk food diet is contradictory to health and can result in under-nutrition. The junk food diet is a very poor nutritionally and is fattening. Junk food puts the woman in a weight gain, then weight loss and then weight gain cycle. It is designed to keep the weight loss industry rich while mentally and emotionally assassinating the Black woman. Additionally, it weakens immunity and gives the cosmetic appearance of health.

Black woman's marriages are attacked and restrained. The Black marriage is a poor imitation of a White marriage. Most Black marriages emotionally dysfunctionalizes the children. This results in assimilation and integration of White culture. Assimilation and integration is destroying of Black culture, Black children and the black family. Black marriages that use White romantic love which is "self-centered" above African "family centered" Maat unions, are diseased.

Africa's gift to the world is "Human Relationship" based on Maat. Black women/men must give this humanistic gift to each other in order to cleanse themselves of Emotional Trauma. Despite the obstacles of this cleansing, nothing can take place without a healthy body. Black people must have a living body to participate in life. If you are on a junk food diet, you are nutritionally illiterate and a part of Slavery Trauma. Junk foods cause physical and emotional diseases. Junk food, drugs, and alcohol are not a part of the African centered culture. To be African centered means you use your talents, thinking, behavior and skills to uplift Black people socially, emotionally, militarily economically and spiritually. Liberation of the Black woman is a cultural and family necessity. The purpose of marriage and any relationship between Black peoples is to serve Maat.

Family-The First Technology of Africa

The first technology (science) of Africa is the family. In traditional European terms, technology means a scientific way to achieve a practical purpose. However, technology is a method (holistic) used to create a family, a community and a civilization. The holistic (body, emotions, mind, spirit) family was used as the basis for all the growth and development of ancient African science and technology. The family was nourished on a diet of natural organic non-GMO foods free of additives, dyes, synthetics, artificial ingredients and preservatives. Black people used Herbal medicine which has no synthetic chemicals or drug. They breath fresh unpolluted air and drank spring water both of which had live bacteria, plants, fungus, minerals, vitamins, and micronutrients. It was a life without Caucasian cultural control or influences.

In chattel slavery, slaves were forced to breed like animal livestock. Brothers and sisters had to have sex with each other and mothers and fathers had to have sex with their own children. The slave master to bread slaves. The object during slavery was to breed more slaves. There was no respect for what was morally correct. Any attempt of slaves to refuse sexual incest or practice Maat or have African cultural-type marriages and have children by God's will was met by the European slave-masters' chemical weapons (alcohol, drugs), biological warfare (diseases such as syphilis) or physical brutality. A child of an African cultural marriage was cut from the pregnant woman's belly in full view of the plantation slaves, the man's testicles were cut off and the child cooked and given to the dogs. This imprinted in the slave's brain to obey the slave master and obey the slave master's God. Today, the child is allowed to be born and then attacked by the chemical warfare (synthetic foods, drugs), biological weapons (AIDs, TB, cancer), psychological weapons (miseducation, jail, recreational sex, abortions, homosexuality, selfishness) and worship Caucasians as a superior race.

One of the primary Caucasian weapons is their theory based fairytale psychology. The Black psychiatrist Franz Fanon stated the greatest tool of the oppressor is the mind of the oppressed. The social scientist Neely Fuller Jr. basically stated that "if Black people do not understand White Supremacy and how it works then everything else in their life will totally confuse them". White Sexism is a tool of Caucasian culture that is used to keep Black people controlled. African culture's sexuality is the tool of African culture that bonded Black people to Maat and God. It teaches that sex was created by God and is spiritual. Sex is a technology of culture and bonds the Black people to Maat. If the Black woman has use make up, put on the White woman's underwear, straighten her hair, wear high heels rings, tattoos, perform perverted sex as if she were white woman then she is still a slave to White culture's sexism. The Black woman is taught to have sex and relate to the Black man as if he were a white slave master. Black Holistic sex starts with a spiritual sharing in communion with Mother Father God and ends with both partners sharing in communion with God. SEE the Cultural Virtues for ideas about prayers or spiritual phrases to before, during and or after sex. Thus, holistic sex is a procreation or regeneration and not a Caucasian recreational activity. A slave's sex starts with lust and ends with a real or imagined physical climax instead of a spiritual climax. The purpose of Black couple's marriage is to be a technology advances the race with children that can solve the races problems. The children should strengthen and uplift the culture, family structure and free the race from White Domination, White Supremacy and White Racism. In contrast, European sexism teaches Black people to marry to satisfy their ego, and romantic love (lust) and use their partner for sexual and social entertainment. The Caucasian institution of marriage and love is theory based. It is a type an emotional prison that is a sexist weapon that divides Black people from the Maat technology of the family.

The African family structure (technology) was built around the Mother-Father God concept. In this structure, each child views all adults in the village as mother, father, sister or brother. For example, the child's father's brother would be called Father Uncle. The child's father's sister would be called Father Aunt. The child's mother's brother would be called Mother Uncle, and the mother's sister would be called Mother Aunt. There are Male Mothers and Female Fathers in the African family. The child's grandparents on the father's side would be called Father Grandfather, and Father Grandmother, while the grandparents on the mother's family side would be called Mother Grandmother and Mother Grandfather. All children relate to each other as sisters and brothers, which makes all children relate to all adults as Mothers and Fathers. The adults have the same parenting responsibility to the child as the birth mother and father. If the child is disobedient, the Elders punish the parents and family and then the parents punish the child.

In the African family structure, an adult (single or married) must have their parents' permission before engaging in any social or personal activities. This family technology does not allow arguments, verbal abuse or physical violence. A husband or a wife that has a disagreement about a social, economic or parenting activity will not argue about the issue. For example, a wife will talk about a disagreement with her husband in a joking manner to the husband's brother and in the case of the woman or the wife's sister in the case of the man who is in disagreement. Then the sister of the wife will confront the wife with the disagreement or complaint that was reported by her sister's husband. The wife's sister may try to resolve the conflict or disagreement between the couple. If the disagreement cannot be resolved on that level, then it is taken to the sisterhood group (age grade) leader or priestess. If the sisterhood group leader cannot resolve the conflict then it is taken to the wife's grandmother. Usually the disagreement is resolved before it reaches the Council of Elders' Queen Mother.

This Black family structure makes every member of the family directly responsible for every member of the family. In the pure sense of cultural and family technology and in the ancient African language, there is no such thing as an aunt, uncle, cousin, stepmother, stepfather, stepbrother, stepsister, half-sister, half-brother or in-laws. Additionally, there are no adoptions because you cannot adopt a child into your family that was born in the family. There are no orphans or out of wedlock children, called bastards. A child is born with a mother and father and is part of a family. The African family structure is holistic while the Caucasian family is fragmented. The use of the Caucasian cave family structure creates individualism, selfishness, dysfunction and destruction. It may sound oversimplified, but a Caucasian couple (male and female) gets married and has a family while two African families get married and have a couple (male and female union). The contemporary Caucasian practice of Black men and women choosing to get married without the families' permission, control or discipline is an outgrowth of slavery and colonialism.

Slavery was started because the Caucasians needed to act out their psychosis by creating assimilation and integration for Black people. Caucasians needed human resources (labor) and natural resources (cotton, gold, sugar, wood, oil = resin) commodities to sell and make money. The Caucasians looked at the African buildings, urban cities, mathematics, chemistry, religion, industry, commerce and thought that this technology built Africa could also build White Domination, White supremacy and wealth. The Caucasian were completely ignorant that African technology is based on the family. The chattel slaves carried the technology in their DNA and music, art, science and family structure. It was intelligence that guided the first cowboys in American that were the Africans from Gambia. They were forced to herd cattle on the Sea Islands off the East Coast of North America. The first contemporary American deep-sea divers were Africans who possessed these skills learned in Africa. Many technological skills were raped from the Black people. Europeans used the profits (money) from over 400 years of free slave labor (European welfare) and 2000 years of Arab, Chinese, East Indian oligarchies that used slaves to build wealth and empires. Caucasians first destroyed the African family technology by divide-and-conquer and splitting the family members apart, selling them to different plantations and different countries.

Ancient African procreation, regeneration, health, art and science were viewed from a holistic communal or family perspective. The African science of nutrition is a family-based technology. It views the relationship of the family of vitamin, proteins, fats, minerals as a family of elements (oxygen, Sulphur, iron, calcium etc.). Elements compose a communal nutrient community. Each element in various combinations creates a nutrient family. Elements have chemical reaction ceremonies for inter-relationship and must work in harmony synthesis, decomposition (reciprocal) or displacement with other nutrients. Inorganic (without carbon) create organic living plants. Living nutrients are designed to speed up, slow down, maintain, and stimulate energy already within "hue-mans." Living people can only use living (organic) energy to stimulate energy for living. For example, a cooked apple (dead) cannot get nourishment from a live apple. People cannot get positive stimulation from dead (cooked and junk) foods.

It is Caucasian superstitious science (theories) that declares that dead food is healthy. Caucasians believe (unscientific ideas) that a live tree can get nourishment from dead soil. They actually believe that plants eat dirt (inorganic dead matter) for food. Food is passive and the body's action upon food is mistaken for energy in the food. The body rushes its own energy towards the food and this feeling is mistaken for energy in the food. Human beings at birth have all the energy they ever will have; nothing can add to it; it can be stimulated or destroyed by junk food, drugs, cooked food and animal flesh as food. Again, food is passive, people must chew it, digest it with enzymes, push it along the digestive tract with muscles, use arteries and muscles to distribute it into the body, and push it out the body as bowel movements.

It is a Caucasian superstition (theory) that humans, animals and plants can only live by destroying something. They created the science myth that destruction is natural in nature. Therefore, Caucasians believe that it is natural for them to destroy Africa and Black people to be powerful and supreme. In contrast, African nutrition is based on the elements existing in a communal family. The elements that make nutrients share (synergistic) interactions. This creates power. Disease is caused by holistic disobedience to Imhotep's health system. Following the health laws allows the body to cure itself of disease by nutrient family interactions.

The African holistic health system has the following principles and requirements:
- ∞ Sex is cultural and a form of spirituality
- ∞ Disease is a cleansing process of the body
- ∞ The Body is self-healing
- ∞ Organic non-GMO raw foods for live people; herbs for medicine
- ∞ Sunshine daily, deep breathing, exercise, trance (meditation), proper sleep
- ∞ Cyclic laws must be followed (i.e. eating, birth, exercise, male/female principles, etc.)
- ∞ Communal cultural life
- ∞ Clean (unpolluted) air, water, soil, food, etc.
- ∞ Maat (means living according to Truth, Justice, Propriety, Harmony, Balance, Reciprocity and Order) in relationships with nature and people.
- ∞ African centered cultural focus

The holistic family cultural concept is applied to dimensions of life. For example, in art the colors were combined in a family. The color "Black" consists of the "color family" if indigo, violet, blue, black and red. In African music, a musical sound (note) consists of a family of sounds of partial tones (sounds). For example, the musical note "A" natural has a family of partial tones that were also called the musical note "A." On the piano, these tones are found in between the black and white keys. In nutritional science, the vitamins and minerals are a family. For example, the Vitamin "C" family has extended family members in a communal network. The nutrient family concept was too difficult for Europeans to understand so they called the Vitamin "C" family, the Vitamin "C complex" (B complex). In ancient African universities, this advanced family science concept was in all fields of knowledge and was too difficult for Europeans to understand so they called an African education a mystery system.

The African family colossal (large stone-carved statues of African families) of men and women united by holding hands or interlocked arms standing or sitting side-by-side to show family unity, were destroyed by the Arabs and Caucasians. The female companion statue was destroyed by cannons or explosives and/or cut off by invading the European oligarchy armies. These invading European tribal oligarchies states did not come into existence until the fall of the Mediterranean countries of Rome and Greece. These Europeans tried to destroy the "hue-man" (human) family concept.

The word "human" (hue-man) comes from the word "hue" which means the color (black, melanin) and "man" which means "thinking" in other words "hue-man" means Black thinking. Thinking is mental and emotional improvising on ideas as a family of thoughts. Melanin is produced by a gland (Pineal) in the center of the brain. Melanin controls the bipolar internal clock (cycles) of all organs, the growth from childhood into adulthood, the time of day you sleep, the growth of hair, ideas, emotions, rhythm, and the human body. The more melanin in the body the more bipolar rhythm and the more an individual is connected to nature, the galaxy and the sun's cycles. The Melanin Solar connection is clear in African science, religion and physiology.

The solar (sun) cycle is obvious in African civilization. The childbirth cycle of African women having a baby every three years is a solar cycle. The newborn child's umbilical cord is connected to the solar center of the child (abdomen) and the child is carried in the solar center of the mother (abdomen). Amon Ra, a spiritual system, is solar-based and the yearly calendar is of solar origin. The African metric (meter) measuring system is solar-based. Eating food was solar-based as the heaviest meal eaten was before the sun is perpendicular (high noon) and the last meal was eaten before the sun is horizontal to the earth (sunset). African games had solar-bases such as the card games (52 cards, 52 weeks in a year, total points in the deck, 364 plus the joker an extra point for the 365 days of the year). The 4 cardinal points of the directional compass are of African solar origin. The breast-feeding of children lasted 3 to 6 years and is solar-cycled. Melanin is highly responsive to the solar cycles energy of the sun and has significance in African "sexuality."

Black peoples "hue-man" nature is totally different from White nature. The digestive system processes a higher amount of nutrients, buttock muscles are more highly-developed, bone mass is 10 times greater, the White Blood Cell count is lower, the ears hear more sound (due to high melanin content), protein is recycled and the calcium requirement is lower. Black people have more fast twitch muscles, non-electric brain and Glia brain cells and nerve messages are sent via water, the body has a lower salt content and the brain processes brain waves faster and the hair is torqued and has more color bands than animals. This means Black people have hair and Europeans have fur (identical to color bands of animals) which is erroneously called hair.

Black people that ignore the melanin factor in family and community (communal), fall victim to the slave mentality and go against the genetic code of their hue-man race. Black people that ignore that they evolved from God and accept the Caucasian superstition theory (fantasy belief) that they evolved from an ape are miseducated. If there is an evolutionary "missing link" between the Caucasian cave people and ape it is the White people. It is Caucasians who anatomically are partial ape and perhaps partial "hue-man". It is Caucasians who have white skin, short legs, thin lips, limp hair, and flat buttocks, like the ape.

The evolutionary theory is merely a superstition fantasy idea used to justify the Caucasian primitive barbaric behaviors towards Black people and other colored people. This White Supreme psychotic racist evolution superstition belief means that Caucasian have to be excused for their crimes against Black people. Caucasians melanin has Sulphur in the center and Black people's melanin has selenium in the center. It is genetically impossible for White people to have evolved from Black people. Caucasians are growing towards more barbaric behavior and are not part of the Black race or the "hue-man" family. Probably more related to the ape family.

The Black woman is a victim of White theory based medical sexism, drugs, hysterectomies, abortions, fibroid tumors, rape, petty rape, chemical castration, birth-control pills, poor synthetic diets and scientific racism. The Black woman is denied her human sovereign rights and is given Caucasian civil rights (rituals). Civil Rights can be taken away by White Congress or the White Supreme Court. They are rituals (privileges) given by Whites (Europeans) to former slaves. Sovereign rights cannot be given by Whites or voted upon or taken away by whites.

The African American people are part of Caucasians military and police forces. They are the most armed Black men in the world, and have military technologically skilled and combat-trained. Militarily, Black people have access and knowledge of a variety of weapons and tactics to protect and liberate his African continent, children, family, community, nations and themselves. The assimilated and integrated Black people stand in awe and fear of white soldiers with the same training.

The Black singers and rappers record music that popularizes sexual lust instead of Maat marriage and family. They promote the White Domination that is destroying Black culture, child and family technology. They are victims of White Supremacy that has mentally destroyed their culture and given them a slave mentality. Black people make enough money from Black-exploitation music videos, records, sports, acting, commercials, movies, and television and sports entertainment to sponsor Freedom revolutions in Africa, America and the world.

The ignorance of the great nutritional science of ancient Africa is destroying the family's future-children. The White corporate own junk food diet has destructively replaced non-GMO organic natural foods with junk foods that look and taste like food and are nutritionally nutrient less and valueless (junk food). The modern processed "food" is GMO, dyed, plastic, test tube grown meat, preserved, bleached, salted and sugared. White sugar harms the pancreas, while artificial sweeteners harm the Liver. Feeding the body poorly with synthetic GMO food feeds the brain poorly. An undernourished brain causes learning problems, depression, violence and fatigue. High amounts of sugar cause irritability, schizophrenia, uncontrolled emotional explosions, confusion and addiction. High amounts of salt can cause waste to stay in the body, depression and mood swings. Junk "foods" are low in vitamins which can cause paranoia and personality problems. These Caucasian processed foods are a weapon used against Black children.

In New York City, a ten-year study was conducted on 803,000 children (over 60% Black) by the University of California, at Berkeley, School of Nutrition. This research was presented at The International Conference on Nutrient Brain Functions hosted by the American College of Nutrition at Scottsdale, Arizona. In the study, the school children who ate school breakfast and lunch on a natural diet got the highest Achievement Test scores at all grade levels and had the highest intelligence gain in United States history. Aside from this, disruptive behaviors and dropout rates decreased dramatically. Additionally, violence, learning problems, short attention spans, suicides, rape and drug addiction had a 45% decrease in 25 studies with over 20,000 juvenile prison inmates (over 70% Black) in 7 different states. Virginia Wesley University, Southern Mississippi University, Johns Hopkins University and California State University conducted this research. Basically, the nutritional research returned the black children to the non-GMO organic natural foods diet of ancient Africa. These studies made three basic changes in the diet. Bleached white flour was taken out of the diet, white sugar in food was reduced by 3 to 5% and all preservatives were removed (including dyes, flavorings). Sodas were eliminated and fruit juices were substituted. Ironically, private schools in Connecticut and New Jersey saw the results and started buying natural food from the New York Public Schools.

There are natural supplements available to prevent mental (learning) and physical diseases of children. Profit-motivated White companies are allowed to mask the nutritional starvation and death of black children. This means no future for the Black family. The corporate own oligarchy of the food industry has no moral concern for Black children. Added to this, the National Academy of Sciences has lowered the recommended daily allowance of vitamins, minerals and other nutrients. This information can be used to lower the amount of money spent on school lunch programs, federally sponsored food programs, and food stamps. This is a strategy used to aid in the deterioration of Black children and senior citizens' health and will increase disease. This is done at a time when the number of children and adults with physical impairments (handicap) and birth defects has been increasing steadily at 10% per year because of junk foods and drugs (World Health Organization Survey).

Nutritional suicide is prevented by the family technology. A holistic family built on the foundations of Maat, emotional, spiritual, physical and mental unity will always seek try to use non-GMO organic foods to nourish itself and guarantee a future. The Maat family will stop destruction and White Domination. Charles Darwin, who founded the theory of evolution, wrote *The Next Million Years* and pointed out that the least creditable feature of White Supremacy is [that] it is criminally foolish. It is foolish to allow the diet to be contrary to nature (processed, GMO) which makes it contrary to life and the Black family.

The Black community in America of the past had a family structure and ate a natural organic food diet. The first contemporary Africans in America (also called Gullahs) were born in 1526 on St. Catherine's Island off the coast of Georgia. The Gullahs and many others had independent family-structured communities in Florida, Alabama, Georgia, and North and South Carolinas in the 16th, 17th, 18th and 19th centuries. They traded with each other and threatened to end slavery because they attacked plantations, destroyed plantation crops and had armies (called runaways by Whites) that freed slaves. General Andrew Jackson used the War of 1812 as an excuse to attack these independent communities. He also attacked them again in 1816 and 1818. Finally, in 1842, General Jessup of the United States War Department told Congress to make no mistake about it: "This is a Negro and not an Indian

War." Thus, he declared "The Negro War." He told the War Department that the runaway Negroes were able and willing to defeat America. If they were not destroyed, they would Africanize the South. The U.S. military attacked and murdered those African Americans, destroyed their families, communities and defeated their armies. The survivors of the "Negro War" were driven off their land and marched at gunpoint to reservation-type areas in Mexico. Some moved to Indros Island and other areas. In any case the survivors of slavery and "The Negro War" still legally have their own land in America.

The Caucasian oligarchy power elite whose economic purpose was to capture southern oligarchies, and land states and resources financed the Civil War (War of Northern Aggression). The power elite capitalist's oligarchy has never been interested in democracy or government. They are motivated by greed to feed their power and psychotic needs. They did not want the Black prisoners of war (so-called slaves) to be aware that they (Black people) were sovereign world citizens and could fight and gain control of American states. Consequently, the Europeans created the lie called the Civil War. The British and Confederates emancipated slaves before the American Union. This allowed them to use the slaves to fight for Caucasians (caucrazians) civil rights. Emancipation kept the slave's unconscious of the fact that the European criminals were fighting over what they had stolen (America, Africa and Africans). Emancipation means transfer of ownership. Slaves were no longer property of individuals. They became property of the federal government (U.S.A.). Emancipation and the Civil War were political devices used to keep the slaves from uniting to form an all Black army and an all Black Sovereign nation within America. This army could have fought and defeated the flea-infested, violent nature, cannibalistic, bed wetting, Caucasians oligarchy criminals.

In 1848, the United States versus Henry Turners' Heirs court hearing ruled that the "Neutral Strip" of 2,961,983.5 acres of land in Louisiana, Arkansas and Mississippi belongs to African Americans. In 1940, the neutral strip of land was again verified to exist as not belonging to the United States. The Louisiana Department of Transportation acknowledged that Neutral Strip on its survey. Historically, it is neutral because it was not a part of the 1803 Louisiana Purchase of land by America. The Black communities legally have ownership of that land and possess the skill, ability and technology to be free.

Also, the 13th Amendment to the U.S. Constitution calls for the elimination of slavery and all incidents of slavery. Therefore, African Americans not allowed a reparational economic base, land or to maintain Black citizenship suffer from an "incident of slavery" and have the legal rights to file claims and pay no income tax. The Black community first must use the family technology to build positive communities, relationships and a healthy diet before gaining self-control.

The technology of the family is not the only thing for freedom; it is everything in freedom. The family is the root from which the strong tree of Africa grew. The Black family tree gave the world science, religion, civilization, nutrition and community. What the ancient African ancestors have done can be done again. What they have achieved can be achieved on a higher level if the family technology is used. It is Black people who must save the future and world from Caucasian destructive cave behaviors. It is stupid for Black people to wait for mother nature's revenge-major changes in the galaxy, saviors, destruction of the ozone, millennium, nuclear wars, collision of planets or stars, climatic changes, etc., to do the job that Black people must do themselves. It is the world's change agent (melanin dominant Black people) that must discipline and correct white people's toxic cave behaviors. It is a human issue that must be solved by humans.

Chapter Two

Health

"When you make men slaves, you compel them to live with you in a state of war"

Olaudah Equiano (1789) from his book
"The Interesting Narrative of the Life of Olaudah Equiano"

White Racism: Nutritional Causes

All past behaviors are current behaviors, just as the study of history is the study of current events. The Ice Age era of Europe reduced the population of the White people. Large mountains of glaciers melted at the end of the Ice Age. Global warming melted glaciers causing massive floods and soil erosion. Massive flooding and erosion caused the soil to be stripped of water soluble nutrients such as iodine, sulfur, zinc, manganese, copper, selenium, magnesium, etc. Aside from mineral-depleted soil caused by melting ice, White people used the nutrient depletion soil for farming of food crops. Today, the corporate own agricultural empire continues to rob the soil of nutrients by their synthetic fertilizers, herbicides, hormones, pesticides, GMOs and machine cultivation farming methods. In addition to this, the totally unnecessary cooking of nutrient-depleted fresh fruits and vegetables further depletes the nutrient value of plants. This makes the nutrients left in plants less valuable. Further, cooking of animal flesh destroys nutrients. The food animals are raised on crops grown in nutrient depleted and poison soils.

Nutrients have an effect on the mind, mood, emotions, and state of consciousness, spirit and physical body. White people assume their nutrient deficient race and civilization are normal. They use their nutrient-deficient body chemistry as the standard for Black people and all races. White people assume that their biochemical personality, moods, emotions, thoughts and behaviors are normal for all races. The White people psychotic mental illness White Supremacy diseases is normal. The nutrient robbed plants and cave life trauma behaviors of violence, ruin, destruction, rape, dysfunctional families, and dependence upon human and natural resources of Black people contradicts their assumption of supremacy.

Glaciated soil lacks many minerals. For example, Selenium is a vital mineral lacking in certain types of soils. White people biochemical personality has an abnormal deficiency of selenium. Selenium deficiency causes premenstrual symptoms, hot flashes, breast cancer, infertility, birth defects, crib death, and liver damage and alters the rhythm and cycles in the body. Cow's milk is deficient in selenium. A diet high in cooked fats causes selenium drain.

Another mineral deficiency of the White race is sulfur. Lack of optimum sulfur causes depression, rhythmic imbalances, irregular nerve impulses and retarded growth of egg and sperm. Sulfur is denatured or destroyed by cooking.

Zinc depletion can cause schizophrenia, infections, retarded growth, fatigue, digestive problems and sterility. Zinc is denatured or destroyed by cooking food. It is drained from the body by ingesting cow's milk, cooked

Tobacco nicotine, cooked marijuana cannabinol, roasted coffee, alcohol and contraceptive pills.

Europe's iodine-poor soil can cause nervousness, irritability, toxins in the brain, low energy, obesity, melanin deficiency and growth problems. It is destroyed by heat, cooking and processing.

Manganese is lacking, which can result in pineal gland irregularities, muscle problems, brain and nerve difficulties and digestive problems. White women with this deficiency can lose their nurturing mother instinct (Mother Love) and ability to protect their child. This may allow them to let their human baby suck the breast of a lower animal (cows, goats, etc.). Excessive sex and high amounts of cow's milk, calcium, iron and phosphorus can destroy manganese.

Many minerals were lost by the many floods of the Ice Age. The absence of nutrients for plants to biologically transmute imbalanced soil nutrients causes soil without normal levels of copper to be harmful to health. Soil that grows plants with very low levels of copper results in depression unstable brain functions and nerve damage responses such as hyperactivity. Inadequate levels of magnesium in the soil can cause irritability, depression, tremors, muscle, nerve and brain problems. A loss of the mineral vanadium can cause low birth rates, blood sugar problems, and high death rates.

Soil with inadequate phosphorus levels can result in feeble minds, mental illness, inability to coordinate muscles, brain function problems and increased aging. Soil with potassium depletion causes high levels of physical, emotional, and mental stress, aging, nerve problems, arthritis, rheumatism and heart problems. Potassium can be destroyed by processing foods, cooking, salt, white sugar, alcohol, coffee, bleached white flour and stress.

The Black people came in contact with White people raised on soil robbed of minerals from the Ice Age and cave traumatized emotionally and mentally ill White Europeans. They were physically imbalanced because of their glaciated and nutrient-drained diets. Emotionally and mentally ill White people believe themselves normal, superior, humanly evolved, and capable of understanding the culturally superior Black people. The White Supremacy mind and cave traumatized White race feel that their nutritionally inadequate brain thinking is correct and perfect. This White Supremacy psychotic mind has become a victim of its own imagination. An imagination that is emotionally and mentally ill. Their brain and body has been nutritionally deprived for centuries and assumes that it is not ill when in actuality, it is mentally ill. A nutrient-deprived brain can hallucinate about reality and intelligence.

Whatever the cave insane mind creates is believed to be sane. Added to this, when peoples cave life experiences were with shadows in the caves it causes them to see or sense horror with Black images. They associate fear with Black as evil. The cave DNA lifestyle caused their conscious and subconscious mind to become an emotionally insane complementary pair. This reinforces its own insanity and labels it sane.

White people cooked animal flesh diet is not a complete protein balance and is depleted of nutrients. This depletion causes mental problems and disease. Cooking destroys the amino acid, Glutamic. A loss of Glutamic acid results in learning and behavioral problems, schizophrenia, senility, rhythmic loss, poor memory and stress. Cooking meat destroys the amino acid lysine. Lysine helps to regulate the pineal gland, growth, activates breast milk, use for infections, skin diseases and herpes the pineal gland monitors acid and alkaline balance. Without Lysine, infections are common. Tyrosine is an amino acid that can be deficient, causing an unstable mind, irritability, and irregular rhythm of the organs and glands. The amino acid histidine is necessary for relaxation, erections, proper child growth and organ rhythm. It is inadequate in White people, who were raised on animal's milk. Black people came in contact with these White unstable personalities from dysfunctional cave families with emotional and mental problems and the White Supremacy psychosis.

Many (perhaps all) of the emotional and mental problems the White race have never been therapeutically treated. This may be a result of their inability to see or admit that they are emotionally and mentally diseased race. The 9th Dynasty of Egypt 3000 BC, White people were described as a miserable race living with a shortage of food, a shortage of water (it was frozen) and always in search of food such, plants, animals or another White person (cannibalism) to eat. Additionally, there were massive diseases caused by nutritionally lacking soil and plants.

White people tend to be emotional and violent. In fact, when White people were first recorded in history, they were recorded in acts of violence against Black people. The Palettes and Mace heads found at Hierakonpolis, an area near the upper Nile River, reported that the Africans were fighting uncivilized groups of White people around 4000 BC. The Palermo Stone reveals that Africans were fighting the barbaric, pagan White people that were trying to invade Africa. It was King Menes who drove out the savage White people in the First Egyptian Dynasty. Since that time in world history, the emotional and mentally ill White people have been using violence, war, terrorism, invasion, peace, to rule, ruin, criminalize and inferiorize Black people.

White people have a deep sense of insecurity about nature and themselves. They still have barbaric hoards (gangs) which they call peace keeping forces, UN, NATO alliances, and USA. These alliances (barbaric clans) psychologically and violently attack Black people all over the world and inferiorize Black people so they can have imagined superiority. White people believe that money is the root of evil. Money is a not evil. Whites use money to be evil. Emotional control over Black people is used to make them feel emotionally secure.

Corporate own White countries have wolf-pack type attack upon Black countries, then they start to attack each other's countries for human and natural resources. The White countries with their corporate own militaries have gang attacks, gang sex (orgies), as well as gang chaos. Chaos seems to follow their insecurity. White people as a group only feel secure when they use violence to control. White countries tend to only unite for violence; then afterwards they fight among themselves. They are cultural, historical, natural and human resource thieves that fight over what they have stolen from Black people. W.E.B. DuBois summarized White countries fighting in World War I as a fight between pirates over the spoils-Africa.

White people are not consciously aware of themselves as a primitive violent group of cave people. There primitive Ice Age genetic heritage causes them to still eat frozen food such as ice cream and to use ice cubes to make drinks very cold. Cold drinks cannot be used by the body unless they are 98.6°F. Therefore, a cold drink retards digestion. They are a form of nutritional violence.

White people will disregard their religious differences (Jews, Muslims, Christians), political differences, (democrats, republicans, communists), ethnic differences (Irish, Slav, Russian) and will unite to watch violent sports such as football, boxing, ice hockey, wrestling, racing cars, movies with violence or violent threats to life, such as circus acts with tight rope walkers, lion tamers, knife throwers, or violent activities, such as roller coaster riding, sky diving, Ferris wheel riding and hunting.

After the violence is over they separate, mistrust, abuse, lie, steal and use each other in a chaos that they call society. This chaos is their superstitious, socialized system of rituals and ceremonies that they alone call "culture." Their culture composed of White Supremacy psychosis, Narcissistic Avaricious Disorder, Cave Trauma Disorder, and Psychopathic Personalities is a culture of equal mental illnesses. Mental illness is democratically shared by each White gang called an ethnic group. White people psychotically label their inferiority as superiority. If the White people use a wooden club to kill a person this is called primitive. If White people put on a suit, shirt and tie and uses a gun to kill a person this is called modern or civilized. The behavior is still primitive, and the tool, be it a wooden club, drone, terrorism, spying, or a gun, is simply another way to be primitive. White Supremacy is simply a tool of an inferior, primitive cave people that is used to make them feel human worth. White people are a chaotic collection of adult delinquents who have children who are also delinquent.

White peoples current, animal meat flesh consumption, dairy, starch centered diet and wrong food combining junk food diet (meat and starch, milk = cheese do not combine with any food) causes them to be mentally, emotionally physically and biochemically imbalanced (perverts). Perverted biochemistry causes abnormal behaviors, emotions, thoughts, and relationships with other races. A biochemically imbalanced White people with a high protein diet, starched centered, and junk foods have a high acid content of blood. Acidic blood will cause high blood pressure. High blood pressure causes decrease blood flow to the uterus and prostate causing the them to weaken and degenerate. The combination of an acidic uterus and an acidic prostate together with high blood pressure may cause sexual problems and weak sex organs.

Animal meat eaters have toxic, poisonous uric acid blood that irritates the brain, nerves, muscles, digestion and especially the reproductive organs. This abnormal, acidic biochemistry irritates the sex organs causing wet dreams (ejaculation while asleep), masturbation, violence, and a need for sexually stimulating music, dance, movies, videos, games, clothes, religious books, etc. This uric acid and acidosis from a starch centered junk food diet irritates the mucous membrane of the uterus and prostate. This acid condition is compounded by food irritants, such as cocoa, alcoholic beverages sodas, cooked foods, caviar, condiments, coffee, onions, vinegar, oysters, chocolate, caffeine, tea, pepper, wheat, salt, oats, mustard and garlic. Black peoples naturally organic alkaline vegetarian diet biochemically balances the body, emotions, mind, and spirit.

The emotionally caused Eating Disorder mental illness of overeating (binges) causes acidic biochemistry. Overeating constipates, resulting in an increase of impurities in the body. Eating Disorders make the body toxic and acidic. White theory science uses their Eating Disorder diseased body as the normal standard for all Black people. The Caucasians' White Supremacy behavior perverts their social activities, emotions, and mind.

White people participate directly or indirectly in maintaining their White Supremacy. The former slave owner Benjamin Franklin once said, "If everyone (Caucasians) is thinking alike, then no one (Caucasians) is thinking". White Supremacy does not have to be thought about or purposely acted on; it is a cultural disease that feeds on Black culture. They have an acceptable mental illness level of behaviors and emotional which they call the normal. And, they have unacceptable behaviors and emotions of mental illness, which they call mental disease. The mental illnesses that were present in the in the caves and Ice Age, Dark Ages and Feudalism are present today. They are weaved and mixed in every aspect of white peoples social, moral, religious, family, sexual and violent behaviors. All past behaviors are current behaviors, just as the study of history is the study of current events. Their behavioral and mental disorders are psychologically protected and reinforced until these disorders are no longer visible to their mind and their mind is in denial.

White people's neuro-hormonal development is slow with limited responsiveness. This causes their bladder (urinate) control nerves to slowly grow to the bladder muscles at age 2 while Black people's bladder control nerves grow to muscle within 6 months of age, allowing toilet training. The complete adult neuro-hormonal growth occurs by 12 years of age in Black people, and between 18 and 21 years of age in White people. This slow development limits the amount of emotional and mental flexibility White people can have. Consequently, White people lack the melanin ability to voluntarily accept holistic therapy and free themselves of White Supremacy's psychotic illusions of emotional and mental illness.

The continent of Africa provided Black people with nutrient-rich soil, vast varieties of fruits and vegetables, which supplied all the amino acids, minerals and vitamins for a normal mind and body. The European soil was nutritionally robbed. Additionally, Caucasians theory based nutritional science and proper food combining knowledge, have a melanin-deficient biochemistry and are civilized in an immature infant culture, which nourishes their emotional and mental illness psychosis of White Supremacy. They are historically and scientifically a racial and culturally inferior race that could be helped and developed if they wanted to change. However, White people do not recognize White Supremacy as a disease and enjoy the white privileges that White Supremacy gives them. White people came out the caves 30,000 years ago this was after all other colored cultures had been in existence over a million years.

Traces of White people's cultural immaturity and violence still exist today. The vast majority of their amusements and activities are focused in violence such as violent children's fairy tales, movies (murders, rape), or stealing, lies, word trickery, marriage and relationship conflicts, cops and robber's themes, one group overpowering another, deception, etc. White people's entertainment has these themes because they were raised in an uncivilized cave culture infected with murder, dysfunctional families, rape, fear, anger, violence, conflicts, wars, threats to life, sex orgies, and social wolf-pack behaviors. White people have difficulty communicating within themselves and to others.

White people because of centuries of nutrient-depleted soil and food, are mentally, emotionally, and physically ill. Chronic undernourishment is more dangerous than the diseases of rickets, anemia, Kwashikora, and Beriberi. Chronic diseases cause personality disorders, violent behavior and mood swings. The victims of undernourishment have slowly gotten the disease state and do not recognize themselves as ill. When this condition (nutrient deficiency) has occurred over centuries and the vast majority have it, the white majority of people believe themselves normal. The correction of chronic undernourishment takes place slowly over a period of 5 to 6 weeks. This is too slow to show an immediate change in nutrition status. This also makes it difficult to be recognized. In obvious diseases such as Beriberi, a Vitamin B hypodermic needle injection will immediately help the tongue and lips feel less sore, the digestive disorders and thinking will clear up. Centuries of chronic undernourishment from glaciated land have been erroneously documented as normal. White people's abnormal behaviors, emotions, and thinking are erroneously considered normal by White people's theory based sciences. And, their religions verify their abnormal behaviors as normal. The study of White people's history is actually the study of emotional illness and mental illness and asocial behavior. White peoples nutritional and historical cave behaviors validate their White Supremacy psychosis as an illusion reinforced by nutritional deficiencies. Their culture, religions and nutritionists are too nutritionally deficient to recognize this. It is similar to this: "in a land where everyone has one eye (Caucasians), a person with two eyes (Black people) is considered a freak". Using White people's theory based psychology traps Black people into a mental illness with no escape.

Destroy the Pineal Gland

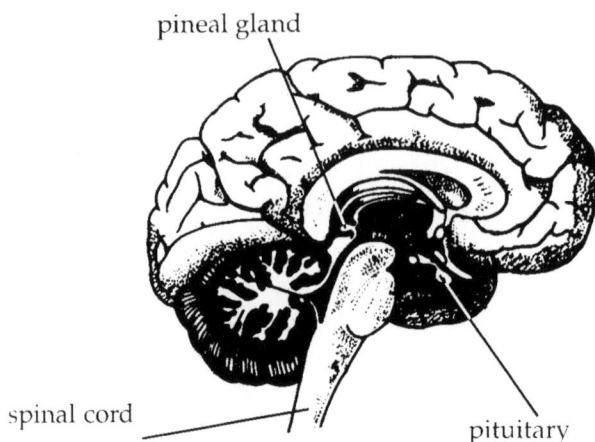

pineal gland

spinal cord

pituitary

A healthy pineal gland secretes melanin. Melanin makes highly melaninated Black people superior to all races. So, it follows, an unhealthy pineal would have an effect upon the Black people's health, emotions, mind and spirit. There are many ways to deteriorate, weaken and/or destroy the pineal gland. This destruction can occur without the knowledge of the victim. In the vast majority of White people's theory based health and mind sciences the pineal gland is omitted. They do not mention of its health status. It is medically clear that all glands can get diseased. The White Racism in medicine ignores the dis-eases and nutrient-deficiencies of their pineal gland. Because, in Caucasians, the gland has the lowest activity or is usually (dead), so it is not diagnosed or treated for illnesses.

The pineal gland is highly sensitive, nutrient-dependent, oscillates, and is biochemically and electromagnetically very active. Drugs and nutrients cross the so-called "blood brain barrier (a theory)" and get into the pineal gland's tissue. Drugs such as sodium chloride, (table salt), concentrated sweeteners, cocaine, alcohol, codeine, fluoride, X-rays, low radio waves and ultrasound waves, caffeine, Librium, microwaves radiation, nicotine, antibiotics, Demerol, Tylenol, morphine, cooked caffeine, Ergotamine, toxic fumes, cooked cannabinol of marijuana, cooked nicotine of tobacco, antihistamines, decongestants, amphetamines, aspirin or Tagamet, can have an effect on melanin and the glands. The pineal gland and melanin get damage from lye and lye-like chemicals (hair relaxers), skin bleaching agents, synthetic tattoo chemicals, chemicals in cosmetics and deodorants, and hair depilatory chemicals. Toxins in the pineal gland can result in degenerative

90

diseases such as arthritis, senility, cataracts, cancer, Alzheimer's, diabetes, Parkinson, menopause, impotence, glaucoma, osteoporosis and arteriosclerosis.

The White people's theory and myths of the "blood barrier" serving as a form of liquid protection against toxic substances is an excuse that stops pineal diagnosis. Synthetic toxins such as drugs, white sugar, cooked saturated fats, GMOs, viruses, genetic drugs, free radicals, and bleached white flour can interrupt the pineal gland's cycle and ability. This can result in degenerative diseases, abnormal growth activity, altered moods, and states of consciousness.

The sensitivity of the pineal gland on many levels is unique. The nutrients stored in the pineal, such as indoles (tryptophan and natural indigo chemicals), histamines; dopamine and norepinephrine (noradrenalin), monitor and direct energy. Synthetic chemicals destroy the monitoring ability. Many synthetic chemicals and junk foods are dangerous. Public drinking water is basically deodorized recycled sewage water. The Fluoride drug in drinking water, toothpaste and all related chemical species such as chlorine and iodine are harmful. Hay fever, allergy or cold medicine with antihistamine can result in slowing down the secretions of glands and the pineal gland.

The junk food diet has dangerous heavy-metal toxins. Many of the dangerous chemicals are in junk foods such as cooked animal fat trans oils are found in cream, peanut butter, salad dressing, butter, whole milk, cheese, potato chips, bread, medicine, doughnuts, pizza, cakes, pies, candy, pastry, catsup, mustard and mayonnaise.

Black people, especially those in large cities, have a sunlight deficiency because they do not get enough sunlight. Inadequate sunlight does not stimulate the pineal gland. This is called "seasonal affective disorder (SAD) but for Black people it can be an "all-seasonal affective disorder." Under stimulated pineal results in depression. Low energy, cravings for sugar, drugs or other stimulants and a vague sense of feeling ill.

The stressing effect of White Supremacy can lead to cravings. Stress causes the pineal gland to be over-stimulated and exhausted. This can result in a vicious cycle of eating disorder, taking stimulants (chocolate, coffee) and taking drugs, that can exhaust the pineal gland. Ironically, this causes Black people to seek security and avoidance of fear by using White people's values. For example, Black people with a "slave plantation servitude mentality" will not visualize economic success unless it includes being in White culture or working for a White high-paying job, getting a White College degree, White peoples expensive junk food and/or earning White people's dollars. Assimilation and Integration Black person sees, success as being in some way white and on the slave master's plantation (living in a white country or using White academic standards).

The under-stimulation of the pineal with inadequate sunlight, junk food and a polluted environment and reduce pineal gland activity. Black people's desire to combat the low pineal activity can cause a craving for junk religions (white Moses, white God, white Jesus, white Muhammad). This nutritionally leads to another cycle of low pineal energy production. The pineal gland becomes weaker and weaker by this cyclic destruction. This lowers the quantity of melanin available and weakens or destroys' a Black person's ability to be African centered.

The pineal gland and melanin directly or indirectly controls many functions in the body such as the cyclic behavior of organs, growth and development states of children, catecholamine production, sleep patterns, energy storage, information storage (memory), genetic information; regulates body temperature, carbohydrate metabolism, bone growth, extrasensory perception, etc. Melanin stimulates the repair of cells, tissues and organs. It acts as an antibiotic, enhances immunity in the liver, converts sunlight energy into vitamin D, stimulates DNA synthesis, influences lymphocyte production, and increases sound and light absorption.

The galaxy sits in Blackness which means it is connected to Black people and the Black "inner space." In White people the galaxy is "outer space". Without optimum melanin levels, Black people sabotage any effort for freedom from White Supremacy. White Supremacy inherently emphasizes White people nutritional values and destroys melanin and the pineal gland (destroys Black people). Without the full use of the pineal gland Black people are puppets for White Supremacy.

The pineal gland masterminds the control of the pituitary, hypothalamus, gonads, and adrenal glands. Black people under the tension and stress of White Supremacy develop a weak immune system and pineal gland. The pineal gland has a defense reaction to dis-ease and stimulates the adrenal glands to produce adrenaline. White Supremacy leads to adrenal and pineal gland exhaustion. The pineal gland's ability to switch the sympathetic and parasympathetic nervous system off and on is weakened. The systems cannot harmonize and all bodily activities become imbalance. The pineal gland stimulates the release of prostaglandin, which defends the body from heart and circulatory disorders. Therefore, an undernourished pineal gland can cause heart disease and circulatory problems. Black people are not taught about the pineal gland or melanin. This helps to control and destroy them through "information colonization." Black people may vaguely know that White people use melanin-stimulating synthetic hormones for suntans without sunlight. But, Black people are never taught that pineal gland extract stops cancer or tumor growth. Black people are not taught that the life span of animals is increased by 25% when given melanin extract. Without an organic non0-GMO natural whole foods diet, the pineal gland is limited. A limited functioning pineal gland makes Black people easier to control, rule and ruin. Black people use their mouth as a tasty junk food way to die.

White corporate own USA and their rich elite Oligarchy running dogs and puppets (i.e., Japanese, Israel, Soviets, Arabs, Chinese, Britain, African countries, India) are constantly researching melanin. The melanin information is used militarily, dietary, medically, for drugs, computer science, sex, genetic breeding and outer space. This information is classified as top secret and not given to Black people. White peoples public and secret melanin organizations of information pirates and thieves of the European, Pan American and Japanese societies own Pigment Cell (Melanin) Research. They held fifteen International Pigment Conferences between 1946 and 1993. The Black people have never held an International Conferences on melanin. There have been very small conferences held in different countries but not a unified conference.

The natural defenses of the body use energy conservation. If tissue, cells, organs, or glands are not being used, then the body will not give energy to the unused tissue or gland. It is a "don't use it, you lose it" philosophy. In some cases, the unused tissue or gland will become calcified (turns to stone). For example, the liver can be damaged the toxic poison of alcohol beverages. If the liver is continuously abused by drinking alcohol, it will turn to stone (cirrhosis). The prostate gland can get damaged or diseased and will become hard like stone (calcified). Many toxic chemicals in junk food, sodas, or toxic drugs will inflame tissue, organs, or glands causing appendicitis, pancreatic, vaginitis, hepatitis, nephritis, prostatitis, and pelvic inflammatory disease. The pineal gland, like any other gland, can suffer the same type of inflammation. The pineal gland will become hard as stone – calcified. White people pineal gland is calcified by the age of 12 or younger.

The highest amount of pineal inactivity and pineal gland calcification is 60% to 80% among White people. Black people have the lowest amount of pineal gland calcification. This calcification indicates the effect of the junk food diet and drugs in Black people, (5% to 15%). Pineal gland calcification can increase as White people continue to use drugs and junk food. A weakened pineal gland aids in the control and destruction of Black people. Black people with dull weakened or partially destroyed pineal glands are waiting for White people's theory science to tell them that they are killing the pineal gland.

White Out Black Culture

"White Out," a white liquid used to "correct" **black** (ink) mistakes made on paper is symbolic of White Supremacy. Nutrition, or the science of how to nourish the body, emotions, mind and spirit is a Black science. However, the majority of Black people are eating a disease-causing junk food diet and they are dying from it. This may make them a "healthy" White person but never a healthy Black person. It is ironic that nutrition is an African-derived word, which comes from the Egyptian word "Menat." Menat means to nourish or nurse. In recorded history, one of the earliest uses of nutrition was recorded in the Egyptian 6th Dynasty. The Amulet of Menat, worn by Osiris in pyramid paintings verifies this fact. Colorful (Melaninated) Black people should eat colorful food.

Color is very important in nutrition-especially for Black people. Nutritionally, "white-out food" that has been conjured up in White people's corporate own synthetic chemical factories-called "food" companies. The White peoples GMO chemical junk foods and drugs factories are interested in profit-not nutrition-and least of all the correct nutrient level for the melaninated, biochemically unique, Black people. It is no accident that most grocery stores sell "food" that "makes you sick" and incorporate a "drug" store section with drugs that suppress the sickness caused by foods that they sell.

White people as a group have not learned how to eat, what to eat, when to eat, how to prepare food or how to combine foods. Food has combining rules based upon enzyme metabolism. Therefore, do not combine sugar and starches; meat and potatoes; sugar and milk; oil and starch; oil and protein; fruits and vegetables; do not drink and eat solid food at the same time because liquids dilute and weakens enzymes. White people follow their cave food combinations. Correct combinations would be starches and vegetables; vegetables and proteins; fruits eaten separately; grains and cereals eaten separately; and never drinking while eating.

Nature's naturally colorful organic food is not as profitable for the corporate own White junk food industries constipating and disease causing bleached white flour, white sugar, white salt, fried and chemically drugged foods. The White people's superstition that white (food) is supreme is based upon the belief that the white race is supreme. Processed bleached white foods are emotionally satisfying for White people but very dangerous and disease causing concoctions.

Black people should avoid processed foods and try to avoid plants that have been hybridized GMO and raised with chemicals such as wheat, oats, soy, white rice, grits, lima beans, chickpeas, black-eyed peas, pigeon peas, carrots, celery, cauliflower, beets, peanuts (bean), pistachios, cashews, walnuts, pecans, and sunflower seeds. It is best to get non-GMO organic foods.

Nightshades, such as eggplant, tomato, bell peppers, asparagus, potato, etc., can present problems because eating them in excess blocks nutrient absorption. Black people's diet should be less than 5% wheat instead of the over 90% wheat. Black people cannot metabolize a starchy high wheat diet. Black people should always eat non-GMO organic natural foods, such as wild rice, short grain brown rice, string beans, collards, mustard greens, okra, avocado, cho-cho, kale, squash, bananas, oranges, papaya, plum, mango, passion fruits, cantaloupe, limes, plantain, red yams, water-melon (eat rind), honeydew, and pears, instead of wheat, rye, masaltarina, amaranth, Quinoa, spelt, Kamut, buckwheat, etc. If you must eat foods that are not organic, then take herbs and/or supplements to help the liver get rid of the chemicals in nonorganic foods such as: Milk Thistle, Dandelion Root, and/or Glutathione, MSM, Methionine, etc.

Black people should eat as natural as possible and as much raw food as possible. Follow the rules of food combining and do not mix protein with starch (i.e., meat and potato, meat and bread), or concentrated sweeteners (sugar) with starch (i.e., breakfast cereals, cake, pies). Black people should combine vegetables with starch, protein and vegetables, eat fruits alone and never drink and eat at the same time (drink one-hour before or after a meal). White people food industry combines foods ignorantly which creates diseases and promotes faulty scavenger cave-like food-combinations.

The "White" food area in the grocery store includes bleached white flour cakes, pastry, cookies, pasta, bread and pizza, snacks, ice cream, milk, dyed liquid/white sugar (pop, soda), potato chips, etc. White "food" can remain on the store shelf longer then colorful natural whole foods. Natural organic foods are alive and will spoil because they do not have chemical preservatives. Therefore, they have a short shelf life, which decreases the stores high profit margin. Grocery stores sell processed "foods" which must be embalmed with poisonous preservatives. Black people that eat embalmed foods are getting sick and are themselves becoming embalmed with dangerous toxic chemicals. The "food" store is in reality a funeral home.

Grocery stores have a "pink" area which is, perhaps the most dangerous. The pink color of the dead animal flesh is caused by their blood. Blood-be it red, clear or gray-is usually 50% sewage (waste) of the animal (this includes fish, seafood and fowl). The animal's meat (flesh) is the most processed food with toxins (poisons) such as arsenic, genetic mutants, radiation, DDT, sex hormones, nitrites, deodorants, herbicides and pesticides. White people as a group have a diet that is high starches, animal protein and cooked fats which prevents the recycling proteins. High protein diets are related to cancer, soft bones and sickling of cells.

The "green" area of the grocery store has GMO vegetable produce and fruit which are chemicalized, lethal gas-sprayed, radiated, processed with

95

synthetic fertilizers, herbicides, antibiotics, sex hormones, origins can be outside the country and follow no health or safety standards and plants cloned with human and animal cells. Plants genetically mixed with animal flesh can cause dangerous genetic changes and reactions in the human biochemistry. Fortunately, vegetables cannot hold high concentrations of toxins like meat. Boiling vegetables (which should only be steamed) causes the nutrients to be washed away in the water or become too coarse to be metabolized. This ritual of cooking kills probiotics and the nutrient value of the food which will "white out" your health resulting in diseases. The synthetic chemicals cannot be destroyed or parasites killed by boiling the plants or boiling the water.

Color is essential for foods and Black people. Nutritionally valuable foods have color. For example, natural oils (olive, corn, vegetable) have a brownish color. White peoples "food" companies destroy nutrients with bleach, antifreeze, radiation, deodorants, heat, and filter out the nutrients that give a brown color, rendering the oil clear. Food that lacks natural color lacks nutritional value. If the food is "whitened" (processed), it is nutritionally worthless. If it is white, don't eat it. It will "white out" your life and replace it with disease and death.

Cooking alters the color of food. Cooking has become an accepted way to denature, devitalize, clone and process food. This causes food to become a synthetic poisonous concoction that destroys to the same degree that it has destroyed. In other words, you destroy the food and the food destroys you. It is nature's revenge. Cooked food was never an accepted dietary tradition in ancient Africa. Cooking allowed the White war mongrel armies to carry their own food supply. Carrying dried meat, beans, rice, and barely increased the army's mobility. Cooked foods have the lowest nutrient content and contain inorganic irritants. Eating devitalized dull colored cooked foods caused Black peoples armies to become weak and sick from the food. Black people that eat, degenerative cooked foods are nutritionally raped.

White people that invaded Africa or enslaved Black people forced the practice of cooking foods upon Black people. This food cooking habit started during colonialism, slavery and the societal disruptive invasions (wars) upon Africa. White people's invasions of Africa destroyed crops, farmers, irrigation and the agricultural trade system. This caused fresh and ripe foods to become scarce, and dried foods such as legumes had to be cooked or sprouted in order to be eaten. Ripe beans, rice, millet, etc. are partially green they are ripe. they should be eaten partially green, not when they are unripe. Unripe dried beans are basically half protein and half starch in nutrient content. When cooked while unripe, they are an improper nutrient combination of starch and protein. Cooked unripe beans ferment and rot in the stomach causing stomach gas (flatulence).

White peoples Information Age began with the "Race War" invasion of Africa. The Race War caused Black people to lose control of land, food transportation routes, human and natural resources, agriculture and their diet. White people developed the cooked food habit in order to eat unripe and rotten foods. Cooking enabled them to eat rotten and partially spoiled foods. Cooking food has caused White people to be emotionally and mentally sick, physically ill, and to develop degenerative diseases.

Cooking food destroys most of the nutrients the quality and quantity of life. Over half the life expectancy is lost by cooking foods. Ancient Africans consumed an over 90% raw food diet, and were free of disease. Black adults had the constant energy of a child, required less sleep, had no rotten teeth, heart trouble, sex organ diseases, emotional and mental illness, colds, childhood diseases, diabetes, high blood pressure, arthritis, and lived to be over 150 years of age. Modern Black people living today with high blood pressure believe they get high blood pressure disease from, picking up paper all day (paper work, administrations, etc.,) while their enslaved ancestors on a mostly organic non-GMO raw food diet did not get hypertension, high blood pressure or stress from picking at least two acres of cotton every day. White people's evolutionary ape-like cousin, the Orangutan monkey, lives on a raw food diet and is free of disease and has a long-life span. The Orangutan's human so called cousin of the White race, eats cooked food and is continuously diseased and has a short life span.

There is no safe cooked food, be it an apple or spinach. All cooked food is anti-life. Added to cooked foods are drugs such as sodium chloride (salt), white sugar, cooking oil or animal grease, vinegar, alcohol, synthetic dyes, preservatives and toxic GMO spices that irritate the digestive tract. Cooked food perverts the taste buds and chemistry of the body. This perversion causes Black people to crave more dead flavorful garbage is called cooked food. Cooking destroys the live enzymes, vitamins, minerals, proteins, amino acids, fats, fibers, water, and carbohydrates within the food. The heat from the cooking process causes food nutrients to become inorganic, addictive, coarse, harsh, abrasive, poisonous toxic irritants, which are deadly. For example, cooked organic calcium turns into a coarse inorganic (dead) type metallic crystallized of sand, which makes it indigestible.

Black people that eat cooked food turn into a cesspool of walking liquid manure. Cooked proteins stick together in broken particles of acid. Acid accumulates in the body and weakens all tissues, cells and bones. Cooked starches turn into an inorganic crystallized sugar and charcoal. Cooked oils turn into trans oils, gummy that makes thick blood, and coat the internal organs causing cells to stick together. Cooked starches and sugars ferment in the stomach while cooked protein putrefies. They are not metabolized but are absorbed as rotten irritants. Dead (cooked) food feeds

97

bacteria. Bacteria create more ammonia, acids, toxic gases, alcohol, vinegars and poisons. Ironically, cooked food junkies season their food with the same addictive irritants the foods make in the intestine such as vinegar and acids (white sugar and bleached white flour make vinegar and acids) and ammonia (animal flesh makes this).

Digestion is slowed down, hampered, constipated and suspended by junk food, cooked food, cow's milk, cheese, alcohol, vinegar, salt, malnutrition, stress, worry, anger, tension, fatigue, fear, anxiety, and frustration. Cooked foods basically causes addiction to cooked foods. White peoples cave trauma and the White Supremacy food experience is a record of White people's current food behavior. Their food history is a record of their emotional injury. Their food experience teaches the White people nothing other than to repeat the past cave lifestyle. Wisdom teaches Black people not the trials and errors of experience. Black people learn through their ancestor's food wisdom. A solution to past food experiences is part of the past event. The future belongs to the teachings of ancestor's food wisdom, not the food cave food experience of White people. A healthy Black person that eats naturally colorful raw food and non-GMO original food can develop the level of intelligence to solve the negative experience of being cultural captives of White people's psychotic superiority complex disguised as democracy.

Catch AIDS, Catch A Cold, Catch an Infection or Catch Ignorance?

Colds, AIDS (Acquired Immune Deficiency Syndrome) and Venereal Disease (VD) based on the Germ Theory and Contagious Disease Theory is a syndrome. A syndrome is a collection of disease that already have names. The collection or grouping of diseases is arbitrarily selected by the drug companies. They usually have drugs prepared for their new made-up diseases, new treatment protocols and machines and laboratory test before they market the new syndromes. Their grouping of diseases is a collection of the natural cleansing processes of the body. The body always cleanses itself. Therefore, the drugs are treating the body as if its reactions should not exist. Sores, warts, bumps, blisters, mucus draining of the nasal passage and lungs, rashes, inflammations, lesions, ulcers or mucus drainage from the genitals are the body's way of flushing out toxic waste and dead cells. This is called a cleansing process or healing crisis. The body uses many different varieties of cleansing processes to free itself toxins. Once the cleansing process is over, the sores, lesions, ulcers, and blisters will heal and the nasal passage and lungs will be clear of mucus and free of cellular waste.

The body uses lesions, bumps, rashes, etc., to cleanse itself only if the bowel movements, Liver, kidneys, urine and breathing action cannot eliminate liquid manure (mucus). Bodily cleansing is what White theory science erroneously call catching a contagious viral or bacterial disease. Catching a disease is superstitious belief based upon the Germ Theory.

Bacteria of all types are present in the body at all times. Contagious bacteria are found in people without diseases as well as those with diseases. The various bacteria populations increase in numbers when they have a fermented or putrefied, food supply and waste and dead cells. When bowel movements and urine fail to eliminate. The bacteria growth increases as a defense reaction of the body. The bacteria feeds on the waste. And, helps to get rid of the waste. A high amount of bacteria, parasites, fungus and yeast are activated when toxins and waste accumulate at a speed faster than the kidneys, intestines, Liver, lungs and bowel movements can keep pace with. Each specific bacterium has a favorite fermented (carbohydrates) and or putrefied (protein) waste that it likes to eat. White scientist label the garbage disposal action of bacteria as the disease instead of labeling the cause of waste accumulations as the disease. White sciences Germ Theory causes them to kill the bacteria and leave the waste that created the over population of bacteria.

Black people can die from White theory base sciences treatments of the disease rather than the disease itself. Drug treatment of a "cold" is estimated to kill over 20,000 annually. A natural remedy for colds is to get bed rest, use herbal remedies, keep warm and drink plenty of spring or distilled water. Usually within 2 days the cold (bodily cleansing) is over. However, most Black people have more belief in White people's superstitions than the White people. It is necessary that Black people stop trying to blame (scapegoat)t virus or bacteria for illnesses they themselves caused. Viruses and bacteria are not trying to hurt the body or are in conflict with the body. They demonstrate that disease is abnormal and that Black people must use food as medicine to be healthy.

Black Assimilationist and Integrationist adopt White people's superstitious belief that a virus, bacteria or germ causes a disease instead of the under nutritional junk food diet is crazy. They deny their hygienic health science, a science that teaches that your food is medicine and medicine is your food. Food in White society is a cooked synthetic, chemically polluted concoctions put together to satisfy taste buds and the crazy germ belief denotes faulty reasoning. African centered Maat common sense tells you that a contagious virus or bacteria is in the blood and can freely travel all over the body. If a so-called contagious disease such as athlete's foot were truly contagious it could travel to the eyes, genitals, stomach or brain causing Athlete's Foot Brain disease. It could start as athlete's foot brain disease then travel to the feet. Contagious diseases can travel freely. Contagious diseases are given names based on their visible location, such as Venereal Disease.

Colds, AIDS, Infections, Venereal Disease and the fear of germs are all part of the Contagious Disease Theory. It is apparent that a person cannot Catch Healthy, Catch Bad Breath, Catch Ugly, Catch A Cold, Fibroid Tumors or Bumps. The White theory based medicine science classified cancer, asthma and pneumonia as contagious and then removed them from the contagious disease list. Lies change, but truth never changes.

The United States Navy proved the contagious disease superstition to be a lie. At the end of World War I, the U.S. Navy had several venereal diseased (VD) infected persons have sexual intercourse with non-infected people. The contagious VD did not infect those free of VD. The Rockefeller Institute of New York City sponsored Dr. Noguchi's experiment whereby he had contagious, infected people attempt to infect others. The results were that the disease-free people were not infected. Historically, Doctor David Livingston (1813-1873), an invader of Africa, no Black people.

Despite the overwhelming scientific evidence and simple use of common sense, Black Assimilationist and Integrationist scientist continue to believe in White superstition theory medicine. Black people die for White beliefs. Some Black people believe that the White Man's ice cubes are colder than the Black Man's ice cubes. Black people are competing with White drugs to destroy themselves. Contagious Diseases superstition is White people's belief. If you cannot catch "healthy" then you cannot "catch sick" or AIDS. It is illogical for a person to be healthy enough to get a "cold" (contagious disease) and then become sick enough to get rid of Colds. You cannot catch the weather – Cold, Hot, Partly cloudy, Storms, Snow, Rain, etc. The so-called contagious diseases superstition theory of Flu (influenza), chicken pox, mumps, measles, polio are proven to be a lie because contagious diseases occur among people with and without immunization shots. They recur year after year because the same diseased dietary practices are used year after year. A close look at a contagious disease theory such as AIDS can nullify this superstition.

An AIDS virus is a particle of a dead human cell. It cannot eat, reproduce, grow, move, attack you or be attacked. It is not a plant or animal, and it is not alive. A virus is not active one month and inactive (sleep) the next, nor does it sleep between 2 to 5 years before it attacks the person. A virus is neither retrogressive (retro-within) or progressive. A virus is dead particles of a cell. Dead cell particles come in all sizes and can pass through the pores of condoms. The body's cells are constantly being produced and constantly dying. Therefore, it is easy to find a particle from a dead cell called a virus that caused a disease. The cells are composed of many organs (called organelles) which are similar to the human body's digestive, excretory, respiratory, immune, circulatory, nervous and reproductive systems. The cell has a melaninated nucleus (brain). The cell's genetic code is with an energy producing cellular organ called the mitochondria. Genetic information is stored on the mitochondrion DNA (Deoxyribonucleic Acid) and RNA (Ribonucleic Acid). It is particles of DNA and RNA that are labeled the AIDS virus. What is called AIDS is a cleansing process of the body and what is called a virus is a dead cell particle that is not alive and cannot be killed because it is already dead.

Sores, bumps, blisters that burst, pus, mucus, and open sores that drain waste contain fluids out of the body are the body's cleansing process. The cleansing process is called a contagious disease based upon White Scientist Contagious Disease Theory. They chemically try to cure, remedy, stop or suppress the body's cleansing process with drugs or surgery. The body gets overloaded with toxins, waste and dead cells and flushes them out the body with mucus fluids via the lungs, nasal cavities, skin and genitals. If the kidneys and intestines fail to get rid of waste and toxins, the body cleanses by using pustules, rashes, vesicles, diarrhea, bacteria, sores (lesions), fevers, colds, sweats, yeast, tumors, etc.

The continuous eating of junk foods, drinking sodas, alcohol, and artificial fruit water, or cooking the oil (smoking) of toxic chemicals of marijuana, tobacco, meat, white sugar, bleached white flour, salt, drugs (legal and illegal), cooked food, and the taking of vaccinations, drugs, and immunization chemicals destroys the immune system. Eventually the immune system collapses and it is called AIDS and blamed on a dead cell particle called a virus. Ironically, Kaposis Sarcoma Disease has the same sign and symptoms as AIDS, just as syphilis has the same sign and symptoms as Herpes.

The change of names for a disease done by the drug oligarchy corporation need to increase profits. They get profits from the treatment of sick people with drugs and surgery. The diseases are the effects of their drugs and junk foods. The Center for Disease Control, the Food and Drug Administration, World Health Organization, drug companies, hospitals and secondary health support industries maintain the contagious disease theory as a fact. If they cannot blame a disease on a virus, they blame it on a bacteria. The drug oligarchy makes profits from the diseases they created. They create and maintain the public's fear of an evil virus and bacteria in order to sell medicines, all types of soaps, antibiotic deodorants, toothpaste, creams, lotions and greases, all of which have not stopped an attack from contagious germs, virus, or bacteria.

Bacteria are present in the body at all times. They are essential for maintaining health and food digestion. Black people have the largest variety of bacterial flora in their digestive systems, which allows them to metabolize food more efficiently. Various bacteria help to eliminate waste toxins, make vitamins and neutralize impurities. A specific bacteria likes a specific type of food to eat. Black people that eat like White people and eats 50% more starchy wheat than they are historically accustomed (should be less than 5% whole wheat). This causes specific bacteria to increase in numbers and become out of balance with the bacteria flora community. This creates a subclinical disease condition in Black people and limits the immune systems protection. Weaken immunity, which alters the cleansing reflex, causing toxins and waste to accumulate, resulting in a "cold" (mucus congestion). Black people constantly catching colds arc constantly committing the same dietary error over and over again.

There are approximately 20 million Americans who have contagious "colds" each day. It is never explained why the contagious bacteria or virus does not kill the remainder of the population or why contagious bacteria does not travel to the feet, brain, genitals or heart, causing "colds" of the brain, genitals or heart. If a "cold" were truly contagious it would destroy the entire body, as there is no medicine to stop it.

Caucasian medical myths and superstition theory science admits that it has no cure for the "cold." This can only mean that the common "cold" should have killed all people. Added to this, White medical theory science tells people they can catch sick bacteria but not strong lively healthy bacteria. Healthy bacteria could cause a person to catch more good health. The only thing a person can catch is ignorance, if they believe the contagious disease theory based on the superstition of the primitive cave culture.

Black people cannot compromise their health and be healthy. They cannot accept part of the White people's health theory science without getting damaged from part of that theory science. The contagious disease theory is a religious belief that supports White peoples fear of germs and fear economically supports the industries that produce chemicals to kill essential germs on and in the body with toothpaste, antibiotic soap, deodorants, feminine hygiene sprays, douches, foot spray, deodorizers, antibiotic sprays, lotions and shampoo. This supports the belief in purified (bleached white) processed foods. White people do not trust nature nor do they trust Black people. Because, Black people are too close to nature in emotions, thought, behavior, spirit and culture. Black and White people may take herbs and eat the same type food. However, black people metabolize herbs and food differently and express diseases differently. Do not mistake similarities to mean sameness. The physical or mental similarities between the Black and White races do not make them of like humanity or like in approach to health. For example, one can identify the many similarities or commonalities between the organizational structure, training and discipline of the United States Military and the African Liberation Armies. However, their similarities do not make them united in purpose, or united as one. They are by definition and belief totally against each other.

There are also similarities between the White religions and Black spirituality and Black reality science, and White theory science. However, they are opposite to each other in function. The health science of Black people moves from harmony to harmony, while the White science moves from conflict to conflict. For example, in a disease process some tissue of an organ may get overloaded with toxins or waste and the body's immune reflex moves to get rid of the toxins or waste. The Black holistic scientist calls this a cleansing process. The White theory base science defines cleansing as the body attacking itself or in conflict with itself.

A person may accidentally put another individual's bacterial fluid into an open sore or the mouth. Bacteria can be transported from one individual to another. The foreign bacteria enter the body and the body has a chemical reaction. This chemical reaction is similar to the rejection of an organ transplant. Holistic black sciences recognize this as a cleansing reaction while White theory based science calls it catching another person's contagious bacteria. The Germ Theory and Contagious Disease Theory beliefs of White people is superstitions. The assimilationist and integrationist black people accept theory beliefs as facts will remain in a disease state and move from one sickness to another sickness. There is nothing to catch but superstitious white ignorance.

White people defines believe their contagious disease theory is a fact and their sexuality is normal. However, disease is abnormal and White people's sexuality is abnormal. Their belief of sexually contagious diseases theory (VD, AIDS, herpes, etc.) ignores facts. White peoples sex behavior is influenced by their races disease condition created by food shortages, Ice Age, soil robbed of nutrients, ignorance, famines and wars.

White people's premature and begins puberty and because they are sickly. A race that is sickly reproduces quickly (early) and plants that are sickly reproduces quickly (early) Black people that follow the White people's junk food diet, prescription and non-prescription drug use and life style also begin sexual activity at an early age. White people have sexual intercourse primarily to act out emotional and mental conflicts and to satisfy feelings of control, inferiority, ownership and power as well as to medicate their self-hatred.

Early sexual activity is a symptom of a sickly race. A race with constant mild-to-severe degenerative diseases is on the verge of extinction. Normal reproductive sex beings approximately between 18 to 20 years of age or later. Ovulation and sperm production normally starts between 14 to 18 years of age. However, a sickly race will have abnormally early ovulation, ejaculate sperm at an early age and have low sperm counts, and early pregnancies beginning at 8 to 12 years of age. Premature reproduction is a species survival mechanism. This species survival mechanism is triggered in sickly insects, animals and plants. This gives rise to the saying that "a plant that is sickly will reproduce quickly." Early sex among a species with degenerative diseases, excessive sex and masturbation activities weakens the sex organs.

Disease such as arthritis, rheumatism, hardening of the arteries, varicose veins, constipation or low levels of testosterone can prevent the orgasmic contraction of the prostate, uterus and vagina. Consequently, men and women do not feel sexually fulfilled and have excessive sex in a vain attempt to find an orgasm. A nutrient-weak prostate can swell and contract quickly causing premature ejaculation. This can lead to infertility, excessive masturbation, and sex intercourse to feel fulfilled. A bodily disease affects the sex organs, which can lead to accumulation of toxins, waste and dead cells in the sex organs. The sex organs can become an outlet for impurities and have a cleansing reaction, which is erroneously labeled VD or AIDS. Added to this, increased sex and premature reproductive ability is a Post Ice Age and Post War species survival response to increased numbers of people.

The Ice Age, cave life, and Wars exterminated a large number of White people. During the Ice Age, Cold Age (Post Ice Age), and cave era famines, ice Age Wars, World Wars, Cave Wars, Race Wars (Caucasian War Against Black people), and Caucasian internal wars (revolts), cause an adrenaline response. Adrenaline is a hormone that the body releases to give extra energy and alertness for a "fight or flight" response and decreases blood to internal organs which provides more blood for the muscles. Adrenaline increases the emotions of anger, disease, stress, frustration, depression, fear, and danger. These emotions are needed to fight the crisis. Adrenaline activate short term memory needed for immediate attention for fighting for survival. The blood supply for the reproductive, digestive, excretory, is decreased, and used for fight or flight survival. Prolonged adrenaline sympathetic nervous system usage can weaken the excretory (kidney), sex organs (prostate and uterus disease), digestion (acid reflux, Crohn's Disease), and the body's ability to fight disease. A typical Caucasian characteristic rebound reaction to famine, Cave Wars, Post World Wars, and Post Ice Age behaviors is an increase in sex and domestic (non-military) violence.

White people's starchy diet can cause sex and violence to increase. It a diet high in acidic foods such as wheat, potatoes, cheese, bread, oats, meat and dairy. Excessive acid foods consumption cause emotional, mental, and physical illnesses by draining the body of nutrients, such as calcium, glutamine, lysine, potassium, magnesium, manganese, Vitamins A, B, C, D, E, K and amino acid. A high acid diet weakens bone, nerve, and muscle tissues, eyes, heart, ears, arteries, veins and brain. Muscles use carbohydrates, not protein as fuel. If alkaline carbohydrates are not available as fuel, then the energy that would go to secondary muscles (i.e., legs, arms, back, etc.) is allocated to primary muscles. Consequently, the individual can lose weight, degenerate, lose muscle mass and immunity. The loss of muscle mass is superstitiously labeled by white theory science as the body eating itself or self-cannibalism.

White peoples starch and meat-centered diet is contrary to the Black people's alkaline diet of rye, squashes, millet, wild rice, sprouted seeds, fruits, etc. Ancient African vegetarian laborers who built the walled cities, temples, colleges, statues and pyramids, ate alkaline carbohydrates that included figs, dates, onions, lentils, barley, millet, yams, plantain, sprouts, pollen, tropical fruits, etc. The cabbage family provided foods which could be used to alkaline the body such as broccoli, green collards, dandelion, figs, kale, mustard greens, sesame seeds, turnip greens, watercress, etc. Ancient Roman, Greek and European athletes, laborers, peasants and gladiators was acidic. A vegetable shortage caused them to start making meat taste like vegetables by using herbal seasonings.

The contagious sexual diseases theory, along with "colds" and infectious disease theory, are a superstitious cave myth created by White people to scientifically hide their race's sickly, diseased and infertility predicament. It is African cultural treason for Black people to assimilate and integrate into White culture and accept the White superstitious belief. African Cultural Ignorance is created by the White corporate own education system that miseducates Black people about health, nutrition, food and disease. Any education in any subject taught by White people is a miseducation. White people have a 10-20 degrees of understanding on any subject that they teach Black people. Their teachers only get bachelorette, masters and doctorate degrees from colleges because they can only have a degree of understanding.

AIDS

AIDS is a syndrome and a syndrome is a collection of disease signs and symptoms Center for Disease Control data indicates False Positive = 83%

THE FOLLOWING CAN CAUSE AIDS POSITIVE:

Alcoholic Hepatitis
Another Retro Virus
Arthritis
Cancer
Clotting Factors
Cold Virus
Cross Reaction
Drugs
Fungus
Hemodialysis
Hemophiliac Blood Products
Hepatitis
Hepatitis B
Herpes Simplex II
Infection

Influenza
Lupus
Malaria
Malnutrition
Microbes
Myeloma
Parasites
Pregnancy
Prior Pregnancy
Semen
Silicone Implant
Toxins
Tuberculosis
Vaccinations
Worms

Wake Up, Eat Breakfast and Die

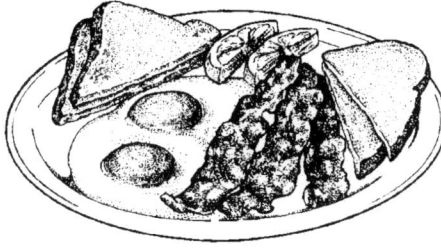

Black infants, babies and children under 2 or 3 years of age cannot eat starches because they do not produce the strong carbohydrate ptyalin digestive enzymes. Carbohydrates (starches)fruits such as wheat, corn, rice and oat or roots such as potatoes or the eating of starchy breakfast cereals cannot be digested by the child. Refined carbohydrates such as a white sugar, candy, cake, pizza, potato chips, pretzels and teething biscuits should not be given to the child. Starches eaten by children become liquid mucus manure that floats in the blood resulting in childhood diseases. Aside from this, a starch centered diet weakens the immune system, and the kidneys, Liver, lymph glands, pineal gland, adrenal glands, and spleen.

White peoples junk food companies and science theory based superstition trained doctors want the baby to fatten up for the profit-making disease journey to hospitals, clinics, and cemetery. Breakfast starchy cereals are usually combined totally improperly. Starches should not be combined with sugar or sweet fruits, as the sugars causes the starches to spoil. Spoiled starches absorbed in the intestine create toxins and an acidic body. Sweet fruits and cereals are an improper food combination. They cause toxins, an acidic bodily condition, that weakens all cells, tissues, organs and bones. Added to this, cow's and goat's milk should not be combined with fruits or sugar or starch. Animal milks are acid and cause an acidic bodily condition. They weaken the heart, bones, tissues and organs. Nonetheless, White peoples junk food industry, dieticians, medical industry, milk industry, and sugar industry tell the black people to combine starchy cereal with fruit, cooked milk and sugar.

Black people are taught to drink cooked orange juice (pasteurized) and eat starchy bread, constipating combinations of sugar, wheat, milk, eggs and trans oil (cooking makes it synthetic grease). Black people are taught to eat bacon (pork belly grease) and eggs (chicken fetus) together. This is improper food combinations. Black folks eat this along with jelly (sugar and cooked fruit) and butter (milk grease) on bread (starch) and a glass of mucus-forming acidic cooked cow's milk. Protein is easily digested between 10 a.m. and 2 p.m. Starch and protein are extremely taxing on the digestive system of the body. If cooked starches are eaten; they would naturally require fermentation to be nutritionally absorbed and should be digested alone or with vegetables. Black peoples natural breakfast diet in the desert was figs and dates or other fruits. The body's Cyclic Laws of digestion indicate that nutrition food should ideally be eaten between the hours of 12 noon and 7 p.m., (food ingestion phase). According to the food cycle food is utilized by the body (assimilated) between the hours of 7 p.m. and 4 a.m. Digested food cleanses the body from 4 a.m. to 12 noon. Ancient Black peoples breakfast was usually cleansing fruits. Until the child has developed a full set of teeth and is capable of fully chewing and mixing the food with saliva, starches should not be eaten.

The junk food starchy breakfast contributes to Eating Disorders. White people have a diseased psychological attachment to food, which their American Psychiatric Association classifies as a mental disease. It stems from the Ice Age cave civilizations and superstition. Eating disorders disease causes the physical and emotional craving for food. It is an addictive habit in which the food controls the person. Food helps White people to bury their true feelings of self-hatred and racial inferiority. Food medicates their cultural delinquency, dysfunctional family heritages, lack of control of self-hatred anger, violence, sexism, helps to bury their history of murdering over 200 million Black people and stealing every technology of African civilization except harmony with nature and other colored races.

White people stuff their babies with food as if the Ice Age and cave lifestyle which had a limited food supply. White people force their babies to eat as often as possible or every two hours and in between meals or suck on amputated breast's rubber nipple. Sucking on a milk-less amputated nipple (pacifier) is negative. The babies try to reject the overfeeding of food by drooling, vomiting, burping, having hiccups, diarrhea, stomach gas and childhood diseases. Over eating causes the babies to become bloated with fat. Fat babies resemble any of the fat cows and pigs going to the slaughter factories. Fat Caucasian babies like fat pigs are only fit to be led to a feeding trough and slaughtered so their fat can be used to fill a can of lard. Black babies are forced to be overfed by well-meaning food illiterate Black parents.

White people have an Eating Disorder which is an emotional and mental illness. They eat emotionally to hide from feeling or to compensate for feeling they do not have. Their Eating Disorder is another means for the dairy, junk food, drug and medical industries to make large profits. The industries cause disease and use the "break-fast" to reinforce the eating disorders. The corporate own junk food industries create a stable profitable over eating Black population with a mental illness called an Eating Disorder. Black people are White food corporation's trained food illiterate addicts that like eat and beg for more. Black people are caged animals that buy their own food and pay rent to live in their urban ghetto economic, miseducated, and unemployable cages.

Food illiterate Black people wake up eat an under nutritious starchy disease-causing breakfast that prepares them for medical drugs and surgery sacrifice and death. They eat starchy cereal bread jelly sandwiches and other type breads called waffles, pancakes, pizzas, or Pop Tarts. These starchy foods turn to sugar quickly and damage the pancreas causing diabetes. High process starch and concentrated sweeteners cause diabetes, low blood sugar hypoglycemic, destroy the kidneys, cause high blood pressure, dry skin, blindness, cataracts, glaucoma, arthritis, inflamed stomachs (Crohn's disease), dry eyes, hardening of the arteries, amputations of feet and legs, obesity, hyperactivity, senility, prostate problems, infertility, incontinence of bladder and bowels, irritability, tooth decay and constantly keep you eating. Starchy foods cause childhood obesity and a sudden energy drop for the Black child while in school (attention deficit). This results in the Black child feeling bored or disinterested in schoolwork. The sugary foods and drinks and starchy breakfast sets the child up to dislike school. The high blood sugar level collapses to low blood sugar levels in the morning hours of school resulting in low energy, fatigue, depression, inability to concentrate and learning problems. Sugar and high starches cause obesity and it is not normal in adults or children. It is a sign of a diseased body, emotions, mind, and spirit. Feeding Black children like they are being fattened up for the slave auction block or an animal slaughterhouse is a crime. A baby eating constantly gets excessive fat cells and bloated. The plaque fat cells (waste) gets into the digestive system cells, tissues, organs, glands and brain. A fat baby is a sick baby. White people's animal farms only force feed them twice a day because its best to bulk up their body. A natural organic foods diet and breast milk are the only defense against diseases and fat bloat, but they are not used. Breast milk regulates feeding intervals and biochemically matches the biochemical personality of the child. A Black child sucking on amputated rubber nipples or bottled cow's milk are eating their way into White People's Ice Age and caves. Aside from this, the child seeking white milk leaves a negative psychological imprint on the subconscious of and they associate with nurturing and love with White people. Added to this when the baby gets ill it is taken to a hospital where all the medical supplies are wrapped in White, and the doctor wears a white laboratory jacket. Consequently, the Black baby associates being made normal and healthy with the White color. In any case, White peoples diet habits are still connected to their cave civilizations eating customs. The custom of fattening the Black child and feeding them a starchy breakfast cereal concoctions along with denying the child Black woman's breast milk presents a bonding problem, nutritional problem and emotional and mental illness problem.

White people's babies who are not breastfed begin to develop mental illness and feel that nature denied them a future and that nature cannot be trusted. This stems from the complete interruption of the breastfeeding "rites of passage". The White mother, raised on food from nutrient poor soil could not continue to breastfeed, so she was forced to have her baby suck on a lower animal's breast (cow, goat, etc.). This has mentally instilled in the baby that nature/mother cannot provide (milk) security or be trusted.

White people's history influences their current personality. A personality that was formed from famines, disease, cave wars, violent women, gangs, constant deaths of dysfunctional family members, hunger, violence, rape, cannibalism and stavation. The constant episodes of starving and then overeating when food was available made life insecure and deficient of higher meaning. Life was explained by superstitions and wars between their many dysfunctional adult and children gangs, good Gods, and evil Gods.

It is this emotionally and mentally ill and deficient White cave civilization with its nutritionally deficient mind and dietary ignorance that is now trying to control the diets of Black people. Further information on diet is in White Racist studies by the Eating Disorders Program at Michigan State University and biased books such as *Managing Your Mind Through Food*, by Judith Wurtman. Aside from the emotional and mental illnesses caused by denying breastfeeding, the replacement of breast milk with animal's milk is harmful. All of this causes physical diseases called childhood diseases.

White people's childhood diseases are normal for them. Historically, Black Childhood diseases are new to Black children and directly related to the starchy junk food and milk diet and White people dietary customs. The diseases are disruptive of the Black family harmony. They weaken the immune system. The Black childhood diseases are usually treated with White people's toxic drugs that cause secondary diseases and destructive to the "so-called" immune system.

White people combine food ignorantly. Their food combinations are cause's the diseases that are blamed on a virus or bacteria. Black parents should fit the child to the food instead of fitting the food to the child. In other words, it is not proper to put sugar, fruit and milk on a starchy cereal to get a child to eat it. Feed the child simple food combinations and do not combine starches with fruit, starches with meat, starches with sweets, or give cooked fruit or a sweet and acid fruit combination. These combinations cause fermentation in the stomach, gas, and manure to form in the stomach and an acidic body.

Allowing the child to be awake past 7 p.m. causes sleep deprivation resulting in brain stress, weak immunity, and attention problems. It is not correct for the Black parent to let children eat (past 7 p.m.) at night, or when the child is overheated, feels bad, is tired, stressed, excited, chilled, in pain or is angry. Help the child work though negative emotions or to relax so that the food will get digested properly. The starchy cereals are usually not chewed but swallowed, and this ultimately causes disease. The child under 3 years of age does not have the enzyme ptyalin to metabolize the cereal foods. Stuffing the child with starchy cereal, cow's milk, and sugar can lead to flu, tonsillitis, colds, learning problems, gastritis, personality problems, mood swings, and hypertension.

The majority of childhood diseases can be treated with herbs and supplements. An enema with catnip and red clover is cleansing, and drinking herbs (alcohol free extracts are more useful) such as Echinacea, gingko, chickweed, golden seal, yarrow, pau D'Arco, peppermint and red clover. Supplements such as Vitamins A, B, C, E, zinc, calcium, magnesium, and digestive enzymes are very beneficial. They are available in candy form such as gummies.

The childhood diseases are the child's sympathetic nervous system trying to defend itself from a poor diet and lack of breast milk. Childhood diseases such as **chicken pox** is toxins released through the skin with pimples that ooze fluid and form a crust in a 3-to-7-day cycle. The child's fingernails should be cut, as the skin is very itchy. **Measles** is a cleansing through the lungs and skin. Usually the child has bumps, a furry tongue, white spots in the mouth and throat and is sensitive to light. **Mumps** are usually swollen Lymph parotid glands in the back of the jaw between the ears. The Lymph glands get toxic from acidic, milk, cooked food and junk food. The glands swell with toxins in an attempt to defend the Black child from the junk food diet. It can be contagious to unhealthy they people 48 hours before the swelling and up to 6 days after.

Tonsillitis is the inflammation of the tonsils caused by constipating food combinations and starchy cereals. The tonsils get sore, swell and there may be an earache, coated tongue and bad breath. **Rheumatic Fever** is an arthritis type condition of the heart and bone joints (elbow, knee, etc.), with pain and stiffness caused by crystallized waste and liquid manure mucus waste. **Flu** (influenza) is similar to mucus congestion called a "cold". It is characterized by a dry cough and dry throat. The body tries to defend itself by ejecting the mucus out into the lungs and nasal cavities and coughing to get rid of mucus. **Asthma** is a type of muscle spasm in the lungs that can be caused by waste in the body and muscles. The muscles around the lungs tighten the chest, which results in wheezing, coughing and difficulty in breathing.

Childhood diseases are accepted as normal. However, they are not normal for Black children unless they eat like White people. Childhood diseases are an early start on the path of nutritional self-destruction. Breakfast is a tool used as a wake-up meal for a dysfunctional life and death. The social factors created and maintained by White Domination place the Black child's health in jeopardy. The book titled *Kids Count Data Book: State Profiles of Child Well Being*, which is a study done by the Center of Social Policy and the Annie E. Casey Foundation, used government statistics and primarily the categories of unmarried teens, birth weight, arrest rates, violent death rate of teens, and single parent households as influences on childhood diseases and dysfunctionality.

The Black parent must put the child on an organic food diet. The National Research Council (Jayne and Williams, 1989) indicates that Black Americans poverty is 2 to 3 times higher than White peoples at all times and the mortality and morbidity of Black Americans is poor and getting worse. White people's corporate own governments created and maintained poverty and social conditions make the Black child dysfunctional.

The idea that breakfast gives immediate energy is a myth. Black people fear that if they don't eat breakfast they will get sick or very weak. Fasting at night while asleep and melatonin secretion helps to create the morning energy, not "breaking the fast" so-called "break-fast". The body gets accustomed to weight in the stomach, intestines and impacted manure in the colon. An absence of the weight and impacted manure causes the Black people to feel the need to eat.

It is not true hunger but the White culturally created appetite that must be satisfied with a starchy breakfast. The food eaten will take approximately four hours to leave the stomach and six to sixteen hours to be metabolized in the small intestine with electrolyte absorption in the large intestine. It is in the small intestine that the energy nutrients are absorbed from the food. In most cases, the drug stimulation reaction to white sugar and bleached white flour is mistaken for the nutrient energy of breakfast. The energy from the food eaten at a 9 a.m. (0900 hours) breakfast will not be nutritionally available to the body until 9 p.m. (2100 hours). At 9 p.m. the body's circadian clock is in the assimilation/melatonin phase. Consequently, the body won't use the energy food breakfast until the next day.

The theory belief is that the breakfast food energy is available to the body at the hour of breakfast. The energy from breakfast food has to go thru the stomach then the intestines and the processed by the Liver and pancreas before it is released, this takes at least 4 to 8 hours or around dinner time. If the constipating junk food diet is followed, then the previous energy from food eaten 1 to 7 days ago is the energy being used during the breakfast hour. In this case, the constipated Black person is using toxic manure, drugs and sugar of previous eaten food for energy. The previous day's constipating food is being pushed along by the weight of breakfast foods. Black people that eat the starchy breakfast concoctions are a human sacrifice for the sick treatment industries of hospitals, clinics, emergency rooms and drug stores.

Previous food eaten requires energy to process (metabolize) and this energy is diverted and drain from other organs and organ systems to increase the blood to the stomach to help metabolize the food. Often the Black feel sleepy or fatigued after eating stimulants because the body is in mild drug withdrawal. Condiments such as spicy irritants, mustard, pepper, chocolate, nutmeg, cinnamon, and caffeine and chocolate drain energy. And are used to overcome the withdrawal and energy drain of sugars, lard, grease, dairy, meat, white flour, refined carbohydrates, etc.

Assimilationist and Integrationist Black people are addicted to White people. They eat White peoples junk food breakfasts and have an emotional illness and physical illness. Junk foods cause degenerative diseases such as arthritis, cardiovascular problems, varicose veins, weak eyes, fertility problems, ADHD, Alzheimer's, senility, weak bones, learning disorders, mood swings, cancer, AIDS, venereal diseases, etc. Black people are eating starchy breakfasts are on a diseased journey to the cemetery. They are having a rehearsal for death. Breakfast should be of cleansing organic non-GMO fruit, whole foods, spring or distilled water and/or organic fruit juice.

Sugar and Spice, But Not Very Nice (Aspartame = NutraSweet, Equal)

All concentrated sweeteners (white sugar etc.) cause brain damage.
Aspartame is an artificial sweetener that is 200 times sweeter than white sugar. It is totally synthetic and is made with a toxic poison called methanol. Methanol is combined with aspartic acid and phenylalanine and called aspartame with the commercial trade name NutraSweet or Equal and Splenda that harms the Liver. Aspartame has Methanol which is an alcohol that damages the Liver and the thymus gland. And synthetic aspartic acid and phenylalanine are toxic to the brain and Liver. It is cheap to make and yields high profits.

The concentrated sweeteners such as crystallized polysaccharides carbohydrates, syrups, and honey are drugs. Their names usually end with the subfix "ose" or start with prefixes "glu or gly". The concentrated powder sweeteners explode when exposed to hot flames. In processing (making) sugar bleaching chemicals such as poisonous Sulphur dioxide, activated carbon or ion-exchange resin are used. Fermented carbohydrates in the body turn into alcohol. Therefore, high levels of sugar makes high levels of alcohol. Consequently, people become sugar drunkards addicted to sugar and alcohol. They crave chemicals related to alcohol such as vinegar (ascetic acid poison). Sugar increases cravings (excitatory) and Ghrelin hormone and reduces satisfaction (inhibitory) Leptin hormone. Processed sugar and narcotics both stimulate the brain's dopamine and opioid centers. This can cause a person to become easily addicted to an emotion, a behavior or a drug. Sugar is put on French fried potatoes to make them a brown caramelized sugar color and a gold mallard color.

Sweeteners cause a craving for salt. And, salts cause a craving for sugar. This is primary reason why salt is in every candy bar. And, sugar is in table salt (sodium chloride). Cheap sugar made from petroleum waste (glycerol) is used in foods.

Concentrated processed sugars causes inflammation of the pancreas and digestive tract (Crohn's disease, colitis etc.) destroys the eyeball (glaucoma), dry eye's macular (cataracts), destroys the bladder's sphincter muscle and skin (urinary incontinence), bowel in continence, damages the nerves (blindness, Alzheimer's) kidneys (dialysis), joints (arthritis), decreases blood vessel circulation (amputation), hardens the liver (cirrhosis), damages the pancreas hormone centers (diabetes), dries scalp skin (hair-loss), decrease blood flow (high blood pressure), dries skin (lotion usage) over stimulates nerves (hyperactivity), ages the skin (anti-wrinkle crème), weakens the prostate and uterus (erectile problems, enlarged prostate, fibroids) causes obesity, loss of teeth, weakens eyes (eye glasses), causes yeast infection and dandruff, and contributes to weak immunity and heart disease.

The U.S. Food and Drug Administration has reported that the common symptoms of aspartame are dizziness, nausea, vision problems, menstruation problems, seizures, malaise and recurrent headaches. The Center for Disease Control has reported that the majority of complaints about aspartame are neurological (nerve damage). Canada, one of the first countries to use it, has noted that aspartame causes menstruation problems, mood swings, numbness and migraine headaches. When teenagers discontinued its consumption for 10 days and the teenagers' migraine headaches, numbness, mood swings, and other symptoms cleared up.

Black Children are not tested for toxic levels of aspartame. The secondary effects or permanently damaging effects known. Aspartame is a sweet way to use Black children as laboratory test rats for the economic profits of Caucasian business. Aspartame can be found in diet foods, chewing gum, wine coolers, sodas, instant tea, milkshake mixes, yogurt, drugs, laxatives, cocoa mixes, cereals, candy, cake, instant breakfast, frozen desserts, gelatin deserts, breath mints, juice drinks, toppings, multi-vitamins, milk, instant coffee and most foods that say sugar free.

Aspartame is used in carbonated sodas in order to use the word "diet" on the label. The word "diet" on the label actually indicates that the soda is part of a diet. It is never specified on the label whether the word "diet" refers to weight loss diet. The consumer assumes that the word "diet" means a weight loss food. Aspartame and other synthetic sugars have never been scientifically proven to cause weight loss. The body exhales toxic carbon dioxide, in order to get rid of it. The consumer ironically buys carbon dioxide and drinks it in carbonated sodas. Carbonated sodas demineralize the body bones and cause cirrhosis (hardening) of the Liver. Sodas contain phosphoric acid (poison lye) which gives a burning sensation to the mouth and throat because of the lye. Lye causes cancer and disrupts digestion. Harmful synthetic sugars are in "sugar free" foods. If a food taste sweet a type of sugar is in it. The Food and Drug Administration only classifies white sugar (glucose) as an official sugar. The word "sugar free" means white sugar is not in the product. "Sugar free" means a synthetic poisonous concentrated sweetener sugar such as aspartame is in the food. Synthetic chemical sugars are addicting and harmful.

The aspartame users have moved from synthetic sugar addiction to synthetic amino acid aspartame addiction. They never get treated for the sugar (sweets) addiction. Sweet addiction (aspartame, white sugar) doubles the disease-causing effects when combined with bleached white flour, white flour, polished (white) rice, salt, (sodium chloride) cooked saturated fats, animal flesh and synthetic chemicals in food. Heart disease, diabetes, varicose veins, senility, coronary artery disease, circulatory problems, cancer and many other diseases are directly related to refined carbohydrates such as white sugar, bleached white flour, white flour, etc. It was not until they were added to the cooked saturated fat to the diet did these diseases increase in the Black population. When concentrated sweeteners are added to the combination of cooked saturated fats, salt (sodium chloride) and hidden synthetic chemicals health problems.

Concentrated sweeteners are synergistic (enhancers) to other synthetic chemicals and hide the chemical taste of junk foods. Books that can reveal more information on the subject are *Sugar Blues*, by William Duffy, *Natural Health, Sugar and the Criminal*, by J.A. Rodale, *Body, Mind and Sugar*, by E. Abrahamson and A. Pezet and *Killer Salt*, Marietta Whittlesey.

White people's businesses use lies to sell white sugar. For example, brown sugar is white sugar with brown caramel color and raw cane sugar is white sugar with caramel color. There are other harmful concentrated sweeteners such as corn syrup, fructose, sucrose, dextrose, honey, etc. Sugar consumption, and concentrated sweeteners cause over 50% of Americans to be hypoglycemic and diabetic while the remainder are prediabetic. Prediabetic means they are diabetic.

The only truly safe sugars are those found within the uncooked raw vegetable or fruit. The herb Stevia is a natural sweetener made from leaves and Monkfruit sweetener made from a fruit do not cause diabetes. Grain sugars such as rice or barley syrup damage the pancreas slowly and are toxic to the pancreas. The sugars ending in "ol" such as xylitol, mannitol, etc. are harmful to the liver. Again, the sweet Stevia leaves and Monkfruit sweeteners are the safest sugar to eat.

The commercial health foods have processed concentrated sugars, improper food combinations and are a type of heath food junk food. There are a large amounts of junk health food and many varieties of sugary sweet foods. The problem with junk health food is they use deceptive misguiding words such as "natural". A few wholesome ingredients are mixed with brown sugar, salt (sodium chloride), corn syrup, aspartame, cooked hydrogenated oils and processed foods. These foods start out being natural but are gradually converted to junk. The Caucasian health movements usually ruin themselves because they are part of the Cave mentality.

SWEET 'N LOW

INGREDIENTS:
SPLENDA (sucralose)
Ingredients:
Dextrose, Maltodextrin, coal tar, use roach spray to cause sugar to spin to the right
Causes:
- ∞ Gastrointestinal problems
- ∞ Dizziness
- ∞ Cancer
- ∞ Seizures
- ∞ Blurred vision
- ∞ Allergies
- ∞ Nerve damage
- ∞ Migraines
- ∞ Weight gain
- ∞ Increased blood sugar
- ∞ Alcohol

Dextrose (glucose, corn syrup)
Causes:
- ∞ Diabetes
- ∞ Cancer
- ∞ Reproduction Problems
- ∞ Digestion Problems
- ∞ Genetic Alterations
- ∞ Mutations
- ∞ Hardening of Arteries
- ∞ Decreased Oxygen to Brain and decrease circulation

It contains traces of Phosphoric Acid (Lye), Sulfuric Acid (Lye), Arsenic, Pig and Cattle Blood (Albumin)
- ∞ 300 Times sweeter than white sugar
- ∞ Increases weight of food (has odorless, tasteless form)
- ∞ Does not have to be put on label

Calcium Saccharin **(made from Coal Tar)**
Causes:
- ∞ Cancer
- ∞ Digestive Disorders
- ∞ Skin Diseases
- ∞ Blood Clotting and Collagen Formation Problems

Calcium Silicate
Causes:
- ∞ Respiratory Problems
- ∞ Headaches
- ∞ Diarrhea
- ∞ Eye Problems
- ∞ Hives

It is used to make Cement and Glass, Aspirin, Food Dye, Cosmetics, Anti-Caking Agent

Cream of Tartar
Causes:
- ∞ Skin Problems
- ∞ Edema
- ∞ Mineral Imbalances

Note: - Can Contain Salt, Dyes, Emulsifiers, Waste, Etc.

ASPARTAME:

Nutra-Sweet

Contains: Wood Alcohol, Aspartic Acid, etc.
(changes into formaldehyde Embalming Fluid)
Causes
- ∞ Alteration in Brain Chemistry
- ∞ Birth Defects
- ∞ Blindness
- ∞ Cancer
- ∞ Genetic Mutations
- ∞ Headaches (Brain Aches)
- ∞ Leg Cramps
- ∞ Menstruation Problems
- ∞ Mental Confusion
- ∞ Mood and Thoughts Disorders
- ∞ Nerve Damage

HONEY

Contains: 70% Fruit Sugar (Fructose)

∞ 30% Sucrose Sugar (White Sugar) composed of glucose (white sugar) and fructose

Causes:
∞ Alters Blood Levels of Insulin
∞ Blood Vessel Damage
∞ Contributes to Uterine Fibroids, Endometriosis, Cystic Mastitis, Breast Cancer, Stomach Ulcers
∞ Gouty Arthritis
∞ Hardening of the Arteries
∞ Heart Attacks
∞ Hyperactivity
∞ Increase Blood Fats
∞ Increases Uric Acid, Cholesterol
∞ Kidney Fatigue and Disease
∞ Liver and Adrenal Glands get larger and damage
∞ Mood and Thought Disorders
∞ Pancreas shrinks and deteriorates
∞ Periodontal Disease (Teeth and Gums)
∞ Strokes
∞ Triglycerides, Cortisone

Alcohol Sugars
∞ Ethylenel glycerol (anti-freeze)
∞ Erythritol
∞ Mannitol
∞ Sorbitol
∞ Xylitol
∞ Isomalt
∞ Lactitol

Causes diarrhea, nerve damage, cirrhosis, upset stomach

Sugar Craving Remedy

*Bilberry (Huckleberry)	increases insulin used for diabetes, heals pancreas
Chickweed	craving
Gymnema Sylvestre	sugar craving
Guggu lipid	help control diabetes
Bitter Melon	sugar craving
Thyme	
Cinnamon	helps control diabetes

1 cup raw stringbean juice = is equal to 2 to 3 units of insulin
considered most effective

Minerals

*Vanadium (Vanadyl Sulfate)   heals pancreas
Chromium   increase energy, stabilizes blood sugar
considered most effective

Yeast Infection Remedies
(Yeast causes desires for sugar)

Pau D'Arco   Garlic

Take A Bite Out of Crime

A diet of raw fruits and vegetables naturally brushes the teeth. White peoples tooth brushing ritual is only needed if you eat slimy, mucus-pasty, fiber less junk foods, cooked vegetables, fruits and cooked animal flesh. The same slimy, mucus tartar, concoctions put a liquid manure coating (plaque, tartar) around the tooth and gums, and in the stomach, small and large intestines, colon, veins, arteries, muscles and joints. The small toothbrush is given the task of cleaning less than $1/10$ of the digestive system (mouth's teeth) while leaving the stomach, small intestine and large intestine coated with liquid manure called plaque. The only thing the toothbrush can successfully do is brush cavities while the teeth rot away from every mouthful of junk food.

The cavities of the teeth actually started prenatally. Black women are the worst nourished, which impacts her unborn babies. Black men a have poorly nourished sperm. White people's myth of telling Black women to eat for two people is responsible for illness. This myth causes pregnant Black women to overeat, resulting in plaque coated intestines, fibroid tumors, cancer, varicose veins, obesity, swelling of the legs and feet, mood swings, personality problems, digestive disorders and weak health and teeth in the unborn baby. Excessive eating of the highly acidic junk foods diet decreases the nutrients from sperm and the fetus' bones and teeth.

Salt (sodium Chloride-table salt) can cause cavities. Sea salt is 7 times saltier. If you eat salt then it will raise the salt level in your blood. Therefore, you would have to raise all the minerals (calcium, magnesium, potassium, iron, etc.) in order to keep the healthy minerals, vitamin and amino acid in the proper ratio with the salt. If you don't raise all the nutrients level then you are putting yourself in an electrolyte imbalance and in a disease crisis. Salt (sodium chloride) is an astringent, bleaching agent and irritant. It causes skin rashes, insomnia, hair loss, kidney disease, heart disease, obesity, tension, and irritants the roots of the teeth. Salt causes waste to stay in your body, edema, cyclic depression, anxiety, migraine headaches and it is addicting. Chemically sodium chloride is a toxic poison. Sodium chloride (salt) is not classified as a food. Sodium Chloride (table salt) has many ingredients added to it, which are not listed on the label. Salt makes you crave for sugar and compounds the addiction to salt.

The concentrated sweeteners and sugar is considered the major problem causing cavities. However, it is processed milled, bleached white flour that causes more cavities. White peoples baked white bread with caramel color looks like whole wheat. Bleached white flour and enriched bleached white flour are synthetic mucus-causing flours that do not have natural organic vitamins, minerals and fiber (roughage). The fiber of raw foods that naturally brushes the digestive tract and teeth, not the toothbrush. It is strictly a synthetic chemical that increases profits for the corporate own junk food industry.

The University of California scientifically researched the bleached white flour ("Science" magazine 93, 1941). They found that animals on a diet of enriched bleached white flour died from malnourishment while animals on plain bleached white flour became crippled, senile and sluggish. The addition of synthetic calcium (or calcium from oyster shell or animal bones, or dirt dolomite) causes acidity, which results in draining the body of calcium. This causes weak bones, bone loss and cavities. A digestive enzyme added to synthetic tricalcium phosphate and calcium carbonate is alkaline and adds phosphate and carbon to the blood, which results in bone loss and cavities.

Ancient Black Africans were over 95% cavity-free without toothbrushes. They used chew sticks and raw non-GMO organic vegetables and fruits to clean teeth, not toothbrushes. White people have an almost 100% cavity rate and constantly use the toothbrush and flossing (ritual). The toothbrush and flossing ritual is a failure. In fact, most of the White dentists have false teeth. They still preach the religion that says the solution to prevent rotten teeth is to brush teeth.

Tooth brushing is a fad (fashion) that is supported by no scientific research. The toothbrush and sugary toothpaste clay increases the profits for companies that sell toothbrushes, toothpaste, dentures, veneers, teeth braces, teeth bleach, teeth plastic, acrylic, mercury and gold fillings, flossing strings, fluoride and sugary mouthwash. Historically, White dentists were allowed into schools to examine teeth and they recommended the toothbrush. A brush salesman, not the dentist, started the ritual of brushing the teeth. Ironically, sugary clay synthetic toothpaste is used and spit out. It is supposedly dirty once it is inside the mouth. It is synthetic clay (dirt) poisonous chemicals, it is probably wise to spit it out rather than swallow it. Natural toothpaste, powdered herbs, or oil can be used to brush teeth and are not harmful and can be swallowed after use. The toothbrush ritual includes the superstition of spitting out toothpaste. There is a warning on toothpaste which says contact the Center for Disease Control poison branch if swallowed. Once toothpaste is in the mouth it is swallowed. In prison, toothpaste is applied to bumps on the face to rid of bumps. Toothpaste is a type of sugary clay dirt candy that sugar addicts enjoy. The sugar in the toothpaste causes cavities and gum disease. Sugary mouthwash is an alcoholic beverage, which alcoholics drink to get drunk. A mouth freshly rinsed with an alcohol mouthwash can indicate drunk driving if you are tested too soon after using it.

The Caucasian toothbrush cannot stop the deterioration of the bones or rotten teeth. It merely represents a medical ritual used to get Black people minds conditioned to being stupid. They have truly taken the bite missing (teeth) out of crime against Black people.

No Laughing Matter

All emotions such as anger, love, sadness, hate, happiness, joy, frustration, depression, disgust, surprise, and fear are connected together in a type of spider web called a neuronet. You cannot have an emotion that functions without connections to all emotions. In other words, you can be in love with a person and simultaneously be angry with them. Emotions are interconnected. All emotions are bipolar and can be used positively or negatively. Some people love to steal (negative pole) and some people love to help others (positive pole). Love is bipolar and can be used for good or for bad.

Laughter and joy are an emotional part of the neuronet. In African civilization laughter was an accepted part of events (funerals, birth, illness, etc.). Laughter is joy. Black people feel the joy of a deceased person going home to the spirit world. Therefore, Black people will shout for joy and laugh during funeral ceremonies. White people label spiritual joy and laughter as foolishness, childish and the stupidity of a backward primitive black people. Black people have been season/behaviorally modified and adopt this White Racist inferiorization and oppression of African funeral joy and wear black clothes and sad faces at funerals. Laughter is a fundamental part of healing and health. Without laughter, the diseased Black people cannot make a truly holistic recovery from an illness.

When Black adults and children laugh, it is more than just joy and happiness. It is a chemical and hormonal activity that stimulates immunity. Laughter creates electrical impulses that turns into a liquid chemical (neurotransmitters). Neurotransmitters are living cells. Laughter and positive thinking actually make protective cells. It is a spiritual, emotional, and hormonal process and helps strengthen cellular immunity and stimulates healing. Aside from this, it is a physical exercise that increases the heart rate, exercises muscle, increases hormone action and increase oxygen use. Laughter increases alertness by releasing catecholamines. The brain secretes endorphins (a relaxing morphine-like molecule) that relax muscles, get rid of pain, lower blood pressure, aid digestion, reduce inflammation, relieve stress and create antibacterial alkaline tears.

Laughter in the Black community helps heal and share feelings, h and bonds Black people. It helps to defeat depression, bad feelings, tension, inferiority, anxiety, panic and conflicts in relationships. Depression and a negative image of oneself can create cells that decrease immunity. This makes you easy prey for disease. Laughter can be used as a type of self-defense. In Black children, laughter is a language that can bridge the emotional and intellectual gap of a child's small vocabulary. Their vocabulary cannot express the child's full range of ideas and feelings.

White cave people are slowly starting to scientifically understand and accept the holistic dimensions of laughter. The Duke University Comprehensive Cancer Center in Durham, North Carolina uses laugh wagons. These wagons are filled with comic materials and pulled in the hallway to spread laughter. In the book *Anatomy of and Illness*, by Norman Cousins, laughter is mentioned as therapeutically important for disease recovery. Laughter truly is not a laughing matter but a hormonal biochemical body language used for holistic health.

Read Labels or Comic Books

Labels are used to lie to the consumer and control the Black American consumer. Historically, Black people that were labeled prisoners of wars were mislabeled "slaves." This was a method of deception was used by White slave owner. Lies are more powerful than truth. Black that are lied to themselves to be a "slave" and think and believe they are slaves. The same White Supremacy mentality that labels Black people as slaves is nutritionally labeling harmful foods as valuable. The nutritional labeling of foodstuffs is not to educate or protect, but is used to control confuse and destroy Black people.

The White corporate businesses own the federal government and the food industry, and the natural foods, vitamin and mineral supplement and nutrition market. They to control the natural foods nutrition market. They have set recommended nutrient daily allowance standards and list the nutritional value of fruits and vegetables and other foodstuffs. They legally have approved 0 to 8.5 grams are equal to 0 grams, food with less than 2m of cholesterol are cholesterol free and 5 calories or less is labeled as "0" calories.

The nutritional value of plants varies according to crops, soil composition, type of seeds, type of rainfall, cycle variant, type of fertilizer and cultivation method. These factors are ignored and a standard value is set for a crop based on a "random sample" (science words for the best guess). Making plant nutritional standard a is theory based science ignorance stupid. For example, there are over five different varieties of red apples. Each type of red apple has a different nutritional value. The soil that the red apple grow in can be different for the same type of red apple grown in a different type soil. The FDA's standardized nutritional value for red apples is applied to the over five different types of yellow and green apples. The standardize nutritional value for apples becomes a tool to treat Black peoples as fools it is lies and the stupidity of White theory based nutritional and calorie counting science. The labels fail to list the dangerous ingredients of the toxic chemicals used to grow and process the foods and the toxicity of the packaging or cans. The Black people's attention is "turned off" to the harm the food does and is "turned on" to the stupid nutritional value. It is a deadly game in which Black people lose health while the food industries win dollars.

The same corporate own government that failed to protect human rights, civil rights and "ethical medical rights" is the same government that cannot and will not stop noise, water and air pollution, oil spills, climate warming, student debt, GMOs, and toxic chemical pollution of foods. This corporate own government is now concerned about the nutritional value of foods. These companies that put disease causing lethal chemicals in the soil, in the water, on fruits and vegetables will never be concerned about nutrition. Food nutritional labeling is a way to protect white thieves and white profits. The label tends to give an atmosphere of respectability to the White crime. Nutrition words appeals to the latest consumer health fad.

The corporate own government and industries have once again completely ignored Black people's unique biochemistry and nutrition levels. They have allowed synthetic food chemicals to retard melanin (pineal gland) production. Both the corporate own government and private companies function to make profits. The only difference is one files income taxes (private) and the other creates taxes (government). Once again, they have decided what is the best lie to tell their "darkies", "coons", "niggers," "colored people," "Negroes," Afro-Americans, Africans in America, and Black people. To them it is automatic to dictate what is best for their Black wage slaves that rent money and rent the ghetto.

White people will not and do not allow African centered consumer scientists, health practitioners, nutritionists, disease treatments or diets to be considered. They control the minds of black consumers. The White corporation lie with Latin words, mathematics, chemical, or nutritional language on food labels. They ignore the nutritional slaughter of Black people. White food corporation are concerned with the correct ritual and ceremonial use of words, which makes White logical sense.

The ceremonial and ritual use of Greek and Latin words on food labels is more important than Black people's lives. Words such as "essential," "dispensable," and "indispensable" are used to confuse and control food illiterate Black people. For example, "essential" amino acids (protein building blocks) are amino acids that the body needs while "non-essential" amino acids the body can make. This it is word nonsense with "Latin words" or "Greek words". The body can make (convert) non-essential amino acids into essential amino acids and essential amino acids into non-essential amino acids.

Synthetic junk foods stops the biochemical ability to convert amino acids such as tryptophan, tyrosine, methionine, Lysine and glutamine are absolutely essential for melanin usage. In White people's diet, these amino acids are not essential. Black people have essential amino acids, which are not essential to White people.

Sunshine is an indispensable nutrient for Black people because it helps food digestion, melanin regulation, and stabilizes calcium. In the white race, sunshine stimulates the diseases and skin cancer in their bodies. Therefore, sunshine is considered unnecessary and dispensable to White people. The words "essential" or "dispensable" are giving a false scientific value to chemically polluted junk foods and fresh produce. Words allow genetically and chemically polluted cow's milk, to be sold because it meets safety standards and lists nutrient value on the label.

The nutritional labeling of food with vitamin, mineral and amino acid content is not easily understood. It is a legal way to give scientific respectability to food that is chemically toxic. A vegetable, fruit or other foodstuffs with an excessive amount of "one" particular nutrient can be labeled as fortified. This gives consumers a false sense that they are getting nutrients. It is the ratio of nutrients in balanced proportions that increase its value. Increasing one nutrient requires all other nutrients to be increased or else the body drains itself of stored nutrients to make up for what the foods are lacking.

It is best to combine non-GMO natural foods to achieve balance rather than let the Caucasian food industry play God by adding synthetic nutrients. For example, cereal protein seeds (wheat berries, corn, ect.) are naturally high in the amino acid methionine and low in the amino acid Lysine. Legumes (beans, peas) are high in the amino acid Lysine and low in methionine. Therefore, the combination of cereal seeds and legumes provides balanced proteins (amino acids). The ratio of synthetic herbicides and pesticides combined with food processing chemicals causes lethal destruction to the human body. No indication or measured amounts of toxic chemicals are labeled on non-organic vegetables, fruits and foodstuffs. Only the nutritional value placed on the label. This accentuates the positive (nutrients) and causes the African American's mind to ignore the negative (chemical pollution). Nutrition labels have become a way to cover up the health destruction (Nutricide) of African people.

The fast food industry does not use nutrition to sell its disease-producing, immune destructive, anti-melanin, constipating, and synthetic junk foods. This industry has never provided educational information that could help the consumer select or combine food properly. They only meet health sanitation standards. The same government that allows food to be chemically polluted is now concerned about nutrition standards that they cannot and will not enforce. It is a case of "the blind leading the blind." It is one white racist capitalist telling another white racist capitalist how to protect African Americans' ethno medical, ethno nutritional and ethno physiological

127

sovereign human rights. Nutrition labeling in the hands of a white racist is another tool of "nutrition restraint" and Nutricide. Nutritional labeling has combined the White Racist Health food industry with the "White Racist junk food industry."

Historically, Black people did not get ethno nutritional rights when Caucasian were eating organic health foods. Caucasians' diets were of non-GMO organic foods up until the 18th century. Then, Black people failed to get ethno nutritional sovereign human rights in the junk food era (19th century to the 20th century). And, now they have failed to get those rights during the current Caucasian health food fad era. The Caucasian diet wheel has made a complete turn and only serves to roll over African bodies.

The current food ingredient labels actually give a vague idea of what the foodstuff contains. The food manufacturers and the corporate own Food and Drug Administration (FDA) have no idea of the true ingredients. They are just as puzzled as to what the food products contain as you are with the Greek and Latin words used to label ingredients. The FDA does not set standards for identification or set limits as to the chemicals used to make ingredients or the toxicity of chemicals used to make nutrients. They are not aware of the medical problems Black people have from eating junk foods lethal chemicals. For example, carbonated sodas contain emulsifiers, artificial colors, synthetic flavoring, aromas, flavor enhancers, glycerin, anti-foaming agents, sodium chloride, caffeine, dirt, foaming agents, retardants, buffers, lye, (sulfuric acid and Phosphoric acid) synthetic sweeteners, preservatives and "optional ingredients." The "optional ingredients" are synthetic chemicals that do not have to be put on the label. Added to this polluted toilet water is used to make soda a liquid.

The soda chemical companies and other food companies' labels amount are chemical make believe, and pretend fairy tale type of ingredient story. It would be better to read a comic book than the ingredients of a soda; at least the comic book is entertaining. If you were to separately eat one of the chemical ingredients of a soda all day you would get brain damage, become sick or die. You can eat a natural food ingredient all day without getting sick. However, an unwholesome food eaten all day such as mustard, vinegar, salt, white sugar, mayonnaise, pickles, black pepper, cayenne, cooked oil, grease, nutmeg, salad dressing, wine sauce, tartar sauce, etc., will cause an illness, because they are not foods.

The ingredient label of natural apple juice (not made from concentrate) would list organic apples or apples (no chemicals or water would be in it). You can read a natural foods label without the help of a Latin, Greek, or science dictionary, or interpreter. Commercial grocery stores and health food stores should have a label (sign) on their building that reads "Caution, the foods in this building can be harmful to your health."

Talking Can Make You Sick

Conversations with supposedly nice, well-meaning Caucasians can cause destructive emotions, anger, boredom, frustration and stress in Black people. Black people's melanin content makes them highly emotionally, psychically and spiritually sensitive. Therefore, Black people can feel Caucasians are deceitfully and emotionally hiding their insecurity racism and hatred. White people dependent on word order or logic to hide their racism. White people have rational (crazy) conversation to put down Black people. It is White peoples try to be emotionless which in itself is an emotion. They have racist emotional and psychological clashes with Black people. In other words, White people feel that if something is emotionless and makes sense to them it must be emotionless and make sense to Black people. They feel their logic has no emotional value. There is no emotionless music, language, food or culture. Each race's music, language and food dish is connected to the emotions of culture. However, white people arrogantly demand that their brand of emotions must be accepted emotionless by Black peoples. This is White racist arrogance. White people's emotional conversation has feelings attached to it. Word order is emotional in different languages. Word order is the sequence of words, a noun followed by a verb, other languages have a verb followed by a noun the sequence of word order. People talk in a word order because feelings are the emotional design of their culture. Cultures create emotions with rituals. And rituals for words come from the culture's emotions. Cave life created word order and word sounds that are emotional. White people's emotions are non-rhythm. They feel they make emotion less sense to Black people.

Black people conversations rely on the emotional concept (picture) of a word. White people's emotions are control by the emotion of the mob called statistics, research, polls, surveys, or the average person theory. Black people typically are in emotional harmony with nature and themselves and are emotionally, honest and open. Black emotions have many levels that are confusing to be felt by the emotion less emotion White people. Many times, Black people's emotions go up and down similar to a songs melody, heads are moving from side to side and bodies are moving as if dancing. White people see this holistic use of emotions and say Black people are too emotional or getting ready to fight each other.

Emotions are used in a cultural ritual and ceremonial feeling that paints pictures. Emotions for White people are assumed to be culture less and emotion less. They do not see how Eurocentric their emotions are. White people's emotions are based on superstition, self-centeredness, cave language, and the collective emotional illness of being psychotic (White

Supremacy is a psychosis). White people tend to focus on a single emotion (fragment) and ignore the total family (colors) of emotions.

Fundamentally, the problem with White people and Black people's communication is the emotionally ill (White person) talking to the emotionally sane (Black person). Black people would have to be "out of their Black mind" and into the White people's emotions to communicate emotionless with White cave people. A Black person "out of his mind" and into the adopted White people's emotions do not see that White peoples culture is in a mentally ill civilization. In any case, White people emotions and conversations are draining to Black people. White emotions have the built-in superiority attitude. They feel that they are superior and have an arrogant insulting tone. They mix right emotions with wrong emotions. They have conflicting emotions they think that important long words. And, black emotions in conversations have the feelings in wrong tone of speech.

White people's conversation is a series of words without emotions. White emotion-less emotion conversations cause Black people to have stress, emotional torture, emotion confusion and it is upsetting to feel and hear. Black people may not consciously be aware of the sympathetic nervous system reaction to White people racist emotional assaults, cause feelings of being made stupid, inferior, or a vagueness and emotional emptiness from White peoples "word salads." White people typically use clichés, socially pleasant emotional sentences, they give the emotional attitude of "I am a nice white person talking to a Negro" or they have the emotional tone in their voice of; "I am not a racist, but I am white and superior". Black people's emotions react to this emotional tone of white superiority. Black people holistically feel the inferiority tone. This white emotional conversation tone causes Black people to use nutrients to defend them from white racism's. It nutritionally requires extra vitamin B6, phenylalanine, yucca, suma, gingko, tryptophan, rosemary, gotu kola, L-dopa, niacin amide, methionine, tyrosine, ginseng and a non-GMO organic foods diet to have nutrients to emotionally defend yourself. Black people have to cope with the subtle emotional energy loss caused by the white people's emotional abuse (unwholistic emotions).

White people's emotional illness of cave trauma is part of their mind, mood, state of consciousness and this emotional illness is part of their conversation and listening skills. Their emotions are diseased. White people's emotional arrogance (I am superior you are inferior attitude), hostile negative emotional temperaments and White Supremacy psychosis diseased is directly and/or indirectly emotionally felt by Black people. White people's emotions are never identified as being as crazy as they are. Their subconscious subliminal superiority emotional attitudes are not examined by them or taught in African centered education or Black Studies. It is obvious that their White racism has polluted their ability to honestly emotionally communicate and emotionally listen. They do not have the ability to turn off their superiority complex.

White people's emotions are not healthy, but part of their emotional illness of Post Traumatic Cave Trauma and White Supremacy psychosis. When a Black person reacts to the implied emotional superiority tone in conversations, White people label the Black person as too emotional, not intellectual and inferior. The normal White people's conversation is emotional oppressive to the feelings, mind of Black people. White people's emotions cause an energy drain. Their emotions can cause drug use or cause the use of alcohol to restraint from taking a violent defense (kicking the white person's ass). Black people use chemically restrain drugs because of the emotional disturbance, anger, and rage caused by the craziness of White people's emotional superiority conversation tone. Some lead Blacks have to use nutritional restrains such as junk foods such as white sugar, bleached white flour, grease, synthetic chemicals, cooked cow's milk and salt to put themselves below the emotional problems. This makes the Black person temperature drop and cools the body, so the Black person says, "I am being cool", they cool down from racism. Drugs numb the emotions, from the pain of hearing the superior emotional attitude tone of a psychotic. The chemical and nutritional restraints weaken the pineal, adrenal, Liver, hypothalamus, thymus and gonad glands and drain the Black person's emotional sanity causing them to act crazy. Ultimately, the effect of talking with or listening to White people emotionless emotional talk can make you as emotionally sick, and lead Black people to levels of emotional frustration. It is a frustration that they cannot explain to White people.

Safe Drugs – Ritual Superstition

Superstitions are deeply rooted in White society and White theory science. In medical science, they practice superstitious cultural beliefs by using animals or Black people as experiments or sacrifices to prove a drug is economically safe for human use. Drugs used on animals are a scientific cultural ritual called an experiment. This ritual testing has been proven to be scientifically stupid by the United States government's Office of Technology Assessment that published this in publication No. 286 929, titled "Assessing the Efficacy and Safety of Medical Technologies" (September 1978).

White scientist do scientific drug tests on guinea pigs when it is known that guinea pigs can eat "strychnine" (a poison that kills humans) without harm. "Penicillin" is an antibiotic that kills guinea pigs while destroying the immune system in people. "Tuberculin" vaccine causes tuberculosis in people while curing it in pigs. "Digitalis" causes high blood pressure in dogs.

131

"Aspirin" causes birth defects in animals. A heart medicine such as "emidin" proved safe for animals while in people it kills and causes digestive and eye problems. Aside from this, a scientific method for converting lower animals, physiology so that it equals human physiology is an impossibility.

When animals are not used, Black people in ghettoes, jails or at government-supported medical facilities are used as experimental sacrifices. Sample sizes of drugs are given Black patients. This free sample allows the drug companies to use Black people as human sacrifices that they call clinical experiments.

Caucasian cannibalism is still being mislabeled as science. The drug corporation use human cells to pervert, freak (hybrid), and stimulate plant growth and growth of test tube animal tissue for burgers and steaks. The consequences of eating cannibalistic plants that have been raised or mated with human or animal cells is dangerous. Human cells used as plant drugs is a clear example of the cannibalism psychosis of Caucasians. If the United States government cannot use the entire Black person's body or the cells, then they use poor people in foreign countries. The U.S.A. pays countries to abort fetuses up to 5 months for organ harvesting or cell use. Sacrifices are used in the scientific "double blind" studies (experiments) in which physically or mentally ill people are given medicine or a sugar pill (placebo). It is called "double blind" because the doctor is not aware (blind) who is getting medicine and the sick person is not aware (blind) whether he is getting medicine or a sugar pill. However, the laboratory workers are aware. Double blind studies are a violation of the sick person's human rights and medical ethics, which states that a doctor must help the sick get healthy instead of allowing a disease to kill them. The drugs companies get poor Black women to sell their eggs. Black people also sell their kidney, eyes, unborn babies, young children for adoption, sperm and blood. Unfortunately, nobody wants to buy Black people's kinky hair or else they would sell it.

Black people are sacrificed for another Caucasian superstitious ritual called a clinical trial. In clinical trials, Black people are paid to use an untested drug. Whether the Black person takes the drug or throws it away is really not researched. Nonetheless, Black people that do take the drug are usually damaged in some way. If the drug is 20% or more effective, then it passes the clinical trial and is sold to the general public. The clinical trial with synthetic chemicals is nothing more than a ritual with no purpose other than to satisfy superstitions. The drugs can go on the fast track and avoid being tested for safety.

All synthetic drugs work by slowing down, speeding up or destroying Melanin. The science of biology and chemistry that they use to make synthetic chemicals are based upon Melanin. The science of chemistry (Kemet-Black-Melanin) is based upon studying Melanin particles called electrons, protons and neutrons. The science of biology based upon the action and reaction cells Melaninated nucleus (brain) operation upon tissues, organs and systems. The language of White people's chemistry and biology uses mathematics. Mathematics is based upon White People's Numerical Theory. White belief based theory science is merely another translation of their belief in White Supremacy. Their White GMO synthetic sugar chemical sweeteners destroys the Black Melanin centers of the pancreas (Islands of Langerhans) resulting in diabetes. The Prozac synthetic drug works by stopping the Black melanin hormone (serotonin) from being used (reuptake inhibitor). The drugs work by destroying melanin. The drugs destroy the ability to Black in mind, mood, and state of consciousness. A White scientist must have a culture before they can choose a culturally based profession. Theory based science is White culturally based. Science cannot exist without the culture of the scientist. People cannot exist without a culture. White science like White culture is a collection of superstitions, rituals, and ceremonies decorated with science words. Their collection of cultural rituals and ceremonies support White Supremacy.

The New Drug, T'is The Season to Be Healthy

Drugs are used, abused, misused and misunderstood. People are trained to rely on drugs to change their poor health to good health, to change our bad moods to good moods, and give a false sense of life (reality). Drugs answer our emotional needs. If people need energy, they take uppers (amphetamines, speed); if they need sleep, they take downers (sedatives and depressants); if they need relief from pain; they take pain relievers. To stay awake people, take wake people take uppers (speeds) like caffeine, and if people want to feel good people become mentally ill by poisoning their brain with alcohol, marijuana, heroin or cocaine. People live in a drug-oriented White (European) society.

In the past, the drugs of choice for Black people have been depressants (downers) such as alcohol, marijuana and heroin. Oppression causes the drugs of choice to be depressants. They are downers slow down the depression. The illegal drugs of choice for white society have been speed (e.g., cocaine and mind-altering drugs like LSD). Over 70% of the White people are drug addicted while less than 30% of Black people are addicted. White people believe they have a good life, and they want to travel the good life faster with speed drugs such as cocaine. Black people have the bad life and want to go through it slower and use drugs to get down below and underneath the hurt and pain of oppression, so they would take "downers" – (depressants). Now Black people are trying to rush through their oppression by taking addictive accelerators like cocaine, energy drinks, meth and caffeine.

The White slave master gave the Black chattel slaves drugs to get more labor out of them. Then, after chattel slavery, Black people advanced to wage slavery (barely enough money to feed themselves, pay rent and bills). Now, the assimilating and integrating Black people have advanced to emotional and mental slavery. They freely volunteer to put on their own psychological chains into White culture and emotionally whip (self hatred) themselves. These are the most dangerous types of slaves because they no longer need the slave master; they have become both slave and slave master. They are now the new assimilation and integrating Black people from Negro-land. These Black people are not out of their own mind; they are out of the white people's mind and a creation of White Supremacy called "a nigger". The end result of drug usage (and addiction) in Black culture is a dysfunctional family of destruction, death and contribute more wealth for the White corporate own governments that promotes the manufacture and sale of these addictive poisons.

Addiction of any type follows a simple step-by-step process. People can become addicted to anything by following these steps. All addictions are not bad or evil. For example, addiction to exercise, natural foods and herbs, good manners, and being truthful are good addictions. Then there are bad addictions, such as drugs, slavery, violence, junk foods, pornography, social media, cell phones, computer games, masturbation, etc.

The steps to addiction are as follows:
Step 1:
  ∞ **Introduction** – to the drug (or negative activity usually by a friend).

Step 2:
  ∞ **Re-introduction** – the victim requests the drug.

Step 3:
  ∞ **Craving** – the person develops a desire for the drug and associates it with pleasure.

Step 4:
  ∞ **Mental dependence** – the victim must have the drug or destructive activity in order to "have a good time."

Step 5:
  ∞ **Physical dependence** –physical withdrawal pains and/or emotional pain will occur if drug use or co-dependent behavior is stopped.

A person can go through these addictive steps in one week, one month or one year. They can take the drug once a day or once a year and still be an addict because the drug controls their life, emotions, mind, and body. A drug is really any substance or social activity that is isolated and concentrated. For example, white sugar, once you take sugar out of the sugar cane plant, it becomes a drug because it is isolated and concentrated. Cooked nicotine or cooked cannabinol is isolated and concentrated by burning the marijuana or tobacco in cigarettes. Alcohol, white sugar, sodium chloride, salt, bleached flour and caffeine are just a few of the many drugs.

If you take the Black people out of Africa culture, then isolate them from African culture (using slavery, oppression and exploitation), and concentrate them in ghettos (urban concentration camps), put them in the social underclass (lower economic class), and White culture's educational (European academics) prisons, it creates an assimilated and Integrated into White Culture called a Negro. The Negro person is the social drug for White people. White people get a drug high from Black people's music, dance, and entertainers (actors, athletes, politicians). They advance their type drug high with Black people's science mix with sex, violence and White Supremacy psychosis. Dysfunctional assimilated and integrated Black people have become the White people's drug. These culturally homeless Black men, children, and women dress up like Europeans, celebrate White holidays which validates White culture is superior and Black culture inferior. Dysfunctional Black people are living commercials for the superior emotional attitude of White people and are White peoples type of psychosocial high. These Dysfunctional Negros socialize with and marry and have sex with white folks. Assimilated and Integrated Black people have become intoxicated on the White Supremacy psychotic high. They are culturally homeless and a cloned high of White Supremacist.

ADDICTION

- Is built into the predatory White society (poverty, rape, crime, violence, self-hatred, dysfunctional family, homosexuality, etc.).
- It is a symptom of White Domination (victims of White Supremacy).
- Social conditions create drug suicides (buy drugs to kill oneself).
- Associated with oppression, Slavery Trauma, Cultural Stress.
- Is a part of Black People's Co-Dependency upon White Domination and White Supremacy psychosis.

TREATMENT
- Must bond to African Culture (defines a Black person's reality, self, solutions).

- Must serve the basic needs of emotionality, spirituality, family, shelter, food, health, job or self-employment, economics, military, and cultural.
- Must provide personality adjustment, not personality change.
- Counseling must be at arm's length, do not touch or force eye contact.
- Starts after detoxification from drug, co-dependent behavior, etc.

STEPS IN TREATMENT
- Bond to Maat, culture, customs, rituals, natural foods, exercise, herbs, adequate sleep, etc.
- Solve needs and act upon needs to destroy White Domination.
- Heal relationship with self, family, children, friends and/or intimate relationship.
- Develop Psycho social and Historical Awareness.
- Identify Problem.
- Design method to change negatives to positives.
- Evaluate Achievements (Rewards, Punishments, etc.)
- Follow treatment schedule, goals, relapse therapy, etc.

Spit in the Face
(The Medical Symbol)

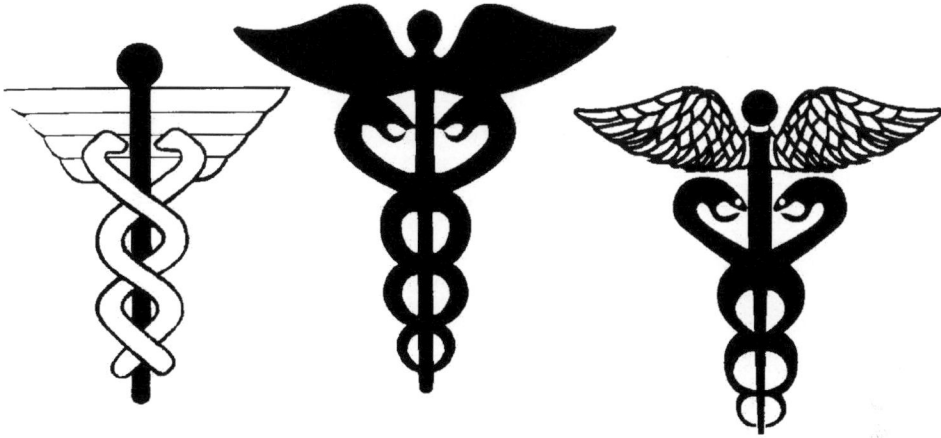

The healing arts and science symbol was created by black people. It reflects the origin of medical sciences, nutrition and civilization on this planet. The healing arts and science symbol called the caduceus, serpentine fire, tree of life or Aesculapius is used White medical many organizations. It is erroneously believed to belong to European medical schools. It is not exclusively a registered trademark, copyrighted symbol or creation of any European White organization. This symbol predates all European civilizations and its earliest usage was part of ancient Africa's religious (spiritual) based orders (schools).

The ancient Africans were the first to use the medical symbol. Greeks and Romans called this African mythological symbol Aesculapius. Aesculapius is the European name for a Black African man named Imhotep. He was an Egyptian doctor. Hippocrates was a student of Imhotep and was called an Aesculapian.

In the Aesculapian symbol, or tree of life symbol, the two snakes (serpents) intertwined indicate the harmonious connection of the bipolar cycles (laws) and the unity of the two great truths (i.e., day/night, female or male, life or death, health or sickness, right or wrong). The crossing snakes are intertwined around a divine Rod, which was carried by Hermes Trimegistus (Greek/Roman word) who was originally called Thoth by Africans. Thoth was the healing attribute of God, inventor of calculus; geometry and the spoken word (language). Thoth wrote the name of King Seti I on the tree of life in the Temple of Karnak. "Seb" the ruler of snakes, (order, cycles) joined the two snakes together to show the bipolar harmony of the

137

two truths autonomic nervous systems sympathetic nerve and parasympathetic nerve (female/male principles of life). The circle at the top of the septer represents the cosmic circle of the whole that contains all creation or the astral (stellar) that has the solar and lunar inside it. This is a sign that the Greater contains the Lesser.

The triangle symbolic pyramid of the tree of life represents the sun being born in the east. The three points (corners) on the triangle indicate God, humans and nature or the pineal gland, pituitary gland, and hypothalamus gland or the heaven, earth and nether world which was also called the Orion Star of Horu. The bird's wings represent the Vulture or Eagle's wings which symbolize the Atel (judgment) or the twin truths (day or night, female or male, etc.). The two wings also indicate the double Horus (order, law, structure, cycles) which are separated and united by the Urem or Rem or Nile River and the city of Coming Forth by Night (city of the dead) on the West Bank of the Nile. Aside from this, the tree of life symbolizes the solstices, equinox and solar opening of the earth (Harris Papyrus).

The snakes, wand, wings and cosmic circle combine to form the tree of life. Trees in ancient Egypt were called Teru and indicate order, structure, academics, rites of passage (schools of learning), cycles the generative principle and woman. The tree of life symbolizes holistic (spirit, emotions, mind, body). The crossing of the snakes represents the crossing of the sympathetic and parasympathetic parts of the autonomic nervous system and primary energy force fields (acupuncture meridians). One snake represents the mind while the other snake represents the body intertwined and tied around God's divine rod (septer).

The symbol is also called the Caduceus and the word "cadaver (body)" is derived from it. Cadaver is a Latinized African word. The tree of life is symbolic of reincarnation as the snake sheds its skin and is born again. In African mythology one snake died (body) and was reborn when the other snake gave it a healing herb (spirit). The serpents (snakes) were given the names of Imhotep's children such as Panakia (pancreas) and Hakia (hygiene).

If the tongue, fangs and deadly sting of the snake are exposed, it represents allopathic medicine. European MD's use this type of suppressive drug medicine to treat disease. This medicine treats symptoms with poisonous to purify the body. When the serpent has its tail in its mouth, this represents naturopathic medicine. Naturopathy nourished immune system in the body and allows the body to cure itself.

Imhotep's Greek/Roman name, Aesculapius, reveals further the African origin of medicine. "Ashe" means human, "scul (school)" means instruct, and "aphe" means snake and the combined words mean "to instruct about the snakes." The Greeks/Romans/Europeans learned from stolen books knowledge of the world's oldest books on medicine, the African books called the *Hearst Papyrus of The 7th Egyptian Dynasty (2000 B.C.)* with 250 remedies, *Kahun Papyrus of 12th and 13th Dynasty (2133 7 TO 1766)* with gynecology treatments and in the *18th Dynasty (1500 B.C.)*, there is medical and physiology information in the *London Medical Papyrus, Ebers Papyrus, Edwin Smith Papyrus, in the 19th Dynasty (1000 B.C.), Chester-Beatty Papyrus and Berlin Papyrus.* Aside from these medical books, there are other African books, which are still secretly held and some were destroyed. For example, Clement of Alexandria A.D. 200 and lamlichus A.D. 363 reported that 42 books on Human Knowledge called *Hermetic (Thoth) Books,* were destroyed or stolen. Book number 37 on Anatomy, book 38 on Disease, book 39 on Surgery, book 40 on Remedies, book 41 on Eye Disease and book 42 on Female Disease are missing.

There are many more African medical books by countless Black African authors that Arabs, Chinese, East Indians, Asians, and Europeans destroyed such as the 40 books written by Ahmad Babo, who was the first Black President of the University of Sankore in Timbuktu.

Ancient European historians such as Dioscorides, Galen and Theophratus wrote and quoted the medical prescriptions that they learned from the books in the library of the Temple (University) of Imhotep at Memphis, Egypt. Hippocrates (who Europeans say invented medicine) quotes the African textbook called the *Carlsburg Papyrus #4*. Many of the Latinized African words, letters, and symbols were passed to the Europeans in 1600 B.C. when Thutmose II colonized Cyprus, Crete, Syria, Babylonia, Kadesh and other Mediterranean and Asian countries.

Thutmose Stela at Karnak contains the "Hymn of Triumph" which states the 110 European colonies paid taxes to Africa. In fact, the European colonies would protest to Africa leaders for not providing enough African soldiers to protect Europeans from other European barbaric raiding hordes of thieves, gangs, liars, rapists, and cannibals. Historically, this contact with African civilization allowed the Europeans to learn of medical science and its African symbol, "The Tree of Life."

In contemporary times, Africans brought to America and enslaved demonstrated that they learned medical science and nutrition in Africa. The enslaved African women and men (doctors) knew the exact medical healing principles of herbs. African doctors were sold as slaves because they were expert medical scientists. These African doctors were used by European physicians and pharmacists until laws were passed that made it illegal (1749 General Assembly of South Carolina).

The African healing art and science symbol has been stolen by White people's. However, the medical symbol, whenever it is seen announces to the world that Africa and Africans are the originators and creators of medical science. Despite the Arabs, Chinese, East Indians, Asians, and Europeans' stealing the African science and destroying valuable books that belonged to Black people, White people remain the most diseased race. White people are constantly seeking cures, drugs, surgery, and technology to slow down their bodily diseases and disguise their disease of emotional and mental illness (White Supremacy is a psychosis). White Supremacy is an emotional and mental illness which causes White people to use any and every means to control human and natural resources of Africa and destroy Black people. White people use peace, nutrition, drugs, school systems, police, courts, news reports, jail, food, science and medicine to control or destroy Black people. The African medical symbol represents not only Black people's knowledge, but is also another means by which White Supremacy spits in the face of all Black peoples.

Chapter Three

Children

"Let us not forget that it is our duty to remedy any wrong that has already been done and not ourselves perpetuate the evil of race destruction"

Marcus Garvey

Born into Diseases

The Caucasian have waged full-scale war against the health of Black babies. Black children are highly melaninated, highly biochemically responsive, highly spiritual and electromagnetically united to the galaxy, sun, moon, cycles, planets, parents, water, plants, and the earth. Each African child has the specific prenatal rhythm of its zodiac sign. The prenatal movements of a Capricorn child are distinctively different from the prenatal movements of a Libra child. Consequently, the zodiac sign and ancestral aura of the child requires that the mother alter her diet to meet the specific nutritional needs of the unborn child.

The Caucasian theory based medicine, nutrition, disease and remedy systems ignore rhythm, melanin and White Racism. Their health practitioners have no rhythm and holistically do not understand rhythm. They ignore the zodiac specific movements of the prenatal babies' growth and development as well as zodiac specific nutrition requirements.

Sound, which is melanin driven, is very important for Black child. A child's pineal gland and ears (the first mature physical senses) are very important. The ear drum is fully developed before birth and translates sounds (light energy) just as the highly melaninated skin can convert light energy into images that are interpreted by the brain as that of sound, smell, touch, sight, psychic energy and extrasensory information. Black people have the highest melanin content in their ears. The prenatal child's ears act as part of the brain. The correct cultural music and drumming should be a definite part of the parent's surroundings and in the prenatal child's environment. This would help to stimulate melanin properly and prevent predisposing the prenatal infant to melanin deficiency.

Cancer

The White doctors, nurses, drugs, hospitals, diet, test standards and birthing techniques are an unnecessary interruption in the prenatal child's rhythm, nutrition and brain function. The child is subjected to cancer-causing ultrasounds. The needles used for taking the amniocentesis fluid (determines whether baby is a girl or boy) is guided by cancerous ultrasound. Fetal monitors that are strapped on the mother's abdomen use ultrasound. The internal metallic devices that are screwed into the unborn baby's head cause inflammations with pus-filled abscesses. X-rays given to the mother cause 50% increase in various types of cancer. Aside from this, the increase in electronic and computer machines has caused an increase in Caesarean Sections (C-Section). C-Section babies have an increase in learning problems. Their biochemical "rites of passage" and bonding have been interrupted.

Sound

Rhythm (cycle laws) is melanin dependent in African babies. For example, pendulum operated clocks can all be started at different time intervals. However, they all will synchronize to one rhythm. This has been found true even if a house were several women live, each having a different menstruation period cycle. They will eventually have synchronized periods and menstruate at the same time. The Black baby and mother will have synchronized heartbeats. Sounds become human cells in the baby's body. Since the ear matures first, sound is important because it produces sound waves that are absorbed by melanin and translate into thoughts, feelings, emotions, spirit and ideas. Babies should not be exposed to sounds of arguments, hostility, fighting, violence, White Racism (cultural insults), and disharmony. Consequently, Caucasian medical principles ignore the melanin rhythmic importance to the baby and mother causing a conflict within the body and towards the mother. Rhythm controls the growth of organs and bones. A baby can grow up to 1 inch in height in 24 hours. Growth cycles (rhythm) are controlled by melanin. When melanin is imbalanced, or not nutritionally fed, a sudden growth spurt can occur internally and/or externally. This can result in sudden irritation in a baby (*Growth Research*, University of Pennsylvania by M. Lampl, M.D., Ph.D.)

Brain-Assault and Battery

Bonding of the child, mother, and father are interrupted by birth techniques of Caucasians. Bonding is the synchronization of emotions and thoughts between two people. Labor is induced by synthetic drugs causing the contractions to be out of rhythm and violently forceful. This results in too much pressure on the child's head. This increased pressure decreases the air, blood and nutrient supply to the African child's brain. The skull is squeezed together too hard causing the bones to collide resulting in a fluid-filled bruise on the top of the head. Drugs in any form (including synthetic food) cause the bones to collide together resulting in dimples in the chin or improper growth such as cleft tongues and lips or dimples in the ear lobe.

Further, Caucasians use a pair of pliers (forceps) or vacuum to clamp and squeeze the head so they can pull the baby out of the womb. This further decreases the air, blood and nutrient supply to the brain. The vacuum pump, which they clamp on the head to forcefully pull the baby out the womb. This drains rhythmicity, electromagnetic energy and nutrients out of the brain and can stop nutrients from getting to the brain. Aside from being unnatural, it is a shock to the baby, beyond any criminal assault and battery. It could be

143

classified according to the United Nations Human Rights Charter as an "assault and battery" with the intent to maim, mutilate and harm for life.

Sex and masturbation is erroneously promoted by White medical science as being ideal for couples and the baby. The total of poor prenatal nutrition, ignorant superstitious medical theory based techniques, violence, and money driven medical activities work to push the baby to a nutritionally self-destructive path. Then the bonding does not occur between mother and child. The baby should be placed on the mother's breast after being born in order to stimulate bonding and placenta release. Bonding for the Black baby starts before conception and prenatal growth. The placing of the baby on the mother's stomach near the breast is an extension of bonding.

Drugs

Caucasian medicine treats a child's birth as if it is a disease process. They interrupt birthing by giving the parents' junk food that retards growth. They give the mother drugs that go directly into the baby's body. Drugs and Caucasian nutritional standards cause the Black baby to try to breathe before being born. In this case, the baby may have a bowel movement and attempt to breathe causing it to swallow amniotic fluid that can have its bowel movement (manure) in it. The baby has a bowel movement before birth due to shock and overstimulation of junk foods and drugs. Drugs retard growth, slow down learning and interrupt the baby's ability to bond with its mother. Drugs cause the baby's immune system to get exhausted and junk foods deplete the immunity as they over stimulate the sympathetic nervous system. They activate serotonin out of its natural cyclic pattern and depress melatonin.

Caucasian – Lowest Humanoid

Black people are the highest on the human development chain. Caucasians are the lowest developed humans of all the races of man. The Chinese, Japanese, Indians, Native Indians are in between Black people and Caucasians on the chain. The Caucasians using a lower, four-legged acidic animal for milk to feed them are closer to that lower animal (cow). However, Black people giving their babies cow's milk or synthetic formula milk are interrupting the biochemical bonding process. Cow's milk helps cows to bond. It may influence a child to bond with animalistic characteristic behaviors or the Caucasian race, but not the Black race. Black peoples alkaline breast milk provides scientifically balanced milk that nourishes the baby, stimulates melanin, and builds immunity. While cow's milk and formula are only good for breeding humans, and building a physical body that can work for the benefit of White Power.

The races of man are classified according to the concentration of melanin, and melanin density. This scientifically measures human mental, emotional, physical, spiritual superiority and inferiority capabilities. There are basically six types of human beings. Black people (Africans) are rated the highest with a number "6." Eumelanin, Pheu-melanin, Pseudo-melanin grades of pigmentation cause the highest-grade rating. The Brown people such as Mexicans, Malaysians and Puerto Ricans are rated "5." The Chinese, Japanese and Indians are at "4" along with Vietnamese, Koreans, etc. Then mixed whites are at "2" to "3" and finally, white people with blue, green and gray eyes are rated the lowest at "1."

Playground or Death ground

The Caucasian culture's playground is made with equipment, which makes the paly area a death ground. They usually have a ground of concrete, chemically polluted sand, asphalt, outdoor carpet, plastic or wood chips, which aside from being pollutants, may include broken glass, urine, fecal matter, fungus, etc. The playground toys and exercise devices can be made of steel or cancerous plastic pipes jagged or razor-edged devices that are hazardous to health. The exercise devices are usually made for monkeys and do not allow all muscle groups to exercise. The toys are unwholistic and based on the Caucasian culture's idea of toys.

African toys were made by Toy Masters. They made toys that utilized the child's learning type, learning style, thinking style, listening style, emotional vocabulary and gender. Toys were made to correct behavior problems and improve the child emotionally, intellectually and spiritually. Toys were cultural learning devices and geared to help the child towards higher growth. The African play activities taught social skills and communal or a sharing activities rather than individualistic or competitive Caucasian play. There were the African games such as Kea (similar to tic-tac-toe), which is played with stones. In contemporary African American history, the Kea type play board was drawn on the ground and shoe heel or stone was used. A game such as "Hop Scotch" has patterns drawn with chalk on the ground, pavement, or in the street, which were patterned after Kea. It had a large chalk drawn play board, which incorporated the symbol of the Sun (Ra) at the apex, pyramid shape inside a square, and symbols of the female and male principle as connecting boxes. This was played with a shoe heel or stone as a moving peg.

Belenin (similar to marbles), Beleta (similar to jacks), Wali (count and capture) and action games such as Kele (chicken fighting) were played. Kele is an action form of Duck Duck Goose with participants jumping in a frog position and trying to push each other over. These games were played by African children until the early 1960's.

Caucasian toys and playgrounds are made so that the child becomes accustomed to competition, military tactics, individualism, and violence. The Caucasian playground toy devices are not organized by gender nor do they reflect spirituality, cosmic reality or have any relationship to family life. Most playground accidents are influenced by the violence and competition. This causes children to violently damage themselves in playground activities.

The Caucasian playground is usually a fenced-in cage of society steel pipes, wood, and wires. Falls and miscalculated play activities can cause permanent harm. No professional athlete would consider training or exercising on the devices or under the conditions that children play. In 1990, almost 80 percent of the children taken to hospital emergency rooms were between 5 and 14 years of age and the other 20 percent of the children were below 5 years of age. The climbing toys and monkey bars caused over 70,000 children to be taken to the hospital. The number of children treated by parents, teachers, school nurses, self-treated, treated by other children or that go untreated would increase the total of playground injuries. The total number of injuries children inflict upon each other on playgrounds has not been determined. The injuries adults inflict upon children that they are helping to play at playgrounds would also increase the total injuries of children. As far as monkey bars are concerned, a safe way to decrease a child's risk of injury is to measure the distance between the bar rungs. If the child's leg is shorter than the distance between rungs, then he will have a higher chance of his foot slipping and inflicting an injury to his body.

The playground lacks instructions for proper use of the devices. The playgrounds do not have warnings for the appropriate distance to be away from the swings nor is any child's exercise safety monitored by another child or adult. The playground devices are usually designed for individual and not for group or family oriented play. The playgrounds do not have first aid kits available. Children can be scarred, maimed, mutilated or injured for life at the caged playground. They should be called a death ground instead playgrounds. Some children are on legal drugs and can be in withdrawal or high (mental illness condition). They can be in Cell Phone or Social Media withdrawal.

The playground and poor health form a doubly destructive combination against the Black child. The child presents its body at the playground and the condition of that body is full of junk food, and nutritionally deprive, with sleep deprivation, along with suffering from social media and cell phone withdrawal. The child is nutritionally crippled. The neuro hormonal and neurophysiological response are degenerates. In other words, the mind and body reflexes are near zero, muscle reflexes are slower or inaccurate, nerves are irritated, mood swings burst sporadically, near-arthritic and rheumatoid conditions and heart failure conditions are present.

The muscles, nerves and brain are below normal and floating in liquid manure and lactic acid waste. The child is carrying around approximately 3 pounds of caked-up toxic manure in the rectum (adults usually have 7 to 15 pounds), which Caucasians calculate as normal body weight. The internal organs, tissues, nerves and cells are clogged and activity-impaired mal-nutrition. Additionally, a low energy hypoglycemic level can strike at any moment caused by the sugary breakfast, junk foods, energy drinks, cooked marijuana cannibal, or dessert or snack or soda or candy. This can instantaneously cause loss of muscle, brain and nerve control. This is directly related to the bleached white flour, grease, sodium chloride (salt), and white sugar, hypoglycemic Caucasian junk foods.

The obstacle courses called playground toys require 100% physical efficiency that the typical junk food diet cannot and will not provide. The Black child is escorted to the death ground nutritionally crippled and asked to perform 100% on a nutrition-less diet. It is a prelude to an accident prepared for them by junk food Nutricide. To make matters worse, the parents, teachers, school nurses, doctors or extended family members are drugged on the tasty junk food diet and do not see the obvious dangers of the situation.

Computer Trained Dogs = African Children

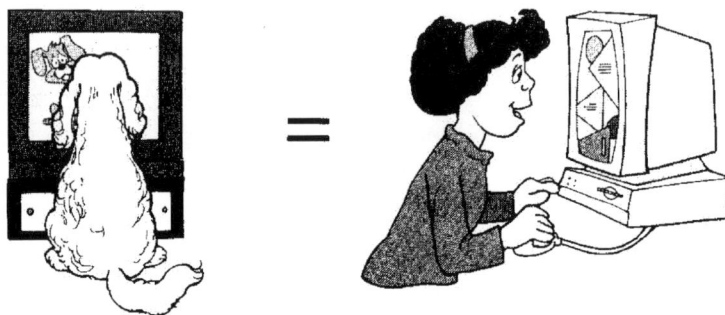

The Black child watches television, text, use social media, and plays games for entertainment. However, the mental and emotional effect of these activities are subtle and yet dangerous. It may be that the games are social engineering and playing the child instead of the child playing the games. The child is assimilating and integrating into White Culture by using computers.

The games with synthetic sounds and music are associated with violence, sex, food and the Caucasian thinking processes. It has been proven by Caucasian physiologist, Ivan Petrovich Pavlov (1849-1936) that by repeated associations with sounds of a bell with a dog's activity. The dog is trained to a desired reflex action can occur. He used sounds to produce desired mental and physical behaviors. In later experiments, he used people. In other words, the abstract synthetic sounds or the computer games can cause thoughts, feelings, emotions and physical behaviors, violence, sex, desire for junk food, Caucasian linear logic, and desires to be part of White Culture = Assimilation and Integration.

Linear logic inducement means that the Black child is trained to think like a white person. Eventually, the Black child will see computers, computer games, and hear the synthetic sounds of music instruments, synthetic action sounds, see computer generated people and associate it with violence, sex, White Culture and junk food. The child will apply white cave thinking and behaviors to Black people. The collective Cave Trauma and White Supremacy psychosis (mental illness) is a part of games (music and television) as well as violence, cave rituals, superstitions, group sex, ceremonies, competition, and social customs.

The Caucasian diseased logic indoctrinates the Black child and adult to view life in terms of inferior versus superior, rule or ruin, win or lose, cowboys and Indians (Native American), sane or insane, crime or police, war or peace, Black people poor, and powerless/White people, rich, powerful, kill or be killed, live or die, violence wins or lesser violence loses, food or famine, master or slave, bad guy or good guy, White beauty or Black ugly, and smart or dumb. In Black logic there is Bipolar (negative and positive) applied to every emotion and idea plus the added dimension of "and or both" three-dimensional thinking. In the white peoples one-dimensional psychotic (craziness) process, a person's feelings get mixed-up inappropriately. The craziness (psychosis) of Caucasian thought mixes feelings together, inappropriately as a feeling sensation. For example, sex, violence, junk food, conflict, love or harmony are mixed together as one feeling. In other words, the normal feeling of love may cause a violent reaction or a feeling of love can result in conflict. This is the primary reason why Black people that act lovingly or non-violently towards White people can get a reaction of conflict and violence.

This same diseased psychosis is programmed in computers, put in video games, and in synthetic video action abstract sounds. Ironically, Black peoples use synthetic sounds in their music. Synthetic sounds do not resemble the natural sound of a musical instrument. A computerized synthetic sound that imitates the authentic sound of natural instrument (drum, piano, etc.) is not to be confused with an alien synthetic abstract sound. Synthetic abstract sounds train the ear to make an association with Caucasian culture, violence, junk food, sex, thinking and reflex behaviors. The sounds and music of African culture are no longer heard by the child who plays computer games.

The computer games, synthetic action sounds and synthetic music sounds are attached to Caucasian civilization's psychosis. Computer games, are derived from Caucasian cultural. They serve the needs and wants of White Supremacy. The former Caucasian slave master's cultural "gifts" (Computer, Social Media, IPhones) to the Black people are used to keep the psychosis of White Supremacy and Black Inferiority alive. The slave master's corporate own government gives Africans the right to vote. Then the Black peoples' political vote is used for their own destruction. The slave master gives the former economic slave (prisoner of war) an education. Then, the

149

miseducation is used to destroy Africans. The slave master gives Black people money. Then money is used to destroy Black people.

It should be noted that 99% of Black people's monies goes to maintain and support white businesses and White government. The slave masters give Black people guns and train them to be police or soldiers. The Black police and soldiers then uses these guns to destroy other Black people. These Black police and soldiers kill Black people in order to defend Caucasian laws (rituals) and order (rituals). The slave master gives Black people junk foods and allopathic medicine, which is used to destroy Black people. Now the slave master has given Black people computer games. These games are used to destroy Black peoples or at least ruin Black people and make Black people assimilate and integrate into White Culture.

Computer games, videos, movies, cartoons and television programs are used by Black people to entertain them, to escape financial, emotional, mental, or physical problems. However, they cause the Black people to escape Black culture and get polluted in Caucasian culture. The computer games cause difficulty in relating to others, boredom, irritability, mood swings, and personality problem. They drain energy from the Black community. The energy spent on computer games, social media, IPhone, could be used to do positive things for the Black family, community and individuals. Instead, the energy is spent to become more Caucasian.

Clinically depressed children view more television, use more social media, IPhones, games, eat more junk food, and are most undernourished. They usually have a melanin deficiency. Black children usually watch 25 hours more television than white children and spend more time with social media, IPhones, and computer games. The digital devices, and television programs arc used to escape oppression and side effects of White racism. Unfortunately, they cause the same problems. This makes being a Black child twice as painful, more prone to disease, and more nutritionally drained than being a white child. The National Institute of Mental Health conducted a 13-year study using 1,200 people, which validated the many mental, emotional, and behavioral problems viewing television causes. It was found that viewing television causes reduced social ability, poor ability to interact and negative moods. This has been revealed in the book *Television and the Quality of Life: How Viewing Shapes Everyday Experiences,* by Lawrence Earlbaum Associates.

Video games are basically structured similar to the arcade games of the 18th century. Black children become addicted to these games, social media's, and the Caucasian White Supremacy psychosis in the games. Their melaninated Black skin identifies them as Africans while their mind, moods, personality, self-centeredness, behavior and thinking process identify them assimilated and integrated into White Culture. These games can help in problem solving of space and movement, sequence in Caucasian logic rituals.

They become carriers of Caucasian, diseased emotions and thinking. The child becomes devoted to fantasy, solo-play and develops an unreal idea of his competence based upon winning against a white acting computer opponent.

The Black child develops competitive behavior instead of the Maat, Black communal, family-centered thinking and cooperative sharing of knowledge and resources. Selfishness is rewarded by a selfish-competitive way of life. In the real world, the Black child loses the holistic African centered ability to interact with real Black people, African cultural artifacts and objects. The child gains a low tolerance of human failure, success, rejection and compromise. Added to this, the Black child (social medias and games-addicted adult) has increased aggressive behavior. He or She also associates synthetic abstract action sounds and music with real life.

The child uses mindless amusement and social medias as fun and increases the potential for doing anything for excitement. They develop the Caucasian emotional, and mental illness that mixes violence with sex or love and cultivates a need to ruin or destroy other Black people. In books such as *Playing with Power in Movies, Television and Video*, by Marsha Kinder, it is estimated that well over 2 out of 3 Black children own computerized Caucasian emotional and mental illness cultural aspects.

The child begins to lose the responsiveness to Maat and the natural cycles of nature, subtle weather changes, natural sunlight variations, slight changes in the taste of natural foods as well as changes in cold, hot, intimate relationship with parents, moods and thoughts. African children begin to react only to mindless synthetic abstract sounds. The sound of rivers, the wind, digestive organs, African music, African drum rhythm (language), trees, and wild life become meaningless. And, Black culture becomes inferior and meaningless.

The Black child is no longer attached to their Black body, emotions, mind, and becomes attached to the Caucasian mind. The Caucasian behaviors of competitiveness, control, violence, sex and destruction are copied by the child. Black children in actuality are not playing the games but the computer games and social medias are playing them – playing them into a tool of destruction of themselves and African Culture. Black children are rapidly becoming the new Pavlov's dog that associates abstract sound with mental, emotional, and physical reflexes which support White Supremacy. They are becoming computer-trained dogs that behave like humanoids (Caucasians can be considered a primitive collection of genetic leftover waste).

Bonding – The Betrayal

Bonding between parent and child connects the child to the parent, world, culture, emotionality, mentality, and spirituality. Bonding defines life and empowers the child. It is a function of White Racist institutions (education, health, nutrition, psychology, sociology, etc.), to destroy or damage the Black sovereign human right to bond. Dysfunctional bonding is a political issue and is used to sustain White Supremacy. Black people that have dysfunctional bonding are easy to assimilate and integrate into White culture and control, economically exploit, and manipulate. A woman who has bond damage is prone to emotionally and physically abuse children. A Black parent has inadequate nurturing skills, and lacks mental and emotional stability. A bond-damaged man is prone to be self-destructive, has poor social skills and has emotional problems.

Bond damage causes men and women to be violent, suicidal, sickly and have a short life span. This human tragedy causes the man to hide his feelings, to be easily agitated and have conflicts understanding and a dysfunctional relationship with himself and his mate. The bond-damaged woman has dysfunctional unbalanced mental and emotional skills, and distributes negativity and thought to traumatizes herself or others.

A damaged emotional bond does not allow the child to complete their emotional vocabulary, emotional attachment, identity, competence, intimacy, concern, and emotional personality. Marriage helps in bonding mind, emotions, body and culture. If the emotional personality is bond-damaged, then damaged concrete thinking and the emotional attachment to culture are distorted and dysfunctional. This is typical Black integrationist and assimilationist Black People. In any case, White Racist institutions continue to emotionally damage Black people causing them to bond with White Culture. They transfer the bond to Black Culture to White Culture. This causes spiritual, physical, mental and emotional illnesses co-dependency to cave civilization.

For example, the original idea of Carter G. Woodson of a Negro History Day is now a White institution (Black History Month) with role models picked by Caucasians. These role models, heroes, sheroes and great African Americans qualify as Caucasian heroes only because they were integrationist, assimilated into white culture, white religions worked for White organizations, served White institutions or organizations or entertained Whites such as Joe Louis, Muhammad Ali, W.E.B. DuBois, A. Phillip Randolph, Madame C.J. Walker, General Colin Powell, LaBron James, Oprah, Michael Jordan, Cornel West, Hank Aaron, Jesse Jackson, etc. Being Black and important is defined only if it relates to Whites and helps to transfer the bond to White culture. The extreme ugliness of White civilization damaging Black people is that Black people have made White Culture their surrogate mother. These Blacks have reality, culture and worldview. It makes Black people emotionally married to white people to have freedom. Unfortunate in the co-dependent marriage Black people become liars, traitors to the race, violent, thieves, culturally castrated and culturally homeless. Black people develop into food illiterates and cultural imbeciles.

Bonding is a necessary emotional and intellectual learning process a type of "rite of passage". The process of developing an emotional vocabulary is the foundation of Black people's maturity, growth, development and contact with themselves and others. Bonding is the ability to synchronize your emotions with someone else. This emotional synchronization starts with the mother, amniotic fluid, and breast feeding. The mother translates the social world for the child. In the mother and child relationship whenever the mother's breathing rate, heart rate, temperature, pH, emotions and or physical movements change the baby changes to compliment the mother's change. This means the baby is in synchronization with the mother which is called bonding. When a man and woman are emotionally synchronized, it is called bonded. Therefore, in a bonded relationship the man and woman are a complementary pair. In a Caucasians relationship, the man and woman are in a battle of the sexes and not emotionally and spiritually bonded. Without bonding, the child is isolated from their culture and Maat. A non-GMO organic food diet and breastfeeding are essential for bonding. A bonded Black child discovers why they are on earth and what their purpose is in life. An un-bounded child struggles to discover whether they are safe enough to survive. The unbounded child tends to be emotionally and physically violent. Black people in Caucasian cultural captivity have adopted white rituals(standards) for growth and development, emotions, nutrition and psychology.

Caucasians are sickly, and for Black people to adopt sick Caucasian rituals(standards) of health is cultural treason and sheer ignorance. For example, the U.S. Public Health Service indicates that over 250,000,000 junk food-eating Americans are in some state of disease while 1,000,000 can be vaguely classified as healthy. In other words, sickness is generally classified as health and this has an effect on bonding. Bonding is a unique emotional and intellectual learning ritual or rite of passage for Black people. White cultural captivity has destroyed, dysfunctionalized or totally impaired healthy Black bonding.

The Black parent and adults have to re-evaluate parenting, bonding, breastfeeding, nutrition and the Male and Female Principles based upon the rapid holistic growth and development of the Black child (SEE Controlling, Understanding and Raising Black Children by Llaila Afrika). Bonding damage and destruction occurs when the Black child and parent use Caucasian superstitious health (theories), bonding, growth and development rituals

153

(standards). For example, the Black child uses words as an instrument for improvisation and rhythmically, the child synchronizes the words with facial expression, voice tone, mood, and body movements. Thinking is treated as a toy and play activity for the Black child. If the child is not rhythmically moving the body and using facial expressions, then the Black child is not thinking.

Historically, movement and the drum were used for instructing and educating the child in school. The Caucasians outlawed the drum, and continued to keep it out of the Black child's education, which caused damaging effects on the child. An education without rhythm is a Caucasian education. The drum, dance and music are a natural part of learning all school subjects and not a separate, isolated, and scheduled school activity.

In Egyptian mythology Osiris taught mathematics with the use of the drum and harp. Learning is a melaninated process. Melanin is a cyclic rhythmic substance that has the highest amount in Black people. Words are rhythmic sounds (phonic). Children associate sounds with body rhythm and senses. Consequently, words used by parents when speaking to children should be sense orientated with words associated with smell, sight, hearing and touch. The adult should perform the child's instructions. Modeling and learning by doing is instructive.

The child views activities as cyclic - each movement has a beginning and an end. For example, the adult tells the child to put on his shoes. The child reacts by putting the shoes on. The child will sometimes put the shoes on the wrong foot. Putting the shoes on is one complete cyclic task while putting the shoes on the correct foot is a separate cyclic task. Consequently, the adult should wait until the child has completely put the shoes on the wrong feet before telling the child to remove the shoes and start over – another cyclic task. In order to avoid this side effect of racism, the adult should demonstrate the activity with the use of shoe/sock identifiers such as a color, number, floor print, letter or symbol codes, etc. The adult should perform the task in a play learning-fashion. "Putting on the shoes" is understood by the child to be a name or label, which is a property of the cyclic task. This is similar to taste, smell and touch being a property of a mango.

One of the side effects of White Racism is that the Black adult assumes that the child has the same thought process as an adult. Consequently, the adult uses adult logic to communicate to a child. This causes a conflict and impairs parent/child bonding. The child thinks from the outside inward while an adult thinks inside outward. In other words, the adult puts together words without associating action or body movement.

The child up to 2 years of age is merely collecting data, such as, properties of events activities, words, spirits, emotions, drumming, music, food, breast milk and adults. The acceptance of this can help to avoid the signs and symptoms of Caucasian-caused bonding impairments. For example, the parent's failure at bonding causes them to give adult instructions to a child. The child does not understand the instructions and acts according to its own ability to comprehend. Consequently, this can result in parents saying to the child "I told you," when there is a failure to communicate. This statement merely pacifies the adults' failure to bond. Other statements often used by parents with bonding impairments are "Next time you will know better," "If you listened to me it would not have happened," "Why is your head so hard?" "When I tell you to do something, you do as you want," "You play too much instead of doing as you are told," etc.

It has to be understood by the adult that the child is processing an abundance of information while doing a task. The child sees colors around objects or senses auras (spirits) and does the task in time (in cyclic rhythm) as opposed to on time (Caucasian abstract). Instructions mixed with play are helpful for the child. For example, Twa (Pygmies) children play at adult reality and the adults play with the child and enjoy the play. The play leads to adult work. The child's play merges with the adult word. The child's thinking is one cyclic movement from spiritual to emotional to concrete to abstract then enlightenment.

A child's thinking may give meaning to events or activities based on the aura-light or emotional, or sensation that the child feels. The adult *must* answer the child within the child's reality thinking. For example, the child may ask "Why does night fall and don't break?" The adult answer could be that the night fell into the ocean. The child may ask, "Who is God's father?" The response could be Ra. The child requires answers that will match its level of understanding. Therefore, the adult answer to questions should not be abstract, scientific or theoretical but more aligned to concrete and action orientation. The acceptance of the child as learning to be a child and at the same time learning to be an adult get complicated. The child will give holistic meaning to events or activities based on what is felt emotionally and what their imagination is feeling about feeling.

The child may say it saw a lion in the kitchen. The adult true or false judgment of the lion's presence in the kitchen is not the issue. The meaning of the child's statement is the issue. The child does not need adult correction or to be called a liar. The child is working through, to and with the rites of passage of idea nurturing and maturity. The child perceives the lion and the maturity of perception is the development of concepts. Concepts change and mature.

Children act upon energy (i.e., lion) and that energy (lion) acts upon them. The child's verbal explanation of psychic, spiritual, emotional, or sensed energy (lion) is not a hallucination, illusion or fantasy, but concrete in the child's logic system. The adult reality has the ability to deal with abstract

155

concepts. Therefore, an adult calling another adult Leo (Zodiac) the Lion or a football team a Lion presents no logic problem while in the child's mind this is confusing. In this lion fantasy or child's warning that a lion is in the kitchen, the adult could go to the kitchen with the child and talk to the lion and ask it to leave or offer it food or chase it away or ask it to protect the house. This would address the child within its logic system, much more realistically than calling the child a liar. The child seeing the lion is an issue of idea maturation and is a necessary step in the experiential learning, practice of idea formation, and the ability of the child to understand understanding.

The child sees the world through the mind, diet, emotion, body and behavior of the adult. Therefore, it is still within the bonding cycles. The child is considered to be connected biochemically with the mother for a year after birth. Incidentally, this mother bond is still apparent in adulthood as music with the same rhythm of the mother's heart beat (usually a walking pace) is the most soothing, best for learning, increases endurance, reduces stress and helps food metabolism. The child's consciousness is an extension of the parent's consciousness in a blended feedback and feedforward system.

The child's consciousness is a function of the Glia brain cells (80%) that dominate the entire brain and the mid-brain (corpus callosum) which unites the right brain (hemisphere) to the left brain. This harmonious mixture of the hemispheres causes fantasy and reality (concrete) to be united in the child's logic system. The Black peoples' mid-brain is larger and has more melanin centers than the Caucasian mid-brain. In ratios of proportion, the midbrain has nearly completed its development and is large. It unites and exchanges hormonal, nutritional, and chemical information so that hemispheres are not very distinct in function. Consequently, language is a function of both hemispheres instead of being primarily a left-brain activity.

Impairment of bonding by poor nutrition and bottle milk impairs the hormonal, nutritional, chemical, melanin unity and exchange between the brain's hemispheres. There is conflict and confusion in fantasy because there are unbalanced mixtures of reality, rhythm, spirituality and play. A child with a dysfunctional, impaired or weak bond, can fear monsters, animals, objects, and can have nightmares that continue into the day. The child is emotionally loss, unfocused, nutritionally restrained without completed holistic bond cycles. Children may verbalize their damaged bond by projecting their loss of empowerment, control, anxiety, isolation, and fears upon objects or animals such as lions. In other words, the child uses its logic system to express the damaged bond.

Children are capable of understanding adult body language, voice tone, mood shifts, facial expressions and not abstract adult logic. Black adults diseased by White Culture may not be able to understand the child's logic or be aware that the child understands them because children have a different logic system. The child lives in the "here and now (present)." Consequently, children believe a dead person is in a different living state. They think that the dead may wake up at night or cannot physically move because they are punished or that death is a result of bad behavior (Karma).

A game such as "Peek a Boo" is a "here and now" game which allows the adult to become conditioned to the child's logic and allows the child to accept the adults "here and now" unity with them. When the adult "peeks" they are here (present) and when they hide, they are an unseen presence (present in emotions) and when they return to say "boo" they verify that life is seen and unseen. "Peek a Boo" is a logic game that demonstrates that life is cyclic and a continuous flow between the living and dead. It also introduces the child to rhythm in speech and the three phonic sounds (peek-a-boo), which develops into number usage and games of numbers.

This and other African games (social skills, learning) are subjected to White cultural values and become fragmented and lose their connection to African culture. Games are an extension of culture. They must be consistent with the culture's Maat morality just as a mathematics, music, drum rhythms, emotions, spirituality or logic are a language of culture. The language becomes diluted, lost and valueless when co-opted by Caucasian cave culture. A White culture's education system defines African social skill learning games as worthless play of primitive peoples.

Caucasian education emphasizes abstract linear thoughts without body movement, emotions, or rhythm (cyclic) or the drum. Their memorizing and discover ideas is a type junk education design to break the emotional bond to Black culture. Combine this with junk food, junk medicine, junk history, junk religion and junk culture and you have created a permanent assimilationist and intergrationist Black servant for Caucasian culture. The Caucasian school education divorces the Black child from the Black community, Maat, family, communal games of sharing and play. Caucasian competition based games can cause depression, self-hatred, addiction to White people, confusion, and anxiety. This cripples the Black child's emotional vocabulary and makes them dysfunctional in African culture and functional in White culture.

In African culture, social skills, learning, games, toys, tools, music and dance allow the child to explore the world. These games, toys and tools gradually develop into adult games, toys and tools (hobbies such as collecting real or toy cars, dolls, jewelry, etc.). Caucasians military type education that stresses the strong over the weak, smart over the dumb, rich or poor, have and have not's, white is right and Black is wrong, either, and/or, fight and flight logic and justifies the White superior position over the inferior Black people. They believe that starting school early (preschool) helps their personality. A white education amplifies the dysfunctional damage done to

157

the Black emotions that starts with the ability to bond to their parents and culture. In African culture the storytellers used in educational and cultural activities keep the parent and child bond intact. African story telling is a living continuum of the importance of fantasy between adult and child. Aside from this, parents who read to and with children help the child to use storytelling and to translate the social world through adult eyes. This increases the child's emotional and reading skills and desire to read. Black children historically are naturally literary. They read words and symbols on that was written on tools, toys, and games. The Black children naturally become adults who read literature on statues, walls, ceilings, floors, coffins and in books.

The lesser evolved White People use of the mid-brain and the conflict or split they have between the right brain and the left brain causes them to define the right mind (brain) as creative, spiritual, feminine and the left brain as evil. Consequently, the right mind that controls the left hand causes the left hand to be classified as evil and is associated with death. The right hand is controlled by the rational, intellectual, conflict-oriented, male or good left brain. Consequently, the right hand is associated with "life" instead of death. This gives to such statements as "if your right hand (life) betrays you, cut it off." White Supremacy psychosis, superstition based science, late development of biofeedback, melanin deficiencies, Cave Trauma and the Caucasians parent and child bond damage causes their ability to help educate others to be a sickly miseducation.

The absence of bonding and the anxiety, mistrust and fear that it causes result in the child being powerless. The child learns to not trust the parent as a source of nurturing and power and as a medium between themselves and the holistic worlds. The bond-damaged child grows to be an adult who fears the holistic healing powers of the body. The child firmly believes that drugs, natural supplements and herbs heal the body and mistrusts African science that states the organic non-GMO food is medicine and medicine is food.

Food naturally nourish healing in the body. Natural plant base supplements and herbs can transform illness to wellness. The emotionally bond-damaged Black child watches their Black parent give up control over their body to a White superstitious theory based medical system. In other words, the Black parent is a slave to White people by using White medicine. The Black bond-damaged adult reacts to situations instead of acting upon a situation to create freedom. The child learns from watching the Black adult that they have no personal power over their life and cannot free themselves from White Domination.

Bonding "rites of passage" emphasize the utilization of emotional intelligence and spiritual ability. The trance "rites of passage" teaches the child when they first awake in the morning to go into a trance state and perceive the coming day. They then learn to change it for the better or avoid negative events. The Trance State before sleep is used to see the spirit world and act upon it and/or with it. Holistic bonding teaches the child to see disease as an alarm that a healing crisis is in progress. No cure, remedy, herb or supplement should be used to stop the body from having a healing crisis. Drugs are to stop the disease from alarming the body of harmful illness. White thinking causes Black people to look for a cure for the body's self-curing process erroneously called a disease. They are looking for a cure for a cure the alarm system is based on white superstitions, science, and myths. Bonding for the child has a cyclic, task-like motion. An example of a bonding activity could be as follows:

1. Be calm, hold (embrace) the child or look the child in the eyes and smile.
2. Ask the child to listen.
3. Give the child instructions in action words. ("Put on your shoes, please," or "Lets go see the lion")
4. Then ask the child to repeat instructions with you. Saying instructions together assists bonding.
5. Model the task or perform the task with the child until they master it unsupervised.
6. Thank the child for his/her good actions.

In the bonding process, the child's emotions, imagination and thoughts sees words as properties of a behavior, words as living actuality and words as truth. They understand that word and action are combined as one cyclic task and one motion. This helps the child conceptualize and bond. The child conceptualizes that creating with creation and form with function are one motion (cyclic). In other words, learning and doing are one cyclic task.

The child's emotions, imagination and logic is the standard for communication with and understanding the child. Their body goes through obvious changes. In some cases, the legs, arms, torso, hands, feet, toes, fingers, nose, ears, eyes and bone structure as well as internal organs may grow out of proportion or sporadically or in synchronized harmony. Growth is physically obvious while mental, emotional, and spiritual development may not be apparent. However, physical growth influences the parent/child bond.

Mental, emotional and spiritual African centered growth is not given importance by assimilationist and integrationist Black parents suffering from White Racism. Bonding is distorted by a White junk food diet. The Caucasian main food groups of dairy, protein (meat), starch and vegetables is forced on the Black child. A child's primary dietary focus should be centered around green starches with raw fruit, raw vegetables, sprouts, beans, raw nuts, raw seeds and supplemented with breast milk. The damaged bond nutritional restraining junk food, GMO diet impairs growth and development. It alters, slows down or stops melanin cyclic utilization. It causes subclinical malnutrition and reduces the brain's ability to emotionally and intellectually function. This makes the child easy prey for White assimilation and intergration manipulation and control.

Bonding Repair Remedies

Bond Damage is a dis-ease and, as such, it can be treated. The accumulation of damaged thoughts, emotions, words, behaviors, moods, spirituality, and relationships, is imprinted in the DNA personality. A bonding, attachment, identity, competence, concern, and intimacy crisis will show signs and symptoms of what appears to be a dis-ease. Dis-ease is merely the body, mind, emotion, and spirit's attempt to rid itself of harmful behavioral, and emotional toxins. The healing crisis may manifest itself by the child (or adult) showing anger towards adult's parents or parenting, rejection of Africentric activities, withdrawal from relationships, confusion, emotional instability, acting lost or being disturbed during nurturing.

This is merely the re-orientation phase of healing. The individual must change their relationships, concerns, emotions, diet, identity, competence, go through a definition of self, parents, culture, and spirit and get accustomed to new African centered feelings and concepts. The bonding-healing crisis will soon give rise to African centered acceptance by the Bond-damaged parent, adult, family and/or child. Added to this, the Bond-Damaged individual must learn to defend themselves from dysfunctional emotions and thoughts constant reinforcement of Bond Damage built into the White Racist institutions, social lifestyle, entertainment media and male/female relationships. Nurturing must be applied while the parent and child or affected individuals go through healing with African centered emotions and thoughts.

Remedy List

- ∞ Carry the infant in a sling close to the naked breast whenever possible. Use a sling to carry the child. Do not use strollers.
- ∞ Do not bottle feed; Breast Feeding is a must.
- ∞ Do not use Caucasian dolls, toys or Eurocentric games.
- ∞ Do not use cages such as playpens or cribs. The Black child is made a prisoner by cribs and playpens. They psychologically can easily accept

160

cage schools with metal detectors, iron bars at windows and police patrols in the building.

∞ Do not use leashes or body harness to walk the child. (This is how dogs are trained.)

∞ Use organic non- GMO natural foods, vegetarian milk substitutes and a vegetarian diet as much as possible.

∞ Avoid nursery school, preschool, day care and other baby-sitting services until Bonding has been established. Use African culturally oriented services and people.

∞ Avoid hospital delivery. Use natural home birth.

∞ Do not play sexual and/or violent music, television programs or movies in child's presence.

∞ Engage in storytelling (read African centered stories).

∞ Play cultural music, put African and African-American artwork and pictures in the home.

∞ No acts of physical, verbal, emotional or spiritual violence or cursing in the child's presence.

∞ Do not call the child's behavior bad or disrespectful; do not call the child bad, stupid, dumb, hardheaded, or a liar.

∞ Sing African and positive African-American songs to the child.

∞ Allow the family to bond with family activities. In some African cultures, the bonding mother and child are alone for up to two weeks and the mother is the only one allowed to handle the child. If the child is handled, it is by a family member. Usually a female family member will assist the mother of a newborn. A family member, as well as the family, are essentials of the bonding remedy process.

Obviously, the remedies chosen from the list vary according to whether the person is a single adult, or married, or single parent or, recovering addict, teenager or whether it will be a group healing process or family healing process. It should be noted that burial of the dead according to African cultural ceremony and ritual helps the person see and feel the bonding in their life. A Bond-Damaged, assimilationist, integrationist Black person is one of the most potent weapons a White Domination can use to rule, ruin and destroy the Black race.

Bonding Disease Stages

There are major and minor sign and symptoms of Bonding Disease. Below are a few generalized symptoms that can help identify the need for Bonding Remedies.

Bonding Disease Stage Symptoms

Acute:
- ∞ Mistakes ancestral spirits for dangerous ghosts
- ∞ Easily agitated
- ∞ Lacks social skills
- ∞ Mood swings
- ∞ Failure to complete cyclic task

Subacute:
- ∞ Opposite sex relationship problems
- ∞ Under reactive to Black culture or African centered emotions and thoughts
- ∞ Under reactive to White Racism
- ∞ All of Acute symptoms

Chronic:
- ∞ Mixes Black culture with Caucasian
- ∞ Confuses spirituality with religion
- ∞ Speaks excessively logical and concrete and does not use spiritual terms
- ∞ Lacks improvisational skills
- ∞ Straightens hair and men cut their hair very short so kinks won't be apparent and calls it neat
- ∞ All of Acute and Subacute symptoms
- ∞ Believes all races are the same or think alike, assimilation and integration attitude
- ∞ Believes all races are the same

Degenerative
- ∞ Assimilation or Integration believes self is one with all races; excuses the Caucasian race's behavior
- ∞ Lacks rhythm
- ∞ Gets angry about negative statements (truthful) pertaining to White people
- ∞ Angers or prefers to protest truthful statements about White people psychosis
- ∞ Dates or has sex with or marries White people and socializes with them in preference to own race
- ∞ All of Acute, Subacute, and Chronic symptoms

Growth and Development of Infants

The Black baby's natural development of the mind, emotions, spirit, and body is suppressed. It is forcefully retarded, twisted, distorted and perverted by forcing the Black child to the very slow White growth and development standards. Black babies who have parents that follow African centered social standards, ethno medicine and a natural or organic, non-GMO diet have children who develop and grow quickly. The Black baby at birth can make eye contact, sit up, smile, and can intellectually participate in life. Its neuro hormonal development is complete at 12 years of age (becomes an adult). White peoples slow retarded adult growth (melanin-deficient) is not complete until ages 18 to 21. Consequently, the Black child is forced to retard and slow down their naturally accelerated holistic growth. This causes subclinical physical and mental illness, emotional reactions to suppression, intellectually antagonistic reactions, decreased nutrient metabolism, ill bonding with parents, family and ancestors and a weak immune system.

Forcing the Black children to follow White health standards and a GMO junk food diet is ethno-medical racism. The amount of emotional, social, and intellectual damage done to Black children and adults by this type of White Racism is beyond estimate. It is reflected in school drop-out, juvenile jails, crimes, drug addiction, violence, broken homes, learning problems, diseases, psychosocial genocide and the nutritional destruction of Black people.

The Black baby at birth is able to consciously make social contact with its parents. Black babies are three to six years ahead of White children in growth and development. In other words, they raise an eagle bird (Black people) to believe that they are chickens (White people). This makes them emotional and intellectual servants to White Supremacy. Consequently, all threats to unify and mobilize Black people is directly defeated by White Domination.

Works by the following authors can be a resource for growth and development, melanin, nutrition and Bonding: *Melanin (Protective Intoxicant Capabilities in the Black Human and its Influence on Human Behavior)* by Carol Barnes, is a three-volume work; all volumes are recommended. *Magical Child: Rediscovering Nature's Plan for Our Children*, J.C. Pearce, *Magical Dilemma of Victor Neuburg*, by J. Overton-Fuller, "*Diet Crime and Delinquency*", by A. Schauss, *Infancy in Uganda*, by Mary Ainsworth, *Ethnological Studies of Child Behavior*, by Burton Jones, *Biological Rhythms in Human and Animal Physiology*, by Gay Gaer Luce, *Specific Health Standards for Pre-Adolescent Children of Three Races*, by Wingerd, Solomon and Schaea, *Problems in the Nutritional Assessment of Black Individuals*, by S. Garn and D. Clark.

Functional Ability

The functional ability of Black children develops faster than in other races. If the child's parents, when the child is on a non-GMO, organic, natural foods diet, herbal medicine and breastfed, it will accelerate the hormonal and biological functions. The functions of the Black child starts decreasing with dysfunctional bonding and the impact of White, GMO, non-organic junk foods. The longer the duration of nutrient deprivation, the more dysfunctional the child becomes.

Functional Ability	African child	Caucasian child
∞ Can make eye contact ∞ Can stop head from falling back ∞ Recognizes parents	18 minutes after birth or sooner	6 weeks
∞ Can hold head steady	2 days	2 months
∞ Can support self while sitting ∞ Looks at self in mirror	7 weeks	5 months
∞ Can hold self-erect	2 months	6 months
∞ Standing ability	2 months	9 months
∞ Can play board games and remove pegs	2 months	1 year
∞ Climbs steps	5 months	13 months

Growth and Development
(Stages for The African Child)

The Caucasian studies of Black children scientifically validate that the Black child is superior to all children of other races. Black children that have had a natural foods diet without parents junk food-damaged sperm and eggs and are African centered bonded with their parents have a faster growth and development rate than Caucasians. The melanin saturation of Black children's nervous system (neuro) and superior control and responsiveness of the glands that secrete fluids (hormones) causes superior and faster growth and development. The melanin-saturated muscular structure responds fast and reacts to growth faster. The Black child has the largest amount of "Fast Twitch" muscles than children of other races.

The child's brain has 12 melanin centers. This allows the brain to transmit, receive and interpret more mental and emotional information. The brain stems melanin clusters or melanin centers are sometimes called chakras. The Black child's intellectual, emotional, spiritual and extrasensory abilities are highly developed. The mother and child bond, is accomplished faster. It starts before conception (epigenetically), prenatally, and birth is a continuation of the spiritual, psychic, mental, emotional and hormonal bond.

Junk food or nutritional restraint causes the child to follow a path of Nutricide and menticide. The synthetic food diet stops melanin from being properly used and recycled. The Black child's reactions to junk food is usually misinterpreted as behavioral problems, genetic violence learning problems, attention span deficient, disease or hyperactivity. The child's defense responses to junk food are erroneously called physical or mental disease.

Stages of Growth and Development

Birth through 2 years of age
- ∞ at birth is holistically aware of itself, parents and fully in contact with the social and physical environment
- ∞ synchronizes mouth and body to mother at a slower, usually unnoticeable pace
- ∞ sensory and motor coordination
- ∞ uses reasoning, logic and memory
- ∞ has ability to respond to slightest variation in the emotional, social and physical environment
- ∞ places esthetic values on objects
- ∞ can be toilet-trained before 6 months of age
- ∞ enjoys rhythm games and activities

∞ feels safe when on a schedule/routine/rhythmic lifestyle

2 years old
- ∞ responds to verbal instructions
- ∞ enjoys intellectual games; will laugh at logic substitute jokes
- ∞ likes to challenge environment, improvise and create different variables
- ∞ forgets task or ideas not in the "here and now (present)"
- ∞ is able to politically manipulate and control the emotional and social environment and others

3 to 4 years old
- ∞ social skills become complicated
- ∞ extrasensory, emotional intelligence and psychic abilities increase
- ∞ has increased vocabulary application
- ∞ does not have vocabulary with adult logic and usage
- ∞ corpus colostrum completes growth; can mix Right Mind into verbal, emotional and listening vocabulary
- ∞ focuses on the concrete and not the abstract

5 to 7 years old
- ∞ enjoys cultural learning with tools, numbers, Trance, spiritualism and dance
- ∞ likes to apply learning to activity immediately
- ∞ samples intellectual and emotional ideas and acts or reacts to them in play or fantasy
- ∞ development of worldview
- ∞ sees adult world as play of adults and plays at adult work, customs, emotions, behavior, rituals and logic
- ∞ likes to disassemble adult ideas, artifacts, gadgets or toys made by adults (child thinks by doing)
- ∞ transitional Bond from Parent to include culture
- ∞ concrete thinking decreases and imaginative and emotional thinking increases
- ∞ thinking becomes action
- ∞ able to reverse reality (i.e., walk on fire without getting burnt)

7 to 9 years old
- ∞ natural cycles of mental, physical, spiritual, and emotional ideation develop cultural meanings of adult

- ∞ spirit world increases in awareness and may have visits by deceased ancestors, strangers, animals and objects
- ∞ seeks clarity about White Racism
- ∞ challenges realty within self

9 to 11 years old
- ∞ selective about types of fantasy, Trance topics and play reality
- ∞ separates word from word meaning
- ∞ uses the mind's emotional and intellectual ability to explore ideas and fantasy
- ∞ experiences other experiences

Development Quotient

Development	African Child	Caucasian Child
Supplemental Eating	Bananas, yams, squash, papaw (with Breast Milk) (*alkaline foods*)	meat, cereal (*acid foods*)
Greets Parents	Musical voice, sounds, claps hands, lifting arms, smile	Similar to mock play of wolves, tigers embraces, hugs (kill's prey) kissing imitates eating prey, lapping blood (tongue kissing)
Toys	Musical, radionics, fruits, berries, plants, stuffed animals	Hunting type spiritual devices, guns, hammers, mathematical
Faces	Family and environment	Face-to-face while sitting with parent
Beating	None – Is too young to understand purpose of beatings	Slapping and beating of infants
Food	Raw grape or orange juice powder herb at 3 months	Meat (cooked or raw), cereal pastry, cow's milk

	No digestive problems	Indigestion, causing burping, drooling, nose dripping mucus; requires patting on back after feeding to relieve indigestion
Sensor motor and Psychomotor Skills	12 months or less Indicates hunger with sound: Cooing and whimper	2 – 3 years or more cries

Growth and Development Through a Child's Eyes

The Black child's growth and development of spirit, emotions, intelligence, physical body and mind have noticeable changes at different ages. These changes at different ages are interpreted and defined by adult logic. This is a mistake that causes a negative effect upon the Bond with the child. The child has to be accepted on its own terms, in its own language and by its own emotions and feelings. Children do not conceptualize or feel abrupt changes at each stage of holistic growth and development because nature has had over a billion years to smoothly perfect the continuous transitions of growth. Abrupt growth spurts in anatomy, emotions and thoughts are caused by a junk food diet, physical traumas, disease, drugs and/or damaged Bonding between Parent and Child.

The child comes from an emotional, non-verbal and hormonal world. Hormones stimulate the chromosome of the male, Y, and is carried to the uterus upon ejaculating sperm, which fertilizes the egg in the fallopian tube. Hormones stimulate the chromosome of the woman, X. The XY chromosomes unite causing fertilization and conception of a boy. If the XX chromosomes unite, a girl is conceived. The hormones stimulate chromosomes and do not possess a gender or sexuality of their own.

In about 6 to 8 weeks during fetal life, the XY chromosome can change to an XX pair. In other words, the slow moving, long living Y chromosome with a missing leg grows another leg and becomes an X chromosome. The Y chromosome is free to change. Incidentally, a change of this sort causes the girl to be born with emotional and mental imbalances and to have sexual confusion.

The child comes from an emotional, undifferentiated state. Consequently, the child's emotional vocabulary must adjust to a concrete and bipolar state of existence. The child tends to touch, hear, smell, taste and see objects, events and people in an emotional (unchangeable) language. The child's emotions understand that the doctor's "bill" is simply a doctor whose name is Bill. This is concrete thinking. An adult understands the doctor "bill" to mean a financial charge for services. This is abstract thinking. Once the child has fixed or associates an emotional concrete property to an object, event or person then it can abstract (change) it. The child's emotions see the world in time (rhythm) rather than on time (non-rhythmic melanin albino characteristic). The Black child performs tasks in time while the adult may come to social events in time (rhythm). This is negatively called "Colored Peoples" (C.P.) time.

The Black child's mind is emotionally centered. The brain is a physical structure that operates with chemical and hormones. It has melanin centers (clusters). The brain's ventricles (open spaces) are filled with continuously moving cerebral spinal fluid (holy waters).

The brain has a force field that physically resembles a galaxy (sometimes called the Third Eye = Horu). This galaxy looks like a cloud and that floats above the pineal gland and hypothalamus in the third ventricle. Historically, the ancient Africans called the fluid-filled ventricles "holy waters" to denote their spirituality.

The 12 melanin centers have properties similar to the 12 signs of the zodiac. The emotions and mind are activities of the brain which is partially in the body (biochemically limited) and partially outside the brain and body (not limited by time and space). The brain's activities are processed through the emotions and hormones of brain cells and calls it intelligence. Melanin is a DNA that bonds all Black people in the seen and unseen worlds. Melanin DNA Bonds to ancestors and unborn children, and plants, waters, earth, animals, weather and united with the Earth's intelligence (Mother Nature).

Melanin allows the child to be in unity with the parents and emotionally synchronized. However, the Black child should have parents that have a natural, non-GMO organic diet and were breastfed and Bonded with their parents. If this is not possible, then the child must have parents who have taken Bonding Remedies.

Melanin makes the brain one functioning sense. There is no split in the brain's neurons and Glia cells. There are brain areas that may have specialized, shared functions. For example, the human eyes are sensors of light (sight), and the brain interprets vision. Without the brain, the eyes do not know what they have seen. The mind sees, tastes, hears and feels with the sensors. You have one sense, the brain, and five sensors.

The Caucasians view life, nature and the mind as in conflict. This is superstitiously how the linear Caucasian brain attempts to be normal. Caucasians see the Right Mind against or opposite the Left Mind, Predator against Prey, Man against Woman (Battle of the Sexes), Good against Evil and Rich against the Poor. This is a symptom of their Mother and Child Bonding damage.

The mind is one. There is only consciousness. Caucasians have divided the mind into fragmented parts called subconscious, preconscious, super-conscious and unconscious. It takes glia brain cells, hormones and rhythm to understand and operate the whole brain. White people do not have enough rhythm to understand the brain or attempt to perform a few simple dance steps. It is a total mistake to rely upon White theory based psychology to understand the Black emotions and intelligence or White Supremacy psychosis (craziness). White people are Bond damaged and have a juvenile civilization and fantasy idea about ideas.

170

The Black child's emotional thinking does not depend upon the intellect. The emotions have their own logic that is separate from intellectual logic. A Bonded Black child's emotional logic is overlooked, and the White child's cave emotional imprint have been forced upon the Black child. This has caused Bonding damage and the perpetuation of White Supremacy.

Black people must follow their own emotional neuronet logic to create a child who is a change agent and a human technology that will defeat White Supremacy. This child will not compromise freedom or Africentric learning. Learning is an emotional process. There are basically three "progressions to learning." *The first stage:* a new emotion is stimulated in the child. The child translates the emotion from adult emotional logic to children's emotional logic. During *the second stage:* the new emotion is experimentally learned. In *the third stage:* the child transposes the emotion and treats the emotion as if it were a toy and uses variations on the emotion either in play or in fantasy. The child uses its own emotional language to coordinate, define and redefine emotions similar to the use of sight to coordinate the senses.

The child sees all of life as emotions and intellectual symbols. All of the child's emotions are attached to the concrete word, fantasy, play and the Parents' Bond. It is important to remember that words are emotional symbols, just as letters, music, dance, fantasy, play and Bonding are emotional symbols. The emotions interpret the world for the child. Bonding is an emotional process.

An adult or child with a disease caused by damaged Bond can be in the acute, subacute, chronic or degenerative stages of Bonding disease. The essential way to understand Bonding and Bonding disease is through a child's eyes. It is the child's emotions as understood by them that leads to the adult emotions. The child's holistic "vision" advances to "supervision" and they must be respected as little "people" not little "children." A child given the freedom to eat any type of natural food will nutritionally balance the diet within a week. The adult needs to read books and take nutrition courses in order to eat a nutritionally balanced diet. A child forced to use adult dysfunctional, emotional intelligence will not use natural hunger.

Mentors

A mentor is a technology of culture and an extension of the family that uses nutritional wisdom for the development of the Black child. Mentors are commonly called a "hero" a "shero," a famous ancestor, educator, athlete, social activist, freedom fighter, scientist, relative or any significant person. Mentors not only serve as role models, and have three primary functions. First, the Mentor is a "coach" that encourages the child's highest [ability] good. Secondly, the mentor is a "Tutor" that instructs in the use of Maat, culture and morality. Finally, a mentor is a "Counselor" that gives guidance on the quality of life needed for Maat ability. Maat ability has a broad meaning and includes talent, rituals, ceremonies, a career, aspiration, family life, community life, business development, leadership and the child's individual concerns. The origin of the Mentor demonstrates its significance in "family-centered" African life.

Mentors have a long history in African American heritage and culture. Mentor in Greek means Divine Teacher. In African civilizations such as the Kush, Ethiopia, Nubia and Egypt, it is explained in mythology. The mythological God name Osiris (his name means guide of the Soul) was a great ruler. Before Osiris was born, the world had no order; there were no buildings and life was crude. Osiris left his country to travel all over the world to teach Maat, the laws of cycles, order, proper worship and technology. In his absence from his children, a highly-developed person was chosen to teach his son Horus the laws of man, God, universe, science, ethics, nutrition, Maat, agriculture and holistic health. The person chosen was named Thoth. Thoth was a God in charge of the written laws of Maat. Thoth taught Maat to Horus. Maat is morals, righteousness, ethics, truth and justice, which includes the divine image of humans, perfection, teach ability, free will of humans and also moral practice in human development. Maat Thoth (Mentor) is also represented by the Kabala, Caduceus, Mancala or Ankh, which means "Tree of Life." The "Tree of Life" is symbolic of the utilization of 12 Melanin centers of the brain, the 12 cranial nerves, the 12 steps of Jacob's Ladder, the 12 steps on the God Shun's stairs, the 12 principles of Metutu, or the 12 cyclic degrees of the Zodiac (attributes of God). These 12 steps plus the Sun God equal number 13.

The "Rites of Passage" of growth and development are degrees, which are called the mystery system and are taught by Mentors. The mentor is basically responsible for the fruit (child) of the "Tree of Life" and is a technology and part of the Black peoples extended family. Sometimes, the principles or steps are combined such as the 7 principles of Kwanzaa or the 7 Halls of Osiris or they can be reduced to 3 steps or levels. For example, the mystery steps could be (1) "Mortal." In this step, there is no "inner-vision" and the application of Maat in themselves and care for the family-centered life, (2) "Intelligence." In this step, the person uses bipolar emotions and intellect to gain "inner-vision" and (3) "Creator" or "Suns of Light" or "Enlightenment." In this step, the person becomes united with the Maat light of God (RA) and receives "super-vision." Mentors and Maat can be used to combat Nutricide.

Male and Female Communication for Family Maat

Emotional and intellectual intelligence is processed differently by the Female and Male. When the Female is in the Feeling Stage, the Male is in the Thinking Stage.

When the Male is in the Thinking Stage, the Female is in the Feeling Stage.

In order to avoid conflicts, arguments, or confusion in talking, harmony is needed between the different stages.

The purpose of communication is to create more harmony, balance, justice, peace (Maat). If the conversation is not serving Maat stop talking.

Female Principle (Cycle Stages)				
Stage	1	2	3	4
Energy	Senses	Feel	Think	Maat (Balance, Adapt)
Element	Earth	Water	Air	Fire

Male Principle				
Stage	1	2	3	4
Energy	Senses	Thinks	Feels	Maat (Balance, Adapt)
Element	Earth	Air	Water	Fire

Grease

The oils, lotion, crèmes, moisturizers, softeners, anti-wrinkle crèmes, powders, bleaching crèmes, rejuvenators, sheep fat (lanolin), and oily concoctions do not allow the skin to breath and clog the pores. It is basically harmful for babies, children and adults. It eventually is absorbed into the blood. Cosmetic chemical companies, solely interested in profit, ignorantly advise the greasing and oiling of the baby's skin. It is the same greased baby that grows to adulthood and greases its body for whatever reason the synthetic chemical company's advertisement says. The grease concoctions feel smooth when touched because the hand slides over the oiled skin. The skin remains dry and unchanged because the skin is nourished and made smooth because of what is eaten not what is put on the skin. Oddly enough, the upper layer of skin is dead and cannot utilize the grease concoction. The chemicals can be fabric-like softeners, bleach, hydrogenated fat, which destroy bodily nutrients and weaken the body. The main cause of dry skin and wrinkled skin is concentrated sweeteners (white sugar). They rob the skin of moisture causing dryness.

The Caucasian custom of greasing their skin has nothing to do with health. In fact, it is mostly steeped in superstition. During the many plagues in Europe, it was believed that open skin pores allowed diseases to enter the body. Consequently, White people stopped bathing with water and started using animal grease to bathe their skin. They used cooked sheep fat, which was believed to be good for the skin because sheep have curly fur. Today, Caucasians use lanolin (sheep grease) in many of their skin care products based on this ignorant superstition.

In the 1600's Europeans used protective alcohol spirit water (cologne) to bathe babies and protect them from evil diseases, this resulted in inflamed eyes, skin and severe pain in babies. Many concoctions were used; even blood (human, menstrual and or animal;) combined with superstitious ceremonies. Today, remnants of the rituals still exist, as a grease cleansing is followed by a spirit mask (clay is used as the mask), then followed with a holy water (skin cologne) rinse or a skin peel (types of Lye), then another greasing. The ancient Greeks used salt, the biblical Hebrews used salt, and Soranus of Ephesus used salt and honey. The Ice Age Caucasian mentality led the Britons, Scythians, Germans, Russians, and Greenlanders to use ice or snow to bathe newborn babies. This damaged the baby's skin and was an emotionally and mentally abusive act.

In ancient Africa, warm water was used to bath babies. In fact, most races of color use warm (not cold) water, such as the Natives of Pitcairn's Island or the Araucanian Natives of South America. Today, the Caucasians add synthetic chemicals, Lye, antiseptics, alcohol and dyes to baby grease.

174

When grease is mixed with water, it is called a lotion. Basically, lotions are emulsified grease floating in water. The antiseptic lotions kill germs and irritates the sensitive skin of the baby. Fossil oils (mineral oil) destroyed oil-soluble nutrients such as vitamins A, D, E and K in the skin and dry it. They cause the skin to peel and chafe and rob it of nutrients. Aside from this, the oil and grease concoctions are absorbed into the blood and travel to the liver and brain. The hospitals grease babies because they do not have time to change their diapers. It is an economic convenience. A gentle massage of the baby's body would help the skin to release its own natural oils. Aside from this, massage is beneficial for the baby's intelligence (increases it) and emotional wellbeing. Good hygiene is all the baby or an adult needs for skin – keep it clean. In the case of fat-bloated babies, the layers of fat and folded fat skin should be kept clean. Greasing the baby like an automobile or metal motor is a way to avoid keeping the baby clean. It is a chemical solution to break the Parental Bond.

In Black peoples Bonding, the mother can sense when the child has to urinate. When the child needs to urinate, the mother lowers the child to a squatted position and the child urinates. Soon, the child learns to signal and attempt to get to a squatting position so it can urinate. Historically, Black people did not use diapers or grease the baby. A child on a raw food diet would not have slimy-paste, gooey-manure (bowel movements), so toilet paper would not be needed. Greasing, toilet paper and diapers are symptoms of a sick White race. It indicates White Supremacy's psychotic fear which has destroyed their mother and child bond. This causes a dysfunctional race with an emotional and mental illness. White people try to make their emotional and mental illness acceptable with cow's milk, toilet paper, diapers and grease. In fact, the White people's abnormal fear and behavior is socially engineered in Black people along with Nutricide.

Historically, White people have a superstitious fear of the weather. This is understandable considering their Ice Age heritage with earthquakes, loud thunder, floods, landslides, huge boulders moving, animals constantly running, food shortages, starvation, diseases, cannibalism, rape, dysfunctional families, no education and no water supply, all of which the Caucasians associate with the weather. They fear the weather, fear God, fear nature, and fear each other.

In fear of the weather, they overdress babies. Babies should be dressed for the type of weather. In the summer, lightweight and light colored clothes. In the winter, the home's temperature should be between 75 and 80 degrees. Summer clothes should be put on the baby while indoors. If going outside in the winter cold, then winter clothes should be worn. Skin rashes are usually caused by putting on too much clothing, which results in sweating. The wearing of synthetic clothes can stop air circulation resulting in sweating and rashes and the microfibers get into the lungs and skin.

Tight underwear and or pants worn by men and women (synthetic, chemicalized cotton) can cause nerve damage, tingling, sweating and fungus growth. It must be noted that the long gowns and full-length clothing of African women and men may appear hot. However, when walking, the clothing creates a type of air conditioning and causes cool air to circulate over the body. The fully clothed African garments are actually cooling. They help prevent dehydration.

If keeping the baby clean and dry is done, then there is no need for antibiotic, antiseptic soap, medicated concoctions, boric acid, starch powder, talcum powder, vinegar, oatmeal or bran baths, greasy, oily, and lubricated wipes.

Using Babies as Toys

Black people can abuse babies by over-handling them. This can occur because babies are abused by being used for entertainment. A baby should not be used to get a laugh or physically manipulated to get reactions. Adults laugh at babies' reactions to stimuli such as sound, light, talk, animals, touch or muscle manipulations. Adults assume these human responses are cute, and make the baby perform circus tricks like a clown or a pet dog. Babies placed in the center of an adult's attention are being abused. Babies put on display like a store window mannequin (plastic dummy) while adults' stare at them, commenting on their physical features and personality, is emotionally harmful.

Emotional abuse is caused by many toys, plastic gadgets, stuffed animals, plastic nipples, bottled milk and noise-making devices are put in their faces or hands. The baby is treated like it is a toy and talked to with non-sense, weird sounds and words while people pass the baby back and forth, and around the room like a remote-control device or a computer game. The baby is forced to endure selfies, loud talking, cursing, harmful LED artificial light (should be full color spectrum), loud music, loud laughter, and disturbed rest/sleep periods. Black babies' livers and immature immune systems, are subjected to the adults, synthetic and/or non-synthetic germs and bacteria.

Usually the Black family members are the only ones allowed to hold the baby. During the first few days after birth only the mother handles the baby and bonding is taking place. A child subjected to dysfunctional emotions of strangers is actually being abused. A baby is a gift from God that requires Maat, deserves the highest good and cleansed spirits in its presence. The continuous display of babies as the center of attention can emotionally cause them to be self-centered and egotistic. They become emotionally conditioned to think that other people or gadgets (toys) must entertain them. They begin to develop the idea that the absence of entertainment brings boredom. The baby gets accustomed to thinking that amputated animal parts and stuffed beasts or computers are fun and normal. They are given an amputated Mr. Potato head or a rubber amputated breast's nipple pacifier or a deformed animal face (Miss Piggy), etc. Eventually, they grow up and accept amputated mannequin body parts in store displays. In stores on display there will be an amputated-human head, amputated breast (modeling a brassiere) or a body with only the hips and thighs (modeling underwear).

The baby is conditioned to accept the mutilation of the human as part of normal life. Mutilated human mannequins (dummies), computer learning games, and toys are associated with fun that gives the self, or ego, pleasure. It is a crazy mixture of human and animal mutilations and amputations and fun that the child gets conditioned to. The destruction of other (mannequin amputations) is viewed as part of getting attention and pleasure. This, along with sexual abuse from watching R-rated movies, music videos, Nutricide and violent films is damaging. Toys, especially Caucasian toys, present a mixture of something to love, destroy and to have fun with.

Silent Guilty – Caucasian Woman

Black people tend to say, "The White Man" when referring to White Domination, Supremacy and Racism. However, the White woman is a co-partner and powerful force in Nutricide. The White Domination, Supremacy and Racism in media does not openly show a White woman's racism. She is as guilty of White Supremacy as the White man. She exploits Black people and inherits the wealth exploited from Black people usually from her family or deceased male. She controls the major stocks in the junk food, medicine and drug companies (usually by inheritance). White women dominate White racist civilization, as there are over 600 million women per 300 million men.

White women's racism is the controlling and dominating labor force in the public schools teaching profession, nurses, news reporters, beauty industry, cookbook and fairy-tale writers. In these positions, she promotes junk foods, cooked foods, White beauty, half nude fashion, and toxic poisonous drug theory based medicine to Black children. Historically, the White woman made prisoners of war (slaves) breastfeed her babies. She raped and helped the White men (buy and sell slaves, beat, torture and hang slaves, taught Christianity) to rape Black women, children and men. She used Black women as homosexual toys and Black men as sex toys aside from preparing slaves' flesh in culinary dishes for cannibalistic meals and rituals.

The White woman educated or indoctrinated White boys and girls to be White Supremacists. She controlled and acted as manager of slave plantations while her husband was away on trips. In machine factories during the World Wars she built weapons used to invade Africa. Her labor helped to exploit, destroy and/or kill African Americans. The White woman still works in junk food factories that make synthetic foods that kill Black people. She directly and indirectly promotes herself as the symbol of beauty and culture by making making Black women inferior.

The White woman as a symbol of the highest form of beauty and sexuality for the Black woman and man is a mixture of deeply embedded homosexuality. She promotes the wearing of clothes that have sexual connotations. The high heel shoes she wears are symbols of perverted sex. The heel on the high heel shoe is symbolically a long erect penis. Historically, the long-pointed toe on the shoe represents an erect penis. The pointed leather toe was stuck into the vagina and/or anus (man or woman) for sexual masturbation. They were erotic decorations and jewelry for the penis like toe of the shoe. She basically dresses in the clothing of ancient White men (dress, skirt, stockings, lace, bikini, high heel and pointed shoe).

The White woman is physically created by her father and mother. Her DNA genes are half man and half woman with a dominant physical expression of a female. She has within her the subdominant DNA traces of the mental, emotional, sexual and physical characteristics of Racism.

The Black man emotionally feels that to be in a non-sexual or sexual relationship with a White woman saves him from White Racism. It is a sexual form of assimilation and integration. In the Black man's act of sexual intercourse with a white woman a subconscious, subliminal, subtle form of mental illness and dysfunctionality exist. The Black man may be consciously having sex with the white woman but he is also subconsciously (subliminally) having sex with the White man. The Black man can be having sex with the White woman to be assimilated or integrated into the White race, to satisfy his need to be loved, nurtured, hate himself, be raped, sodomized, protected and/or possessed by the white man. If the Black man is having sex with the white woman what is he doing emotionally with the DNA of the White man within the white woman? He is in an emotional, homosexual relationship with the white man through the sex act with the white woman. He emotionally and psychologically becomes the white man's homosexual "nigga boy".

The Black person in the act of sex with the White person escapes White Supremacy and emotionally hates themselves. The White people in this White Supremacy dominated world controls all rewards and punishments and the military, money, social media, computer spying, schools, sports, news reports, history, medicine, food, pollution, capitals, resources and stolen African lands. Therefore, they are the adults and all Black men and women are their children (subjected to White rituals and their system of rewards and punishments).

Consequently, in the Black/White sexual act Whites are adults and Blacks are the child (boy, girl).

A Black person that has sexual intercourse with a White person (homosexual or heterosexual) is satisfying a psychotic, dysfunctional desire to be assimilated and integrated and loved by white people. It is a cowardly act. Instead of picking up a gun and destroying White Domination, Supremacy and Racism, the Black man picks up his penis and emotionally and mentally destroys himself. Black people's sexual intercourse with White people is a form of self-hatred. Black/White integration sex indicates that they seek freedom through the act of sex.

The Black man that has an intimate bonded relationship with sex with a Black woman is practicing Maat and healing relationship dysfunctionality. Sex is a political, emotional, military, economic, social and spiritual language of a culture. It is not simply a physical reproductive or regenerative activity. Black people's sexuality is a holistic (spirit/mind/body) cultural language that Blacks use to serve Maat.

A Black person having sex with a White person is emotionally in subconscious self-hatred, assimilating and integrating into the White race and masturbating a mind. A dysfunctional Black person is one that is not free to practice African culture at all times and in all situations. A Black person's lifestyle, family, culture and the continent of Africa has to be free of White domination and able to defend itself and attack its enemies for the Black race to be free. Therefore, any sex or marriage with a White person merely represents another form of Black dysfunctionality.

The crazy sick part of the Black person and White person sexual intercourse or marriage is that the White person exploiting the dysfunctional social situation of the Black person. The White person gets a sexual thrill from the Black person's sexual hatred, denial of a Black relationship and subliminal hatred of his own race. White people get animalistic, exotic, erotic sexual arousal from the Black person's symbolic sacrifice of their inner self identity and race. This makes them safe from their negative Blackness curse and lost lost their fantasy of achieving Whiteness. In many ways this sexual dysfunction compliments the inner emotional, cultural and psychological dysfunction. The Black person's racial assimilation and integration fantasy sex or relationship union is also destroying Mother Africa and African culture. In any case, this White/Black sex or marriage is a way of committing emotional, mental, spiritual suicide and African cultural castration.

It is often said, "The hand that rocks the cradle controls the civilization." In other words, the White woman is the foundation for White Supremacy all over the White Dominated world. The majority of the Sunday school (religious school) teachers are White women, so she is the primary

179

teacher and reinforcer of White racism to her children in news reports, fashion, beauty standards and politics (outnumbers White male voters).

The White woman may meekly or gently hide her guilt. However, she enjoys the benefits of White skin and lets the White man take the total blame for her crimes against Black people. The White woman creates and sustains the fantasy image that the White mentally, emotionally and physically weakest man on this planet is the most powerful. The White woman is a companion and co-dependent partner in the maintenance of White Domination, Supremacy and racism. She does any and everything that is required, by any means required, in order to be the Supreme White Woman even if in the process it means destroying the White man.

The emotional and mental illness, which defends White people's juvenile inferior civilization works as a paranoia. Paranoia acts on the assumptions that the emotions and the mind creates. Added to this, the White people have a phobic (fantasy fear) reaction to their own phobias (exaggerated, illogical fear) combined with a melanin deficiency and divided brain that lacks enough harmony to think holistically. The White woman is by no means half-guilty of White Supremacy, but fully guilty of the crimes she has inflicted against Black peoples.

Historically, it was the White woman who castrated the Black men while they were being hung. It was the White woman who made Black babies drink cow's milk so that her White babies could drink the Black woman's breast milk. It was/is the White woman who did not allow Black children to bond to their parents. It is the White woman who teaches White Supremacy and Black Inferiority. The White woman lacks the mother instinct and does not and will not allow the Black woman to nurture her children and race.

The White woman in American political elections has the majority of votes that can control the government. Her inherited stock controls the major wealth (power elite) of the country. White woman displays her lack of respect for Black Maat culture by putting her sexual immorality and sexual perversion in television dramas called soap operas. White women have perverted nature, perverted bonding and perverted the Mother instinct in order to hold claim to the White Female Supremacy emotional and mental illness. The White Supremacy characteristic of the White woman causes her to be in denial and to avoid being responsible for her racist behavior. Rather than cope with her own fantasy/joy of being the supreme woman on earth she puts her feelings on the White man and tries to tell Black people that she is not as angry, violent, sexually perverted, phobic, paranoid, devious, self-centered, and as racist as her White men.

The White woman has a dependent and competitive dependent relationship with her White man. The White race's fantasy of White Supremacy teaches them to be dependent in order to be intimate. They are intimate only because neither one of them can operate White Racism without the other. One of them may feel dependent upon and exploited, while the other feels taken advantage of. The solution to this dependency is another form of dependency called control. It is similar to the left brain and right brain bonding together by the mid-brain. In this case, the White woman and man are bonded together by their emotional and mental illness, which controls the relationship. Control is one of the paranoid phobic aspects of their emotional and mental disease (Cave Trauma, Narcissistic Avaricious Disorder, White Supremacy Psychosis).

Whites need to control Black people with diet, medicine, democracy, terrorism, childbirth, breastfeeding, psychology, socialism, jails, religion, schools, jobs, drugs, food, sex and violence. In this way, the White people feel that they won't be dependent on Black people's civilizations, science, social systems, resources and land. In reality, White people are dependent on Black people's culture, God, science, resources and land. This is an obvious contradiction, because control and dependency in the mind of the emotionally and mentally ill is a mixed feeling (mixed with sex and violence) and is confusing. Within the White emotional and mental disease, it is taught that intimidation helps to confuse (double talk, word trickery) Black people. This is a way to be superior. Intimidation could have been learned from the Ice Age in which the weather, animals, cannibalism, food and violence intimidated their very existence.

The White women continue to enjoy the fantasy benefits of her emotional and mental illness while they pretend to be innocent of White Supremacy. White women use their sexuality to sell junk food, cooked food and drug medicine to Black people and at the same time creates the fantasy image that she is superior in mind and beauty. Her guilty behavior claims her while her White Racist words indict her. White women are guilty and have committed a sin against the mother instinct—the instinct that says nurture, nourish and protect all children. Instead, she commits crimes against Black children.

Maternal Impressions

The White myths and superstitions before birth surround impressions (epigenetics). In health matters, it is best to leave Black health concerns to Black African centered scientists and leave White people's health concerns to White people.

Epigenetic Maternal Impressions are the impact of the parents emotions, behavior and mentality, spirit, environment, or events upon an unborn child. The ancient Greeks believed that a mother could make her baby a genius, artist or warrior by looking at mathematics, art or pictures of military battles. If Epigenetic Maternal Impressions are solely mental, then

181

the impression of chattel slavery upon Black people would have produced more Black people wanting to be slaves or total warriors against slavery and White Supremacy.

The White slave master used Epigenetic Maternal Impressions to his advantage. Often, the mythological reason that White people gave for a Black woman giving birth to a white baby was that it was caused by her looking at too many white clouds in the sky. White people's myths and superstitions are guarded by religious books, such as *The Bible and Koran,* which were rewritten by political, Caucasian racists. For example, in the book of Genesis, in Chapter 30 verses 29 to 43 it says that placing different colors of rods in front of Jacob's cattle caused them to have various colors.

Trances / Meditation / Daydreams

The trance state of consciousness can be considered a type of self-hypnosis. It has always been used in African civilization. Among African Americans, trance is used in Church. Black people in church while singing, shouting, and dancing go into a trance and get possessed with the Holy Spirit (or Holy Ghost). Black children naturally use trance when they go into a daydream state. Trance, Meditation or Daydreams are activities of the brain called the subconscious. Trance increases learning ability. Trance, vision, possession states or conjure have been used by Jesus the Christ, George Washington Carver, Nat Turner, Denmark Vesey, Malcolm X, Harriet Tubman, Martin Luther King, Sojourner Truth, Marcus Garvey, etc. Trances take on the characteristics of the culture of the person. For example, African culture would have a ritual or ceremony to prepare the Black person for the trance and a closure ritual/ceremony to acknowledge the messages received from the trance. There are basically two types of trances—the isolation (self-centered) and the full awareness (communal-relationship with the environment).

The isolation type meditation requires that you lose contact with the physical and social environment. In this separation or disconnection with life around you, you become only aware of yourself. This is a popular meditation approach because of crowded over-populated city life, high use of technology, social media, constant texting and cell phone talking, high tech/low touch (intimate physical contact) or extrovert attitude and behavior of modern society. This approach creates a meditative space state with a separation between the social and physical environment that allows you to reconnect with self. This trance allows an inner journey into the silence of the body, mind, and emotions. It is believed that all life started in silence or in the non-senses. This type of trance allows the contact with silence or non-senses. This can be a "self-centered" trance if used from a White cultural perspective.

However, Africentrically, it places the communal person in the center of a family centered life.

The full contact, or being aware of the total social and physical environment around you. You do not isolate self but, allow self to be communal with all of life, such as air, sun, moisture, trees, birds, insects, other people, water, breathing, the blinking of eyes, the sound of hearing sounds, the pineal gland's vibrations, and heart beats. This is holistic attention to internal and external life. In this approach, you meditate within the world and do not isolate yourself outside the world. This gives life to the world that gives life back to you.

Black children as well as adults naturally use trance. Children easily drift into a trance, which is called daydreaming. Daydreaming is a mild state of trance. It is not a structured or an educated use of trance. It should be taught in the education curriculum called the "Rites of Passage." The child should be instructed that during the trance (daydream) they are not mentally or emotionally in their body and can experience unseparated existence merger of the past, present and future. In the trance non-senses solve problems, communicate with other spirits and with ancestors living as well as dead. Black children should be instructed that there are appropriate times for trance. Further, the Black child should be told that trance is natural for Black people and that their great ancestors used it before and after studying or doing any activity. All Black children's so-called toys have cultural meaning and many of the musical or spiritually shaped toys contacted the trance state of the child. Play activity which is social behavior learning should include trance activity.

Trances can be done while sitting on the floor, standing, drumming, singing, jogging, walking, lying down, or dancing. Trances are a functional part of life. They can be done by isolating yourself from activities. It can be a healing activity and self-uplifting activity. Deep breathing and slow inhaling and exhaling are essential to trances. Breathing through the nose very slowly is necessary. If standing or sitting in a chair, the legs should be at least shoulder width apart. And if standing, the arms should be relaxed at the sides, or if sitting the hands should be placed in the lap. Erect posture, back upright, not slumped over and eyes either closed or eyes open and focused on a object or straightforward. You can visualize an Ankh or crystal or color or use African music to focus attention or use silence. The object is to go beyond the mind's limitations into the non-senses.

The trance state may need nutritional support. There are herbs such as Gotu Kola, Catnip, Iboga, Gingko and Yucca, which can be used. Also supplements such as Glutamine, B6, L-Dopa, Tyrosine, Tryptophan, Dopa Bean, Melatonin, or Niacinamide can be used. Trance helps to utilize bipolar emotions to create a healthy mind and healthy cells in the body. The

183

deliberate inferiorization of Black trances by White civilization has taken away a vital nutrient for health. Without the use of trance, Black people become culturally deprived. The beginner in trance-learning should go slowly. Perhaps, a two-minute trance and then gradually increasing according to the child's or adult's ability.

Chapter Four

Craziness

"Not only must we teach Black people how to use food nutritionally, but we must teach them to do it within the context of their own culture."

Dr. Alvenia Fulton

Gang Warfare

Gang warfare is the normal behavior of the White race. The White race's gangs are built on a foundation of dysfunctional (abnormal) cave families that form loosely united cave gangs. They have elite oligarchy gangs called International Bankers, Wall Street, Multinational corporations that terrorizes people that do not think like them and destroy the ecology of the earth with chemical pollution. Their gangs attack Black peoples' human and natural resources.

The gangs do invasions to make conquest, then they begin to fight each other over the stolen profits. A deep sense of insecurity about safety, victories, sex, nature, God and themselves causes the gangs to attack each other. They call their gangs governments, ethnic groups, alliances, religions, the United Nations, public schools boards, drug companies, the Food and Drug Administration, Congress, the military, the criminal justice system, the Department of Health Education and Welfare, banks, corporations, the Stock Market, social clubs, police, food companies, entertainment media, computer companies, etc. White people's elite gangs attack Black countries and Black peoples and through pretend information (propaganda, fake). The gangs propaganda make the world and themselves believe that the attacks are to free people and spread democracy. The gang attacks gain emotional security from their insecurity and the Cave Trauma disease of the inner self.

The largest White gangs are a collection of clans, which they choose to call a civilization. The gangs so called governments are a neurotic group from cave civilization and the Ice Age. Historically, the cold climate of cave civilization was filled with aggression, war, violence, and disease. Their dysfunctional behaviors reflect and mirror White Supremacy diseased minds. The collective White mind that controls the junk food and medical drug companies (hospitals) is a mind that is aggressive, violent and at war with itself. In order to remedy the problems of the health field, the problems of White Supremacy have to be solved. White domination, White Supremacy, and White Racism are the shield that maintains and protects the deeply infested emotional and psychological dysfunction.

The gangs' Cave Trauma that shaped their inner psychosis (craziness) is different from White Racism. White people's Domination/White Racism/White Supremacy operates as a separate disease state with its own set of psychotic (crazy) structures. Black assimilationist and integrationist march, sing, write, vote and give speeches to teach White people that they are White Supremacist has no curative emotional and psychological effect on White people. It is the same as teaching a drunk person about being sober— they are too drunk to understand. So it follows that teaching White people that their junk foods, miseducation, special education programs, GMOs, police force, games, news programs, Black television programs, employment policies, predatory loans, vaccinations, White psychology, and drug medicine is destructive to Black people will not help the White people become less racist. A turtle cannot teach an eagle to fly and an eagle cannot teach a turtle to swim. Black people cannot teach White people to be humanistic and White people cannot teach Black people how to behave Black. Only the assimilating and integrating Blacks think they can teach White people. White people need psychotherapy treatments for their White Supremacy psychosis and Post Traumatic Cave Disorder. They need treatments not talking and teaching, marching, voting in new people to offices, and equal opportunity programs, etc. They need treatment for their addiction to their disease of being supreme and treatment for the disease.

The corporate elite oligarchy's degenerative food causes degenerative diseases. The synthetic concentrated food such as bleached white flour, white sugar, cow's milk, grease (lard and oil), synthetic chemical additives and sodium chloride salt causes clogged arteries and starves the body.

When the White owned junk foods, industries, chemicals and drug medicines cause the heart to be injured or stop, it is called heart disease caused by a virus or bacteria or a gene, or a dead ancestor's DNA. When the concentrated foods damage the brain, it is called senility, learning disorders, mood swings or depression. Concentrated foods dry the skin, nerves, bones, muscles and brain. Concentrated drugs dry the eyes, it is called cataracts or glaucoma. The drying of all concentrated, processed foods and drugs dries all skin, bones, muscles and nerves and damages the reproductive system, causing fibroid tumors, prostate cancer or sterility and incontinence of the bladder and bowels. The physical diseases are caused by White Supremacy and Cave Trauma disease of the White people, and is reflected in their thinking and behavior. Their thinking creates concentrated junk foods, cooked foods, synthetic chemicals and poisonous drug medicines that they use advertisements to psychologically force upon Black people. Treating or trying to change the White Supremacy that mask (protects) their inner Cave Trauma disease has no effect upon their obsessive-compulsive craziness of Narcissistic Avaricious Disorder.

The obsessive neurosis of a normal person is quite different from the obsessive-compulsive craziness of a White Supremacy psychosis and Cave Trauma Disorder of White people. The White people's obsessive-compulsive mind tells them to think the way they think, because they must think the way they think in order to think. If this sounds crazy, it is crazy. The White Supremacy mind gets pleasure from thinking the way it thinks, and the pleasure it gets is also a Cave Trauma craziness, which is called Narcissistic Avaricious Disorder get pleasure from thinking they are superior and pain from knowing they are not superior. Their mind is in conflict and at violent war with itself. It is their diseases fighting each other to create another disease. They are in denial that they have a cluster of diseases.

White people live within the contradiction (conflict) of their minds. White Supremacy is merely a reflection (mirror) of that conflict. It is the mind of Cave Traumatized White people that must fantasize reality and simultaneously deny reality. There are approximately 5 billion people in the world, 4 billion are colored and 900,000 million are White people (600,000 million White women and 300,000 White men). The majority of the colored people in the world are Black or mixed Black races. In less than 2,000 years White people have murdered at least 200 million Black people and at least 50 million Natives in India, in the Americas, Australia, Caribbean, Alaska, etc.

White people have not faced the reality of their mass murders or subhuman cave barbaric behavior. Their mind is constantly on trial and declares itself guilty and innocent at the same time. The White people's corporate elite oligarchy junk food industries have murdered millions of Black people with diabetes, heart attacks, hypertension, high blood pressure, cancer, White Racism, mental illness, depression, suicide, tuberculosis, etc. Added to this is the murder of Black people with syphilis, AIDS, sickle cell anemia, legal prescription drugs and illegal drugs (23% of the people that take Valium die, at least 25% on illegal drugs die, 5-10% of Black soldiers commit suicide).

Corporate owned disease (health) industry has caused mutilation of Black people with surgery, drugs, vaccinations and inoculations. For example, the German Measles/Rubella causes arthritis. Flu Shots cause paralysis. Measles causes the nerves to be damaged and burn the brain encephalitis. Whooping Cough Vaccine drugs cause convulsions, fevers and brain problems. Insulin drug use leads to amputations and blindness. Tetracycline drugs used by Black people causes bone problems. Antibiotic drugs weaken the immune system and birth control pills cause cancer and other maladies. White people's profit-making junk food gangs, medical gangs and drug gangs are killing White people and killing Black people. The deaths are blamed on the "obsession" with money. Money is supposed to bring security. The White mind is insecure and "compulsively" wants more security (money). They are obsessive compulsive, White Supremacy and Cave Trauma Crazy White people. Their mind in conflict with itself will never find security. Security craves security to satisfy the need for security in order to be secure from a mind that is insecure.

Each White corporation business gang is in conflict within itself, which means it is mentally and morally corrupt. For example, the Food and Drug Administration allows unsafe drugs to be used and is asked to police (morally control) the Drug companies. Drug companies test drugs and do not test drugs on a speed track. The tested drugs and untested drugs are unscientific, questionable, they use wrong dosage, and fake test results. The Center for Disease Control's research indicated that 80% of laboratory test results are questionable or wrong and 20% could be loosely considered correct. The American hospital-certifying agency approved hospitals as safe for the sick while the Department of Health Education and Welfare declared that over 66% of hospitals are unsafe for sick people. They government demanded that the dangerous Hospitals be closed. However, the government's certifying agency let them remain open. The United States Surgeon General's Nutrition and Health research declared that junk food causes disease. The Food and Drug Administration allows disease causing junk food companies to continue to manufacture and sell harmful junk foods. If one corrupt gang organization is used to correct another corrupt gang organization the problems are not corrected. Each gang merely mirrors the mental disease of White Supremacy, Cave Trauma, Narcissistic Avaricious Disorder, Psychopatic, Personality Disorder. All these disorders combine to create a new diseased. The new disease has no title or label other than it is the nature of being a White person.

Cell Out- Genetic Racism

White peoples biological and chemical rituals and ceremonies that they call "Theory" is based upon beliefs not science. Their scientifically normal standards belief for all human races are based on the beliefs and theories of biochemistry. What little science they do use is stolen from Africa and called a Caucasian discovery. Hippocrates, the "father" of White people's
medicine, stole from the African textbook called *The Carlsburg Papyrus.* Other White thieves, such as Galen, Theophrastus and Dioscorides wrote and quoted the medical prescriptions from the Temple of Imhotep and the African textbook, *Papyrus of Moscow.* Their Caucasian founder of nursing, Florence Nightingale, did not contribute to the nursing field. Actually, the Black woman born in Jamaica named Mary Seacole is the founder of that field. Her techniques and treatments were stolen by Florence.

In 1852 Mary Seacole was instrumental in saving residents of Central America (including Panama) from a cholera outbreak. Mary Seacole helped stop the 1853 yellow fever outbreak in Jamaica. In 1854, during the Crimean War that England, France and Turkey fought against Russia, the War Department of England used Mary Seacole's healing ability to save soldiers' lives on the battlefield. Florence Nightingale was present at the battle but was too sick to work. Nightingale was of some help to White soldiers and at the same time she was infecting soldiers with syphilis. She eventually died of syphilis. The White people's so-called scientists have recorded the behavior of thieves, liars, acts of unprovoked violence, murder and disease warfare against Black peoples. This is historical criminal behavior combined with

189

their modern, contemporary, criminal behavior of stealing wealth and knowledge from Africa, stealing human beings (slavery), global war and terrorism against Black peoples, rape of Black women, boys and girls, destruction of Africa's libraries, art, buildings and culture. They maintain their emotional and mental illness of Cave Trauma Disorder and White Supremacy psychosis. Their physical behaviors indicate that they have a hereditary genetic DNA disease.

The White race is now stealing the DNA information from the Black people's DNA and human cells. In fact, they now have patents on the cells in Black people's body. Their copyrights get them money for the scientists with human cell patents every time a scientific laboratory uses cells to test or help diagnose illness. Genetic discrimination DNA markers based upon theories of disease history is available with no way to keep it private. An individual's parent may not have the criminal mental or physical trait or characteristic, but since it is in a Black person's genetic DNA pool it allows White people to use that information to genetically identify criminals and racistly discriminate against Black people. This is genetic and DNA White racism. In other words, White people can scientifically hate the very cells in a Black person's body because the cells are theorized to predict Black people are prone to violence and have a criminal mentality.

Black people are labeled genetically violent and discriminated against. White genetic engineers can change Black people's cells by using deactivated viruses as carriers of White characteristics that they want in the Black behaviors. In this way, Black people will become designed slaves to serve White's supremacy. This is chemical cannibalism. Genetic drugs are the new weapons available to Cave Traumatized White supremacists are now using genetic DNA drugs to inferiorize and dominate Black people. Dr. Leroy Hood, a geneticist at the California Institute of Technology, claims that the genetic revolution will change White people's drug medicine. In fact, it was reported in *Reader's Digest.* Volume 139, Number 833, September 1991, that the National Institutes of Health has already done genetic transfusions at their clinical center. It is obvious from White people have not reached their highest level of barbaric behavior. Cave Traumatized White Supremacist will always see Black people as inferior and servants for White civilization.

Caucasians, through the use of genetics, re-edit your gene DNA codes (genetic designer slaves), splice your genes with bacteria or an animal's cells, and place their programmed cloned GMO cells into your body. The Black genetic DNA codes cells will be replaced by White GMO genetic codes or synthetic cells. Black people will be White people inside their bodies with Black skin. The Black world community will eventually be a programmed community of cloned DNA GMO CCI (Computer Generated Images) of servants of White people in search of a White master. It will be a cell out of Black civilization.

Mental Illness is Entertaining

Mental illness is when the mind can no longer move from one thought to another freely. The mind gets stuck in a thought process or an emotion. A mind rigidly holding onto a thought or an emotion that is against the health and well-being of the person or others is sick. In White civilization, a mentally ill person is anyone who is against the white standards of behavior or thoughts (white way of life). While in Black civilization, an individual who fails to practice Maat or is emotionally imbalanced reflects the failure of the village or ancestors to create wellness. Consequently, a Black person too "left minded" (logical individualistic, analytical = Caucasoid). Would be told that they were not in their "right mind (spiritual, creative)". Black people should be aware of the subtle emotional and mental illness within the White cave trauma society. In this way, Black people will not have assimilation or integration infection which makes them desire to be White.

White peoples emotional and mental illness causes them to think that violence can be solved by violence. This similar to thinking ignorance solves ignorance. It is white people thinking that putting an illness in their body with vaccination drugs cures the body of illness. The germs cannot protect themselves from other germs. If germs were very successful they should be fighting each other to find which germ can kill the body. If the germs kill the body they kill themselves. In any case, White people's belief based(theory) science of killing germs is stupid. There drugs that destroy suppressive or stop the body from working (antibiotics, aspirin, histamines, cold depressants, etc.) are believed to help the body to work. For example, the Food and Administration in 1991 approved the use of treating bladder cancer by giving the sick person an infection. The germ Mycobacterium Bovis (BCG), which is found in abundance in tuberculosis disease, was given to people with bladder tumors (cancer). This type of science treats an illness with an illness is part of the foundation of their cave mental and emotional illness. The acceptance of this science theory (belief) concept allows the mind to be conditioned to accept theory science as "pure factual science". This type of thinking is a mental illness. If this science is accepted then it becomes easy to accept mental and emotional illness as entertainment.

White people's cultural clichés help to support mental and emotional illness as entertainment or science. For example, a cliché such as "money is the root of evil" is a mentally and emotional illness concept. Black people's money, Chinese money, Native American money, etc., was never the root of evil nor did it cause evil among them. It is Cave Traumatized White people that are evil (emotionally and mentally ill). White people use money as an extension of their culture supports their mental and emotional illness. Money is not a living thing that can cause or create good or evil. However, White people believe that they are not evil but their money is evil (mentally ill). This is thinking psychotically and supports mental and emotional illness as entertainment. It is probably correct that they put their evil picture on their evil money. Pictures of slave owners (to own a person is a mental illness), bandits, pedophiles, thieves, terrorist, rapist and opium and marijuana addicts such as Hamilton, George Washington, Benjamin Franklin, Thomas Jefferson etc. are on White people's money.

White people deny, block out, hide, shut off and cover up Cave Trauma Disorder feelings. White people are in denial and subconsciously know that they are inferior to Black people and Black civilization. Their denial and lies to their emotion causes feelings of anger, violence, paranoia, murder, fear, love, pleasure, anxiety, sex, and excitement. Within this mental and emotional illness is the inability to separate feelings. All feelings are the same or are redirected or may not be felt at all. Consequently, in the White mind feelings of love are mixed with violence. This mental craziness is in their movies, sports, children's fairy tales, games, news reports, social medias, computer games and religions.

White people's inferiority reflex causes them to block out feelings without understanding why. White peoples feel a need to be in control, dominate and inferiorize Black people and that feeling is the same as the cravings felt by drug addicts, food addicts, sex or violence addicts. Their emotions and feelings are not understood or labeled correctly. Their crazy emotions can stimulate feelings which maintains crisis behavior. Their emotions create a need to create events, or social situations, or an issue, or war, or violence in order to stay in control. It is an outgrowth of "self-centeredness" instead of Black "family centeredness." In White male centered civilization "self-centeredness" everything (events, Black behaviors) is either for or against them. There is a lack of acceptance or understanding of where their rights end and Black rights begin. Black sovereign human rights cannot be understood by White People's Cave Trauma Disorder mentality. They use linear thoughts to talk to themselves and listen in communication ("double talk," "talk with a forked tongue,") which is the confusion of mixing truth and lies. They act on their paranoia within themselves and with other people. Paranoids act on their emotional assumptions while sane people evaluate assumptions before acting. Direct communication would require honesty and an acceptance of their crimes (massive murders, extermination of peoples, stealing of Human resources and natural resources, slavery, colonialism) against the continent of Africa and Black people.

White people emotionally believe their civilization to be highly developed, so there is no need for them to consider the rights of other civilizations or Black people. Anything outside of White superiority does not exist. Since White people believe themselves to be the only highly educated people that know and understand everything.

If it were true that the White people are the supreme race, then other cultures (African) are irrelevant because White peoples' collective mental and emotional illness and mythology(beliefs) verify that they are the most evolved, powerful and developed race. They think that gadgets, such as machines or computers, indicate superiority in their civilization. Advanced civilizations have the ability to get along with other races, ecology, nature, provides for the elderly, children, values human relationships and does not pollute nature. It is proven that White civilization does not and will not have that ability.

If White people are responsible for what has happened in their civilization and what they have done to Africa and Black people, then they must be blamed for global warming, wars, and pollution. Everything that has kept them in wars, invasions, exploiting the poor and inferior is totally their fault. White people's cultures are inferior because of the murderous and destructive environmental actions they have committed and continue to commit against Black people. They constantly are making wars and exterminating of natives of North and South America and of Australia, the Caribbean, etc. Despite their stealing of human and of natural resource, of other peoples they continue to believe that their superiority has happened because they made it happen without massive murders, rape, slavery and stealing of human and of natural resource. White people believe their superiority requires them to be in control. They believe that White people have always been in control. Therefore, everything is "just and honorable" that White people have done to be in control. At one time in history, they called the slaughter of Black and Red peoples a part of White "Manifest Destiny." Manifest Destiny is merely a pleasant term for their mental and emotional illness. The "Manifest Destiny," belief translates to mean White people are in control.

There is doubt that communication can harmonize or unite the Black and White races because Cave Trauma Disorder and White Supremacy psychosis does not allow them to see other races or cultures as equal or superior. There is no line that marks a separation between White inferiority and White imagined superiority. This is caused because White people do not perceive Black people (or other colored races) to have sovereign human rights. They see Black people's rights as something that is granted by violence (war). White people linear-communicate (confused crazy inner conversation) within themselves and to themselves. It must be noted that White peoples' inner conversation is with "double talk" or a "forked tongue." White people as a group lack respect for Black cultural boundaries. In other words, they see everything superior about Black culture as a gift from White culture, and within their mental and emotional illness everything and everyone becomes a possession. They imagine themselves to be the center of the world. They constantly describe social activities, and even entertainment in terms of their mental and emotional illness and value structure (cosmology).

The center of White entertainment is violence, murder, sex and emotional and mental illness. The absence of this type of entertainment is called boredom. Black children playing computer games and using computer's logic from childhood to adulthood assimilates and integrates them into White craziness. Consequently, Black people spend their life escaping Black culture and become culturally homeless by using drugs, sex, food, sex dancing, changing jobs, playing computer games, using social media, getting divorces, watching movies, television viewing, physical exercise to build muscles, social media gossip talking or listening to gossip talk shows, going to parties, dropping out of school, sex addiction, shopping, spending money or taking trips in their cultural captivity. It is White cultural captivity that Black children and adults live their life.

White people and the Black people that follow them participate in more fantasy than their children's fantasy world of cartoons, videos, social media, texting, computer games, movies and television. Adult White people consume more-make-believe fantasy stories (i.e. movies, fantasy sports, social media, computer games, television programs, songs, books), use more games with good-is-White, evil-is-Black themes, use more recreational legal and illegal drugs to help make mental fantasy, have recreational sex which is 90% fantasy and live a life where they fantasize White civilization as superior and the continent of Africa and Black people are inferior.

Fantasy is entertainment and sports entertainment is a mixture of mental and emotional illness. The fantasy is so concrete in the White mind that it is real and no longer considered an emotional and mental illness. Like concrete, it is thoroughly mixed and cemented in craziness. It is an emotional and mental illness to eat a process concentrated food diet that causes disease, then eat the same diet while in the hospital in order to cure the disease with poisonous drug medicines.

The central focus of the white fantasy stories is the good guy-versus-the–bad guy themes. The bad guy is anyone who opposes or is fighting against the good White people or good White civilization. The person fighting against the good White people has the major theme of stories has a character that is has a personality defect or is evil or has a mentally illness or wants to destroy the world, or is a savage or bloodthirsty, sex pervert, seeks revenge or is power hungry, lives in an imaginary world, has unreal fears, and it is never a person without mental problems or has a legitimate right to oppose the good White people. Usually, the fantasy type computer games, action movies, detective stories, books, cartoons, television shows, or drama devotes the major part of the time to justify why the White "good guy" should exterminate the evil person who opposes him. This helps to reinforce the White myth that they are noble and may have a few defects but in their hearts, are they good people. This myth that white people are the good people supports them being the supreme race. It is a reworking of the Savior or Hero coming to save the world from the evilness of the mentally ill. Evilness is a form darkness (blackness= the Black race) in the character. They use a mentally ill bad person for the main character to entertain you in their stories. Mental illness is entertainment for white people. Mental illness is "darkness" which is a form of Blackness that indicates a mind without the "Light" of God's goodness and love.

The Black parents' choice for their children is to teach the child Maat, to use trances (daydreams as a form of mediation), to sense the spirit presence of ancestors and to find joy in African culture. Black adults who choose the mental darkness of the mind themes of White people's entertainment stories, computer games, television shows, movies and novels are confirming the dark arts (evil=Black people's brain) are evil and need to be exterminated like the dark skin Carib and native Americans and black skin Africans. If an adult Black person thinks about Black sovereign human rights, Africa for African people at home and abroad, or are about opposing (fighting) White domination, White Supremacy, and White Racism they are the putting themselves on the extermination list.   Therefore, white people naturally fantasize that there is something genetically wrong with dark skin or black skin people. White people know that Black skin people must be crazy to think about defeating white people. Black people question their sanity because white people said that only crazy uncivilized people want to fight them. White people's mental illness based entertainment is used to condition the mind of Black people to believe that they must be crazy.

In news programs mentally ill person is used to entertain the audience's attention during the programs. It is assumed that a mentally ill person has committed murder or a crime and needs to be put in jail or executed. It is assumed that white cave people are not crazy and do not have Cave Trauma. News programs (actually history shows) constantly pick a crime such as murder, rape, brutality, illegal businessmen (drug pushers), robbery, assault and battery as evil when in actuality they are activities of the mentally ill. Consequently, mental illness is viewed as evil and a crime that needs to be punished. White people believe all crimes must be punished which included run way slaves. The run-away slaves were punished for stealing themselves. And, Black people that are social activist or opposed to the white cavies are label mentally ill and need to be punished and one day that will escalate to extermination by solitary confinement or three strikes (three crimes) are given life in jail. The Black child never sees the massive mental illness of White civilization. White Cave Trauma and White Supremacy psychosis is not clearly stated as a mental illness, it is just racism. Racism is projected to be a temporary attitude problem. However, anyone fighting against the White domination and White cultures control is clearly stated as having some type of mental problem. A Black child will accept the crazy logic that criminals are mentally ill if they fight racism. They will not see the so-called normal thinking White person as a having a mental illness because white people are sane. White people have practice racism against Black people for over 2000 years. White people make Black people assume that only a few whites have an attitude problem called racism. Their attitude problem cannot to be corrected by laws, songs, marching, speeches and protest because it is their civilizations deep psychological problem(craziness). Mentally ill White people do not need songs, laws, marches or speeches, they need therapy. It is not a crazy attitude it is their civilization's way of life for white people to constantly hate Black people. The Black child will not conceive or believe that it is normal for Black people to constantly fight the mentally ill White race.

Epidemics, Lies, and Diseases for Money

Epidemics are based upon the Germ Theory belief which is the basis for the Contagious Disease Theory belief that means diseases spread and affect many people at the same time in a particular area. However, the vast majority of these diseases are created and supported by theoretical epidemic beliefs. The diseases are caused by the process junk food diet, legal and illegal drugs, vaccination drugs, corporate destruction and pollution of land, air and water. The vaccination/inoculation drug business combined with the medical drug business makes profits from the diseases caused by the chemicalized GMO junk foods industries. They sell vaccination drugs, inoculation drugs and drug medicine to cure the diseases that they cause. They make profits from selling the junk foods and the double their profits when selling the cures and triple their profit when charging money for hospital treatments, surgery and drugs. Obviously if the diseases spread then ALL the doctors and nurse's families, children and their children's friends and school mates along with those people that they come in contact with in grocery stores, gas stations, at movies, clubs, public places, churches and amusement parks would be infected and die. USA congress indicates that taking vaccinations are an unavoidable necessary harmful risk. They have made it a crime refuse to take the vaccination drugs. Drug companies cannot be sued or be held responsible for the harmful effects of   vaccinations. And to make matters worse the medical industry uses beliefs(theories) not facts to sell their products. People are murdered by a belief. The destruction of farmland and water cause the disease epidemics. And, corporations are not held responsible for causing diseases. None of these businesses will take the responsibility for the epidemics, mutilation and medical human sacrifices that they cause. The Black consumer is led to believe that diseases, germs, bacteria, and virus (Ebola, etc.) are a natural way of life. Keep in mind that normal white people work for the predatory loan companies, Wall Street Bankers, drug companies, the courts, jails, junk food industries, fake news shows, schools etc. It is normal white people that are protesting normal white people. Obviously, the problem is that normal white people are upset with normal white people for being normally mentally ill.

Epidemiology Theory is a belief based science that does not have repeatable scientific proofs to document its findings. John Graunt founded the theoretical belief science of epidemiology in 1662. He had published the Europeans' first book on the subject, *Natural and Political Observations Made Upon the Bills of Mortality.* He wrote that more White men died than White women and that one-third of the White children died before they reached the age of five. This theoretical belief based science is unscientific and fictitious. It has been criticized by theoretical epidemiologists such as Alvin R. Feinstine, Professor of Medicine and Epidemiology at Yale University School of Medicine in 1901 and in the 1980 Presidential Address to the American Heart Association's (AHA) 53rd Scientific Session by the Ex-President of the AHA and Thomas N. James, M.D. Kurt A. Oster M.D. in November wrote an article, *"The Decline of Common Sense and the Ascent of Computerized Nonsense in Medicine."* This article scientifically pointed out the stupidity of theory belief based science and its vast errors.

Epidemiology theories are used by insurance companies to compute disease, "risk factors." A "risk factor" has many meanings. The "risk factor" theory has not caused an improvement in heart disease care. A "risk factor" differs from one report to another. Insurance companies use theoretical mathematical statistical reports that cannot be applied to human life. This statistical theoretical data cannot be applied to observations on Black people's natural diet without a measure of melanin levels and the use of holistic science.

Epidemiology theories use data from public records which they put through complex theoretical mathematical manipulation. For example, from the advice (opinion) of insurance companies, epidemiology theories concluded that "risk factors" such as smoking, heavy alcohol drinking, obesity, disease history of parents with a processed food diet high in cooked saturated fat and cholesterol caused heart disease. This advice was given to the public without scientific proof. It was never reported to the public that this advice was merely a theoretical mathematical deduction and that this belief advice may or may not be of any help or could actually cause disease. The theory declared that a change of diet (lower in cooked fat and processed GMO) would be of

little help or no help. Further, it was not advised that within six months of a lowered cholesterol diet the body rebounds to its high cholesterol level. Additionally, it was not advised that people with type A blood usually have a higher cholesterol level. It was not advised that Black people tend to have low cholesterol levels and a different DNA biochemical personality.

The use of the belief of theoretical standards to judge disease in Black people can result in Black people being considered as having a normal cholesterol level when in actuality they are sick. Black people's undiagnosed sickness progresses further before the White theoretical belief standard recognizes a disease. Black people have to be on "mental alert" and must be constantly aware of the White source of theoretical advice. If the advice is given by a doctor, scientist, an actor, athlete, medical organization, insurance company or the food business, it is still advice (opinion, not scientific). Advice is simply a non-scientific opinion. Aside from this, medical groups change their theory based advice from year to year.

In 1950, the normal theoretical serum cholesterol level was arbitrarily guessed at 150mg. Then for some emotional reason, it was changed to 300mg. Then in 1980 the American Heart Association gave theoretical belief advice that the cholesterol level should be 220mg. Caucasian theory based science does not take into account the bipolar cyclic laws and Circadian cycle of nutrients, hormones, organs, emotions, thoughts, or the human body. In holistic African centered science, the daily circadian cycle and bipolar cyclic nature of cholesterol's monthly, and yearly cycles is included as a factor. The specific circadian cycle and bipolar cyclic levels are different for children, men, and women. Highly melaninated Black people have sensitive and responsive circadian rhythms and bipolar rhythms (cycles). Caucasians with the lowest melanin levels are not cyclic oriented and their theory belief science ignores cyclic factors. White epidemiology relies on theories and advice, mathematical opinions, and belief based theories. Thus, this field is another tool used in the destruction of Black people.

198

Facts about Health

Africans can see the lies and misconception about Caucasian health and medicine by looking at the facts:

Fact 1:   America's worst drug takers are probably physicians. According to a series of articles appearing in the New York Times in mid-1975, the percentage of physicians on hard drugs (heroin, opium, cocaine) was over 19 times greater than the number of people among the general population addicted to the same drugs.

Fact 2:   Numerous surveys, tests, and health evaluation programs have consistently revealed that America's "medical professionals" are no healthier than the average American. Yet they are allowed to give advice on health

Fact 3:   Compared to the general population, over 23% more American physicians (including heart specialist) die of heart and cardiovascular problems. Cancer deaths among physicians are 12% higher than the general population.

Fact 4:   "Whenever doctors go on strike, throughout the world, the same result occurs: The morality rate drops. The first strike was in Saskatchewan, Canada, in the late sixties. The second was in Los Angeles, where, according to Professor Milton Roemer of UCLA's School of Public Health, the morality rate during that strike dropped by 17 percent. The third strike was in Columbia, South America, where the morality rate dropped by 37 percent. The fourth strike was in Israel when, during an 85-day strike, the morality rate dropped by 50 percent. They discovered the last time the morality rate dropped that low was over 20 years ago at the time of the last doctor's strike."

Fact 5:   Annual physical examinations procedures and test are harmful to health.

Fact 6:   Hospitals are dangerous places for the sick because of extreme exposure to other diseases, processed GMO foods served, radiation, and inactive, and lying in bed decreases immunity to disease and weakens the body.

Fact 7:   Most operations are harmful, and are unnecessary.

Fact 8:   Medical testing labs reports are scientifically inaccurate because they use theory belief science and opinions.

Fact 9:   Many drugs cause more problems than they cure because they have over 40 side effects that outnumber the curing effect. (Doctors prescribe drugs "sold" to them by salesmen who use questionable research data.)

Fact 10:   The toxic radiation X-ray machine cause diseases and are dangerous.

Fact 11:   Over trillion dollars was spent on so-called "health care". (If Americans would stop doing #5 and #6, health care expenditure would drop

Fact 12:   Over 250 million Americans have one or more chronic disease condition.

Fact 13:   Only one-and-half percent (12) of Americans are regarded as healthy by the US Public Health Service. This means that over 982 % have some type of illnesses.

Fact 14:   About one billion visits are made by patients to physicians, clinics, and emergency rooms every year in the USA. That is about six visits per Americans.

Fact 15:   Over 10 million Americans suffer such side effects or adverse reactions from drugs and medicines administered by physicians each year that they need to be hospitalized.

Fact 16:   One in five Americans spend time in the hospital for treatment every year.

Fact 17:   Over 100 million Americans suffer from high blood pressure.

Fact 18:   Chances are better than 95% that your arteries are partially blocked by plaque. Almost every American child over 4-years old has arterial plaque formation. Over 45% of Americans die from heart disease or cardiovascular problems.

Fact 19:   More than three out of every ten Americans get cancer. Eighty percent of these people suffer death attributed to cancer.

Fact 20:   Cancer and pneumonia are the number one cause of death among children.

Fact 21:   Over one in three Americans suffer from some form of allergy.

Fact 22:   Over half 60 % of Americans are obese. Americans are malnourished despite overeating processed chemicalized hybridized GMO junk food.

Fact 23:   Over 50% of Americans suffer from chronic digestive orders.

Fact 24:   Over 30 million Americans suffer from ulcers.

Fact 25:   Over 60 million Americans suffer from hemorrhoids.

Fact 26:   Nine out of ten Americans suffer from more or less clogged colons. Constipation is a wide spread disease.

Fact 27:   Over 20 million Americans suffer from asthma.

Fact 28:   Over 50 million Americans suffer from chronic sinus infections.

Fact 29:   There are over 30 million diabetics or near-diabetics in America.

Fact 30:   Over 20 million Americans have psoriasis (a skin disease) diseases: rheumatism, gout, and bursitis.

Fact 31:   Over 50 million Americans suffer from arthritis and related diseases: rheumatism, gout, and bursitis.

Fact 32:   One of five hospital births in America is defective, about half being brain defects.

Fact 33:   Almost every baby born in America has been polluted before birth by poisons processed chemicalized hybridized GMO junk food, fluoride water, and drugs in the mother's bloodstream.

Fact 34:   Over 20 million American children are mentally retarded or handicapped because of brain problems caused by the effect of radiation and the polluted air, water, soil and vaccinations. The chemicalized junk foods, chemicals in makeup and cosmetics, alcohol, energy drinks, coffee, and poison drugs from in the mother's bloodstream affects the unborn babies.

Fact 35:   The 5th leading cause of death is misdiagnosis, prescription and medical errors.

Fact 36:   The average age of death of doctors is the same for general public and people they treat. *Dissent in Medicine Nine Doctor's Speak Out* by Robert S. Mendelsohn M.D. *Confession of A Medical Heretic* by Robert S. Mendelsohn M.D.

Fact 37:   Due to weaken immunity caused by processed foods, chemicals in water, the air, soil, environment, and radiation this causes young people to die from mild diseases such as asthma, etc. The death rate in America which includes suicide deaths has increased for White people between 30-45 years ago.

Blood Letting

The White civilization's bloodletting (making a person bleed by cutting the skin, vein or artery), superstitions, ceremonies, and rituals and the impact of Post Traumatic Cave Disorder and their primitive Ice Age culture DNA genetically influence their behaviors. Historically the celebration called Christmas, use a white sugar candy cane with a red stripe on it that symbolizes the dripping of blood on the shepherd's cane (candy cane). In the past, they use a bloodletting symbol called a barber's pole because early barber's performed bloodletting to cure headaches, "colds and flu," sex problems and to do physic readings (fortune telling). White scientist use blood for their scientific studies, preventive medicines (pus peddlers use vaccinations and inoculations), laboratory values, tests for venereal disease on blood. This indicates that Blood test, rituals, and ceremonies are still in their genes.

It is a characteristic Post Traumatic Cave Disorder to choose blood science rituals such as the blood marrow in bones. In African centered sciences such as those of Dr. Imhotep, they used hair, skin, breathing, pulses, eyes, acupuncture, water, crystals, colors, metals, magnets, body sounds (auscultation) and other modalities to diagnose and treat diseases. Blood can indicate personality typse such as A+ blood type person is impulsive, B+ is emotional, AB+ is introverted, A+ and 0+ are outgoing or socially gregarious. The use of blood is a crude, primitive form of science theory practices. However, the Cave Traumatize Ice Age DNA genetics, leads white scientist to value blood over other forms of diagnosis.

In White people's history of cannibalism, eating animal flesh, the eating of the raw heart of murdered enemies, butchering one another in violence as well as drinking each other's blood, drinking menstruation blood to cure diseases was a standard custom. Blood has symbolic meanings. White people are attached to blood rituals and use blood-red carpeting, red lipstick, rosy red cheeks, red women's panties, red cars, say a soldier sheds his blood for his country, or that Jesus Christ gave his blood. White people put symbolic blood (catsup) on food and pizzas. They admire predators who kill and cause blood to spill. The color red resembles the fires of hell(evilness). Red symbolizes the evilness of women which caused man to commit sin and loose his ability to live forever. The symbolism is red; therefore, women wear red to confirm their low status of being sinful and too mysterious in emotions and sexuality and created sin. The White woman uses sexy red finger and toenail polish, red underwear or light red (pink) clothing to symbolize the spilt blood of a woman captured as prey to use as a sex commodity. They roll out the red carpet to welcome guests; blood is spilled in defeat or if there is an economic business loss you are in the red. They bond relationships by mixing blood from each other's fingers, called a brotherhood bond. Blood means violence to them and red represents a color of action, sex, power, food and excitement. The White culture is so entrenched in symbols of blood that their mind cannot and will not see it. They are in a state of denial about their attachment to symbols.

White people love each other with the muscle that pumps blood (the heart). They use blood scientifically to indicate their relatives. In African Divine Kinship relatives were related by God. Therefore, when an orphan slave child arrived at the slave quarters on the plantation they were immediately adopted by a family and became a part of that family. The child and the adopted parents became related by Divine Kinship through God and not related by blood. White people are related by blood not by God. If a White person has a negative relationship or dispute or argument with another White person they say there is bad blood between them. If they get sick they put medicine in hypodermic needles and inject it into their blood. To prevent disease, they put pus inoculations in their blood. They force feed the sick with white sugar and water that is put in the blood.

If a White person has one drop of Black people's blood in then they are considered Black or a mulatto. The value of blood has any sort of psychotic meaning place upon it. In order to get married you have to do a bloodletting (blood test). If you want to attend their public schools or foreign travel or get some types of jobs you must do a bloodletting (blood test) and/or get a vaccination or inoculation into your blood.

An animal's blood cannot make you healthy, spiritual, intelligent or save you from White Supremacy. Black peoples' blood was used in European (Caucasian) rituals and ceremonies, during slavery and colonialism. Bloodletting in the form of puncturing or cutting open the skin while being hung, using whips to cut the skin and draw blood, castration and other forms of bloodletting amusement was used on Black children, pregnant women and young girls as well as men. The book, *Race and Civilization* by Frederick Hertz, can give insight into the cannibalism of Caucasians.

Cave superstitions White people classify dark red blood as evil (bad) and white bright red blood as good to eat. White food experts tell people to stop eating toxic red blood meat and to eat the toxic light-colored blood of fish and poultry blood is safe. The blood of any animal is at all times half filled with waste. In the body one quarter of the blood cells are dead, one quarter are dying, one quarter are new cells and one quarter is waste and carbon dioxide. The half of the blood is maintaining the functions and transporting waste and nutrients at all times. In the case of about to be slaughtered animas fear of death causes the adrenalin hormone to be released into the blood, organs and muscles and this poisons the carcass before death. The animal's cooked blood, pus and adrenalin hormone give animal flesh its taste. If people were eating meat for protein then the blood and pus could be soaked out of the flesh. This would leave a bland tasting white grayish meat. The blood could be soaked out of the animal's flesh in salt and water. Whether it is raw or cooked the blood, pus and waste gives good taste to meat eaters.

The white people labeling dark red blood (blood without oxygen) is evil because it is close to the color black. Bloodletting meant that they were letting the evil blood bleed out and restoring health. White people's belief that white blood is pure is part of their white supremacy psychosis. Bloodletting practices helped reaffirm the craziness of White Supremacy and black people inferior.

The Clan's Diseases

White civilization has not evolved beyond the status of a collection of dysfunctional clans. White civilization has been controlled by clans such as the Duponts, Gettys, Rothschilds, Waltons, Rockefellers, Krupps, Gates, Hesses, Mellons, Hunts, etc. These clans use feudalism to manipulate and control themselves, dysfunctional families and Black people. They may label their clans as feudalist, capitalist, socialist or democratic governments, kingdoms, corporations, multinationals, republics, and empires or nations. When a few elite oligarchy white families unite, they are erroneously called nations. However, they are clans that support and protect each other under the disguise of a nation government or corporation. Their relationships are built on clan ownership and power. The social structure starts with a family then clan (combination of families), to tribe (combination of clans), to kingdoms (combination of tribes) and then to empires (combination of kingdoms).

Black people's extended family society, based on Maat and humanistic relationships (ecology). It develops into complex Maat human structures such as tribes, kingdoms and empires. Caucasian dysfunctional families are based upon mistrust (backstabbing), selfishness, rape, homosexuality, cannibalism, superstition, individualism, fear, drug addiction and individual ownership. They have not been able to develop beyond elite oligarchies of clans which they call governments. This is reflected in the American economy in which elite oligarchies of families (clans) control over 80% of the wealth resources and power.

White clans base their definition of clan, tribe, kingdom and empire on private ownership of land and resources. Thus, a British elite oligarchy clan controls resources in England are called the a country and government. A clanish government that controls land in Europe is called a kingdom. Caucasian kingdoms that control lands in Africa are called an Empire (e.g. the British Empire).

White civilization has never and can never develop past the clan state. Their clans have never ecologically shared compassionately with the major population of White people. They have failed to adapt to a harmonious relationship with people or the environment.

The Eskimos (Civilization of Man and Woman = Inuit Native Americans) mastered their climate. Their severe cold climate did not make them thieves, dysfunctional, violent or mentally ill. White people are maladaptive; they do not adapt and are consumed with self-hatred and "nutritional restraints." "Nutritional restraints" are the lack of nutrients provided by plants and utritionally poor soil, nutritionally lacking edible plants and a junk food diet. Nutritional restraints stop the body, emotions, mind and spirit from using its full range of actions. It limits the brain's functions. The Caucasian's nutritionally deprived brain is genetically in conflict with the mind. Their deprived malnourish brain creates dysfunctional families and clans called society.

White people cannot see, accept or understand basic sovereign human rights of Black peoples. It is totally wrong for the White racist public school (educational plantation) teacher to teach a Black boy or girl unless they have been treated for White Supremacy mental illness. White teachers (educational overseers) subconsciously transfer their cultural values and biases, cave trauma illness and White Supremacy psychosis to the Black child. Their cultural captivity of the Black child imprints on the child's mind the inferiority. A humanistic White teacher would automatically refuse to teach Black children and would demand that Black people control their own African centered curriculum and non-GMO organic school lunches. The White Supremacy of clans and feudalistic behaviors of Whites will not let them see the harm being done to Black people. Black people are legally forced to attend public schools base upon European culture.

The over $20 Billion a year Special Education business has introduced over 20,000 cave trauma white psychologists into the schools, White psychologist and Black assimilationist psychologist with Supremacy psychosis and immoral and unethical "lifestyle choice" ideas. These White beliefs and ideas about homosexuality, drug use, free to explore their sex organs (masturbation), and free sex as a lifestyle choice have caused an increase in violence, homosexuality, suicide, imprisonment and drug addiction. Only 1 out of 10 Special Education students graduate. The teachers and psychologists have classified children that react to oppression, cultural captivity, White Supremacy psychosis, and malnutrition as mentally ill and make the children into drug addicts Ritalin hyperactivity drug causes drug addiction, cancer, cysts and tumors of the liver. The non-addicted children are forced to socialize with emotionally and mentally ill dysfunctional addicts. This causes the non-addicted child to become dysfunctional and develop co-dependency mental illness. The non-addicted student becomes dysfunctional to function with dysfunctional people. The non-addicted child feels that uncontrollable emotional outburst and emotional abuse are part of a functional relationship. In adulthood, they will emotionally manipulate other people to be dysfunctional in order to have a functional dysfunctional relationship. This is the reason that co-dependence addiction is worst that the drug addiction. If there is to be a change in the cultural captivity of public schools or school diets it will be Black people that directly cause the change. No race knows white people better than Black people. Black people have been with white people as slaves, as soldiers in their wars, in sexual and religious activities, in schools, prisons, sports entertainment jobs, government jobs, politics, social protest activities, and servant lifestyles, participated in segregations, integration and developed an understanding of cave people (Source: Citizens Commission on Human Rights and FDA). If Black people do not know white people by now they will never know them.

Black people must change their diet to non-GMO organic natural diet and dis-ease treatments to natural remedies instead of using allopathic drugs. White peoples junk food diet and drugs has directly and indirectly caused AIDS to be twice as high among Black women compared to White women; asthma is three times higher in Black people than in Whites. Breast and lung cancer is higher among Black people. Diabetes is three times higher among Black women. Seventy-five percent of Black women have fibroid tumors as compared to 33% of White women. Infertility is at least twice as high among Black people. Depression is at epidemic proportions. Lupus is highest among Black women, and over 60% of Black women are overweight. The junk food diet and drugs weakens the health of Black people and increases their susceptibility to diseases. These facts have been compiled from data supplied by the Minority AIDS Project Los Angeles, CA, Asthma and Allergy Foundation of America, National Black Leadership Initiative on Cancer, Bethesda, MD, American Diabetes Association National Service Center, Alexandria, VA, Black Psychiatrists of America Association, Oakland, CA, Association of Black Psychologists, Washington, DC, America Fertility Society, Birmingham, AL, America Dietetic Association, Lupus Foundation of America.

The hoodlums of the corporate owned medical oligarchy clans (i.e., organizations, associations, certifying agencies) and public hospitals will classify a Black people as mentally ill who has Sunlight deficiency, yeast infection, melanin deficiency, food allergy, hypoglycemia or chronic fatigue syndrome and send him to a psychiatrist. They do not help Black people with a disease; they merely prescribe toxic suppressive drugs that will suppress symptoms until the body deteriorates or dies. It is the DNA nature of White clan cave society and drug medicine that creates diseases and death among

Black people. A book that can be used as a resource is *Dirt* by Terance McLaughlin.

Change the Name, Not the Behavior

The improved changes that have occurred in civilization among the various races were of African origin. Africa is the acknowledged cradle of the world's first civilization, scientists and spiritual peoples. It was Africans who introduced the modern developments to the world. For example, in the Americas (before the invasions of Christopher Columbus) the Africans introduced the system of bureaucracy, government, apartments, orchestra, music, pyramids, naturopathic, medicine and kinsmanship to the natives. In China, the African man Fu Hsi of the Divine Dynasty introduced Yin and Yang or Horu and Falcon head social system. In Japan, Africans introduced the religious system of which Karate is a minor part.

Africans sailed the seas long before Caucasians and introduced astrology, culture, language, science, banking, textiles, architecture, agriculture, chemistry, mercantilism, mathematics, the wheel, the arithmetic use of zero, the fire stick (matches), paper, navigation, etc., to other civilizations. Everywhere Africans went they improved societies and helped to uplift people by initiating constructive changes. African culture is the custodian of change and have nurtured change among others. If there is to be another change on this planet it can only be an outgrowth of the initial change that Africans implemented. Change is a biochemical melanin stimulated issue.

Early African Trans-Atlantic and Trans-Pacific traders introduced the fruits such as the orange that came from south and Indo China, grapefruit (pumelo, forbidden fruit, shaddock) from East Indies, papaya from America, pineapple from Brazil, mangoes from Asia, bananas from India, avocado from central America, lemons from Himalayas and Burma and lime from Burma.

The White race is not about change and only make improvements in their barbaric behavior. They can only react to the artifacts or material things of change or steal the products of change; they cannot create change. For example, Africans changed the Caucasian diet by introducing different types of foods and tried to change their disease condition by introducing hygienic medicine. Despite the African foods and natural medicines, the White people clans of barbaric cave people on a meat-and-potatoes (starch) centered diet. They are still a sickly race. They are clan's people with mob violence, mental and emotional illness, dysfunctional families and mob sex.

Historically, mob sex and breeding sex orgies were a central focus of their race. Sex breeding orgies are usually a confused mixture of mothers, daughters, fathers, sons, relatives, male and female casual acquaintances, friends, animals, strangers, homosexuals, married and single people, young

208

and old who may or may not have venereal diseases. This mob sex can be random or scheduled and is usually called free sex, adultery, sex out of wedlock or permissive sexual behavior. It is merely an extended form of mob breeding founded upon White selfish individualism of clan identity. It is a dysfunctional characteristic of their clan societies. Selfish, individualistic societies that have not mastered harmonious human relationships.

White people have not been able to escape gang sex, the Cave and Ice Age mentality, White Supremacy psychosis, full moon, sexual activities, honeymoons, romantic moonlight, etc. White people as a group have emotional and mental illness characterized by self-hatred. They used and use bathtubs for sexual purposes and historically related cleanliness to a form of superstition. White people that bathe used the bathtub for murder, clairvoyance and sex orgies. Others used sheep fat (lanolin), pig, dog or cattle or rotten animal grease to bathe with *(The Bath,* by D. Von Furstenberg).

White people's mob sex, or permissive sex is a part of their society and has not historically changed and is constant. The name has been changed but the activity remains unchanged. In order to change any part of their society they must change their DNA and overcome self-hatred and stop recycling self-hatred. For example, they kink (curl) their limp hair, thicken their lips, tan their skin, shave their legs, buy buttock pads or inject plastic and wear brassieres, use makeup to add color to their pale skin, imitate Black people's dances, music and slang words because they hate themselves. They cannot change the diseases and deaths that they cause with junk food and drug medicine until they make a DNA change.

They changed the names of diseases periodically. However, the human body has not changed nor has its disease reactions changed. Health and disease is easily understood. The human body is a small universe. There are plants, bushes and grass (vegetation) on the skin (topsoil) of the earth. There is vegetation on the skin of the digestive flora (which means vegetation). There are animals and insects that live around the vegetation in the body. There are insects that live around the body's flora except in science they are called bacteria. The evaporation of the waters in oceans and lakes causes water to go up to the sky where the temperature is below freezing. The water vapor turns to negative charged snow, then the fluffy light snow rises higher into the sky and clusters together which forms positive charged hail. The heavy positive charged hail starts to fall and collides into or merges with the negative charge snow that makes energy (lighting). The same thing occurs in the body. The negative charged cells collide with positive charged cells, which makes energy for your body to function. The body is not difficult to understand it is the medical drug practitioners that are difficult to understand. They are into a name change hustle.

209

They change the names of disease in order to keep the change (money) out of your pocket so they can put your change (money) in their pocket. Why do they change names of your body's functions and organs to Latin or Greek names? You don't speak the languages, and they don't speak it. By changing the names, you become ignorant and now need them to translate the Latin/Greek name for diseases into English names. You have to pay medical practitioners to be a translator. These medical hustlers use the name change game to get your change (money). Again, the human body is easy to understand. Feces (waste) than can pass out of the body must go back into the body. Blocked waste goes into the kidneys (causes High Blood Pressure), eyes (glaucoma, cataracts), arteries (varicose), muscles (rheumatism), mouth (tartar and bad breath), arteries (atherosclerosis), etc. Whenever the waste relocates into the body the name of the waste is changed into a disease name. Therefore, the ill person has to change medical specialist, change drug prescription, change to another series of test and x-rays. This keeps the change (money) moving to the medical hustler's, pocket.

White people are consumed by their fantasy superiority in medicine and constantly recycle diseases of body, mind and spirit. They would rather restore (recycle) or rehabilitate trash (waste paper, plastic, glass, aluminum) than rehabilitate the African continent. Caucasian synthetic junk food corporate clans (companies) are not interested in recycling (restoring) Black people's health. They are more interested in recycling trash, drugs, crime and disease addiction. The clans of synthetic food companies, are not built to meet the ethno-nutritional needs of Black people. Food companies only respond to profit, not nutritional needs. They use the economics of stupidity. Their Supply and Demand Theory is the corrupt economics. If you do not have money you cannot make demands (eat). Therefore, you do not get supply (food). If you do not have money you starve.

White people's theory based fantasy economy that has not changed and repeats recycling economic failures (i.e., recession, depression, inflation, bankruptcy, etc.). If the Black people eat chemicalized synthetic GMO food they nutritionally starve their bodies into a disease state. White people recycle their behavior of violence and change the name of their behavior to manifest destiny, exploration, war, slave codes, colonialism, religion, nutrition but remain a juvenile violent civilization.

White people pacify themselves and say they have evolved (changed) from a monkey and will continue to evolve (change) to higher heights. Historically, they evolved to their highest level with Greek civilization and have not changed or improved since that time. Change is melanin mediated. The more melanin a race has the more able they are to change and create change. Melanin converts or changes energy, be it mental, emotional, physical or spiritual. White people are melanin albinos and have the least ability to change.

Change is sometimes related to karma. Karma is a philosophical definition for a reaction to an action. It is believed that white peoples, previous negative behavior caused them to be barbaric, mentally ill and enslavers of Africans. It is assumed that Africans' previous negative behavior of thousands of years ago caused them to be enslaved. In other words, everything is paying for a past negative karma. It is illogical to use Karma to explain that past negativity caused the water to become polluted, air to become polluted, fertilizer poisoned soil, hybrid and cloned plants, animals, and insect's extinction. Karma helps White Racist to justify racism.

Black people's Maat principles explains the relationship of all to the many. The ability to use Maat to improve, establish, understand and create change is a melanin event. It is stupid to look to white people with the lowest amount of melanin to change or relate to change. There is no historical evidence to indicate that white people have changed their relationship with Blacks. The history of the White people's clans uses of junk food to destroy Black people is evident. White corporate elite clans control the land which makes them control the foods and control the people. It is Black people that must change and use non-GMO organic foods and plant base medicines, or else Black people will be a sick and polluted tomb on a path of destruction.

The white food corporations have controlled black people through changes in diet or behavior. White people have told Black people what food to eat and not eat. There are many types of edible grasses. However, Black people are forced to grow in their front lawns and yards grass that they cannot eat and grow in flower pots plants they can not eat. Black people grow grass that only cattle can eat. Black people are taught to believe that the only food worthy to eat is the food the former slave master grows and eats. Black people do not grow edible Dandelions and or Poke plants in their lawns or yards. These plants can be eaten in salads or alone. The young leaves of the Maple tree and or Ash tree can be eaten. However, Black people do not grow these trees and if they do they will not eat the leaves unless told to by white people.

White elite clans control dietary behavior and social behavior. The ultimate control of Black people has had a change in name but not in results. For example, slave codes, home rule, states' rights, Jim Crow (separate but equal); civil rights and curfew laws are designed to keep Black people in physical or mental slavery. This sustains the slave and slave master relationship. Curfew laws (new slave codes) are temporary rules that make it a crime for children to be outside after 10 p.m. Violence and behavior in schools result in arrest and/or fines for the parent and a criminal record for the child and adult. Adults and children unable to pay fines can be imprisoned.

School criminal records lead to violence, underemployment, unemployment, crime, drugs, employment as cheap slave or prison labor and the criminalization of Black children. Children's felony crimes cause the need to create more laws that are easily violated. Once a criminal(felon) the Black person is not allowed to be around know felons which means their family or friends and in some cases their own children.

Black people maimed, mutilated, shot or injured in violence become organ harvest candidates. The organ harvesting is the selling of hearts, kidneys, lungs, corneas of eyes, bone marrow, prostates, genital parts, digestive organs, arteries, aborted fetus, veins, eggs of females etc., is a profitable business of the corporate elite. The Americans for Medical Progress Educational Foundation indicates that in order to double the profits of human organ harvesting, there are plans to cut kidneys in half. Added to this are ethnic junk food companies that sell harmful, chemicalized, processed black-eyed peas, collards, corn muffins, sweet potatoes and turnip greens weaken and destroys Black people's health. This helps Black people to become unable to survive physical injuries which makes them organ harvest candidates. White society has changed the name of their White supremacy and have maintained the behavior of slave master and slave relationships.

Fight to Pieces or Eat to Pieces

The mental and emotional signs and symptoms of Caucasian cannibalism are still present in their culture. They continue to have "pretend" meals of human and raw animal flesh. For example, they eat the pretend flesh of the gingerbread boy, animal and human shaped cookies and cereals, vitamin shaped people such as Mr. and Mrs. Flintstones and the symbolic blood dripping from the Christmas sugar candy canes. The Caucasian women continue to symbolically use blood to attract a mate by painting their lips (red lipstick) and claws (red fingernail polish). They continue to eat bloody flesh such as half-raw beefsteak and liver and symbolically pour red blood (tomato catsup) on animal flesh. The irony of this is that the White Race is too psychotic to comprehend their mental illness and too defensive of their inferiority to accept any constructive criticism or therapy or discipline. To attempt to reason with cannibalistic psychotic Whites is the same as doing an African dance without the drum or having a logical conversation with a drunk or drug addict in a stupor.

Confrontation dialogue with Caucasians often leads to violence. Historically violence is the behavior that White culture uses towards Black people, Native Americans, Indians, Koreans and other people of color. Historically, Caucasian violence and fighting among each other was barbaric and unorganized. Typically, when White men fought each other, they would bite and eat pieces of flesh from each others arm's, face, legs, stomach and would gouge out each other's eyes. They would bite off and eat pieces of ears or noses, mutilate testicles, and fingers, which basically amounted to mutilation and cannibalism. Usually after fights body parts, pieces of fingers and flesh would be found on the ground. Defeat was often followed by the further mutilation of the defeated or eating the defeated's heart.

The French attempted to put some law and order to fighting and the British attempted to use the laws of Kingsbury. However, each clan had its own chaos and victory by all means was the only rule for fighting. Fighting resulted in the loss of body parts or life. It is the same with their disease-causing allopathic drug medicine and GMO junk foods. These foods cause Black people to lose pieces of their body (heart, kidney, uterus, prostate, teeth, liver) or their entire body (death).

Crazy White Folks

White Supremacy is a mental and emotional illness that is a psychosis. A psychosis is a total break with participation in the real world.

Black people have been defending their bodies, emotions, minds and spirits from White Racism and in some cases, have become infected by White Supremacy psychosis. White Racism means the power to inflict White Supremacy. White Supremacy is the belief that the White Race is superior without any evidence to support the belief except lies and their diseased imagination. Understanding the nature of the psychotic White mind helps a Black people to defend themselves against a white-dominated world contaminated by White Supremacy psychotics =crazy White folks.

There are nice, kind, caring, sensitive and humane people with diseases (i.e. cancer, fibroid tumors, arthritis). Being nice does not stop the disease. There are nice White people with White Supremacy disease. Being nice does not stop them from being a White racist. Their niceness is mixed consciously and subconsciously with their emotional and mental illness. In other words, they are still crazy.

Psychotic Whites do not accept what is real. They accept only what is imagined to be real and believe what their imagination sees not what their eyes see. They believe, then see and only believe what they see. The nature of the crazy White mind means that sanity cannot be trusted; only insanity can be trusted. In many ways, insanity gives security because it never abandons the White people's DNA.

Historically, the Ice Age was icebergs, earthquakes, land collisions making loud thundering sounds, unstable weather with floods and an unstable breast milk supply which disrupted or destroyed the bond between

213

mother and child and nature. Cannibalism was rampant along with rape and orgies compounded by diseases and nutrient deficiencies that caused mental and emotional illness to be a normal way of life. The White mind in the past and present has emotionally created superstitions to explain and protect their mind from emotional, psychological and spiritual inferiority. These superstitions may have been needed during the Ice Age. However, the Ice Age and Cave Trauma mentality is still genetically part of White civilization. Their emotions and minds show the signs and symptoms of an untreated mental disease.

A healthy, untreated mind may progress from "anxiety" to "neurosis" and then "psychosis" (insanity). However, the White mind has never been psychologically treated for emotional and mental illness and has degrees of psychosis (craziness) that do not lead back to a healthy mind but back to another type of diseased mind. Their fantasy illnesses weave a thought path based upon the mental craziness of Whites as normal. Sigmund(Sick-man) Freud, a European pioneer on the state of the White mind describes the White crazy mind as possessed with sexual conflicts, self-hatred, anger, violence, in conflict with itself and with its parents and siblings and deficient of love. He essentially says the White mind is created to remain constantly in conflict with good and evil or sanity and insanity.

White mind scientists basically say that the White mind is evil or the mind is good and must overcome its evil to self-actualize (to be good). The basic ingredient of the White mind remains a conflict in a marriage of good against evil or sane against insane. Needless to say, the Caucasian mind scientists never explain the White race's disease of White Supremacy and Cave Trauma. Their scientist are too crazy (mentally ill) to accept or see that they are crazy (mentally ill). White folks have episodes of sanity and are superficially sane in many of their mental activities. This sanity collapses if the mental disease of White Supremacy and Cave Trauma is forced to be focused on. They have situational sanity that is united to incomplete thoughts combined with fragments of White Supremacy psychosis.

The White mind lacks a beginning path. Their mind sees itself as evolved from an animal mind state. For example, evolutionist theory scientist Charles Darwin wrote that Whites did not evolve from the human kingdom but the animal kingdom. Whites believe they started millions of years ago as a one-celled slime creature that lived in a cave in the sea, then evolved (changed) into a fish, then a reptile, then crawled or walked to a tree, then became a white skin hair less ape, then climbed or fell out the tree and became a White man. They believe their minds still have the combined thinking ability of a one-celled slime creature, a fish, a reptile, a white skin hair less ape that grunted a few times and then started walking. The White minds still have primitive qualities. Their White mind must be controlled or it will destroy them in order to satisfy the primitive desire to have sex with themselves (masturbate) or their mothers and fathers. They believe in competition and raping their brothers or sisters. They believe their minds to have taboos, superstitions or conflicting (competitive nature) desires and see the world and all animals and plants as in conflict or fighting for food to survive. They believe their minds cannot be trusted—this is an emotional and mental illness.

White mental illness is constantly moving to and from emotional sanity episodes based on emotional insanity. Insanity that runs from a deep belief that the mind will destroy itself in order to satisfy primitive desires. Insanity is co-dependent on sane and insane thoughts that produces more insane thoughts. Their minds protect their insanity. The trust of insanity creates more fear and conflict and mistrust of sanity. Their fantasy and theory based psychology brings comfort to them because in the real world they are insane and inferior to Africans, Chinese, Indians, Japanese and Natives in North and South Americas. This diseased mind sees conflict (good fighting evil) in harmony and harmony in conflict. This is a disease that consumes itself to be itself. The degree of White Supremacy disease is chaotic, then psychotic or neurotic.

In mental illness, there is order and basically three levels. A sane person can freely move in and out of emotional levels, but an insane person gets frozen in a mental state and cannot move out of it. A creative person may use levels of emotions and thoughts to write a novel, or create music or dance or paint art but knows when to use them, and when to stop. The insane person has lost that ability and are trapped in a mental prison. A temporary, mental imbalance is an "anxiety" which is when you get nervous over something real. For example, a person can get anxious about buying a new house. This is a normal stressor and "anxiety" is a normal response.

"Neurosis" is different. A neurotic person imagines unreal dangers about buying a house. They over-amplify the problems of buying a house and get extremely anxious over an unreal association with reality. For example, a drug addict is "neurotic" because he is addicted and has unreal beliefs about the drug and himself. He may believe he is in control and not addicted (can stop when he wants) and at the same time knows he is addicted. A "psychotic" (White supremacist/racist) person imagines that he has bought the imaginary house and believes that he is actually living in the house and will pay the monthly mortgage with imaginary money. This is a psychosis, a total break with the real world. Any attempt by Black people to demonstrate, march, sing, vote, pray, protest, educate or give healing therapy to a racist White Supremacist will cause a defensive reaction. The defense reaction causes fighting back with abusive mental, emotional, or physical violence and more varieties of craziness. The psychotic White Supremacist are no longer

215

capable of solving the psychotic problems that their diseased crazy minds have created.

The White race experiences cave trauma pain from a history of self-abuse, the deliberate murder of 200 million Africans, the enslavement and the colonizing of Africans. At the same time, White Supremacist get a pleasing sensation from masturbating their craziness on Black people. They continue to fornicate all over the world with images of superiority over Black people with movies, violence, chemistry, wars, games, fantasy sports, history, education, biology, politics, medicine, television, radio, colors, music, computers, laws, religion, money, disease, starvation, crime, ecology, nutrition, jails and sex. They satisfy their psychosis by using all activities to make Black people appear inferior. Whites are a juvenile civilization of thugs that entertains itself with ignorance, sex, disease and violence. The White Supremacist lives in the nation of "imagination." Consequently, they demand Black lives to physically, emotionally and psychologically mutilate and sacrifice to their inferiority.

White Supremacy is a mental and emotional illness built on a deep mistrust of nature, God, self, other races and their own race. The crazy Whites direct their illness at something they can see, weigh and measure, called Africans. The White's crazy mind cannot measure or quantify their mental illness. Their craziness is sustained by acts of violence, and by ruling or ruining (destroying) Black people. Black peoples are put in an inferior social position posture by an inferior White race.

A race is measured by its products such as art, science and human relationships. Whites have no sane human relationship with Africans. Whites have demonstrated that they cannot own or create peace, love, spirituality or a harmonious relationship with Africans. Whites recreate what they are inside their psychotic minds. For example, Whites make assimilated and integrated Black people feel honored or blessed that White people have accumulated vast research and knowledge, military power and wealth. They do not acknowledge that they stole the knowledge and wealth from ancient Black people.

Their mind is in conflict with itself. Their minds are violent with superstitious beliefs. They want to destroy the evil part of their mind. So, they re-direct their violence towards Black people that they fantasize as the bad, inferior, and evil part of their mind. They assume that by stealing a statue of God, they have become God. They fantasize that by stealing Black people's resources, land, knowledge, culture and religion, makes them sane. White people are victims of their own insanity. The whites' psychosis lives on conflict (competition) with nature, people, God, life and competition with sanity.

White people's excessive-conflict-and-competition psychosis justifies the murder of over 200 million Africans with their theory of evolution. The mistakes, conflicts, murders, slavery, cannibalism, chicanery and exploitation of African land and Black peoples are explained as a part of White people's process of evolution. White people's enslavement of Black people is merely a step in their self-actualization and manifest destiny towards White Supremacy.

Competition (conflict) requires that one individual wins and the other individual loses. Competition is not a family, communal or people-sharing concept. Whites have their insanity in competition with their sanity and in this competitive (conflicting) state, if sanity wins, it wins insanity and if insanity loses it loses sanity and remains insane. White people are in fear of insanity and hide from insanity in hopes of becoming sane. Sanity causes a fear because it means that White people must accept their juvenile cultural inferiority and stop ownership of the continent of Africa and America. In a sane state, they would no longer be in power. Their sanity requires their oligarchy pirate relationship with China and Japan that helps them inferiorize Black people.

Whites will hold onto their insanity because it is a safe, secure state for them. They have learned to defend insanity with logic, wars, racism, religion, money, education and the mutilation and destruction of Africa and Africans. To call an insane white race anything other than crazy (insane) is to support and nourish White Supremacy. Whites make insanity pleasing and attractive by using violence and sex as an attractive cover (package) for the pleasure they derive from being insane. If this sounds crazy, it is because it is crazy. This is White craziness and cannot sound any other way. A conversation about soccer or baseball will sound like a conversation about soccer or baseball. So, it follows, a conversation about White insanity will sound insane.

White psychotics think that they can escape White Supremacy psychosis(craziness) by reading the autobiography of Martin Luther King or Malcolm X or watching free speech television, joining integrated groups or collecting postage stamps of Bishop Tutu, Joe Louis, George Washington Carver or Marian Anderson. This is the same as a drunk alcoholic or high cocaine addict reading a book about a sober or drug free person and thinking that that will somehow make them sober or drug-free. White Supremacy is a mental disease that makes any brief episode of sanity a horrible experience. Sanity is worthless because it does not give the White people any White Supremacy power. To be a White Supremacist you have to be insane.

The White brain and Black brain may look alike but are melanin and biochemically different. White people are mentally divided and conquered by their cave trauma insanity. Black people that socialize in a White Supremacy society become divided and conquered when they are not African centered.

Whites are divided as a people. Whites do not trust each other or each other's governments. They maintain police to protect themselves from each other. White countries maintain armies to protect their corporate owned countries from other White corporate owned countries. This universal white behavior starts in the White mind. Historically, whites arrested slaves for stealing themselves. In the White mind a slave that ran away (escaped) from the plantation was stealing themselves. Consequently, they were captured and punished for stealing. This is insanity.

Black people that violently fight for freedom and liberation from White Supremacy are violating White people's freedom and are arrested and punished for crimes against freedom and liberty. It is a crazy White mind that can conceive of a crime of stealing yourself or violating your own freedom by wanting your freedom. They have equally and democratically distributed White Supremacy psychosis to all Black people.

Food Terrorist

Caucasians use food shortages caused by famines or climate change as a way to intimidate or seize control of people or governments. This is called terrorism. When food is used to control a people, it is food terrorism. Food control is called marketing. Marketing is the manipulation and control of food for economic profit. Marketing is the fantasy concept taught in all Caucasian colleges. Marketing requires the fantasy of supply and demand on the free market. Invasion is a word that means to capture, steal, exploit, control or take by force (violence). Invasions result in capital gain that means White power. White power means White Supremacy.

The power of White elite corporate businesses to control the food of Black people is White racism and the violation of human rights. It is nutritional terrorism. Food terrorism is another tool of White Supremacy that serves to exploit, dehumanize, disenfranchise, create diseases and destroy Black people for the economic profit of the White oligarchy. The White oligarchy destroys food supplies with their clans of thugs called the United States of America elite corporations, pharmaceutical cartels, the United Nations and other oligarchy capitalist running dogs such as Britain, France, Russia, Japan, China, etc.

The White oligarchy of food terrorist invasions of Africa is designed to make the continent of Africa and its people food slaves. The terrorist captures the land, then uses the land to grow GMO foods. It then switches the Black people to GMO foods that cause diseases and dependency on drug medicine. Black food and chemical dependency required the White Supremacist to create Black people peasant class of landless laborers. The food terrorist learn the fantasy concept of supply and demand and free market to manipulate people to have mental and dysfunctional behavior. They market GMO junk food to Black people and maintain that the food does not cause disease. is not destructive to mental, physical and spiritual health. Food terrorists use food to control the rate of population growth and access to power.

Food-dependent Black people are triage. It is a socially accepted form of genocide whereby the extremely injured/sick are allowed to die while the slightly injured are saved. However, triage can be used with institutions, the poor, businesses, services or a race of people. In the Caucasian triage system of food terrorism, the Black people are made weak or diseased from GMO junk food and the chemicals used in agriculture, and drugs are left to die while nutritionally stronger Black people live.

The triage disease and death causing system is built into the fantasy supply and demand and free market scheme. The marketing policy of the corporate junk food businesses causes Black people to stop eating millet, rye, barley, wild rice, manioc, beans and other seeds in favor of cheap wheat. White corporations sell wheat at cheaper prices than any other grains. This forces poor Black people to avoid other grains. In other words, they no longer buy from Black farmers; they buy from White farmers. Black people have become wheat-dependent. The Black farmers cannot compete with the rich multinational food terrorist corporations. They abandon their farms and do not grow local crops. African land is then used and abused by chemical fertilizers, pesticides and GMO white corporations who grow "cash crops" such as peanuts, cotton, sugar cane, rubber, cocoa, etc. The African's animal livestock industry is made wheat-dependent. Africa's land becomes enslaved. Africans on the undernourished GMO wheat (bleached white flour) dependent diet in cities become violent and fight each other while Africans in rural areas nutritionally starve.

It is an institutionalized, nutritional, terrorist tactic to use Food for the Hunger Programs, United Nations Care Packages, food relief agencies and religious food programs to addict Africans to GMO junk foods. The junk food is believed to stop the diseases that it causes. The White corporations use food to manipulate social problems, strife, disease, epidemics, conflicts and decrease populations (exterminate). They disguise their food terrorism as "food gifts to the hungry." They are giving a "gift" of disease and death to the hungry.

The food terrorist's processed chemicalized GMO wheat-centered diet increases acidity in the blood. The diet of animal flesh, chicken fetuses and milk is highly acidic. The high acid content of the blood is destructive to the bones, nerves, tissues, reproductive system, glands and the brain. It destroys vitamins, minerals and proteins. Eating large amounts of acidic GMO white rice, GMO sugar and processed GMO wheat flour degenerates the pineal gland.

Aside from this, the Chinese sell plastic rice to Black people. It is cheaper than GMO rice.

Processed (bleached) GMO wheat flour becomes manure at the beginning of the 30-foot digestive tract. It slowly travels along the digestive tract, spreading pollution throughout the body. Food should become manure at the end of the digestive tract not at the beginning.

The acidic GMO junk food diet causes chronic physical, emotional, and mental fatigue. Acid foods are constipating. Constipation is the leading cause of melanin deficiencies and causes 90% of all diseases. High acidity causes an increase in bacteria, infections, white blood cells, fibroid tumors, high blood pressure, impotency, high cholesterol, venereal disease, hyper-sex drive, colds, learning disorders, heart trouble, kidney stones, violence, allergies, cancer, degenerative diseases anxiety, nervousness, fear, anger, and cravings for junk food, drugs and sugar. Historically, White food terrorists caused diseases that caused slaves to be physically handicapped.

Physically handicapped Prisoners of War (POW slaves) were sold at cheap prices at "Refuse Slave Sales." Many slaves became physically handicapped or deformed because of undernutrition caused diseases, work related accidents, self-inflicted injuries or severe torture. For example, slaves on slave ships often suffered from Vitamin D and Vitamin C deficiencies, which caused blindness. The slaves would become blind because the eyeball (cornea) would dry up. Many slaves would arrive to the Americas blind, crippled, crazy or dead.

"Refuse Slaves" were sold and used for medical experiments, circuses, or sex experiments with animals. They were used to demonstrate methods of torture or punishment and helped to perpetuate a fear of Whites. It was cheaper to use a Refuse Slave.

A slave master's fear-inducing torture demonstrations included tying each leg of a slave to different horses, then making the horses run in different directions, which pulled the legs off the body. Pregnant slaves would have the baby cut from the womb and fed to the dogs. They would scalp the head of a male, or hang him by his penis, or boil alive a slave. For a "joke" a slave would be placed in a barrel that had nails driven in the sides then rolled down a hill, causing puncture wounds to his body and eyes. The slave master considered this funny.

In addition to these barbarous acts, slaves were made crippled by the food terrorist diet. Any slave who was too handicapped or diseased to be sold at the Refuse Sale was sold at the "Scramble Sale." The "Scramble Sale" was a two for the price of one sale. The slaves sold at the Refuse and Scramble sales today are called organ harvest sales. Instead of selling the entire slave they sell parts such as Black peoples' kidneys, eyes, livers, genetic cells, aborted baby parts, melanin, bone marrow, and other body parts for experiments or transplants.

People in civilizations are trained from childhood to adulthood to like and dislike certain foods. Food selection is culturally controlled. Each race has a different ability to digest food and taste food based on melanin content of the taste buds. Tasting food is a different biochemical reaction and action that is based on melanin concentration of the taste buds and the body. In other words, Black people do not taste food with the low degree of taste sensitivity as White people. The taste sense is bonded to the culture when the child is bonded to the mother.

In White Supremacy society, food tastes are trained and food selection is controlled by food businesses. The food terrorists select the foods that will be eaten and grown. They select the likes and dislikes of foods. In other words, food illiterate Black people are brainwashed food addicts that are programmed to eat junk food by the combined forces of White Supremacy psychologists, chemists, infantile cartoon characters, teachers, religions, color therapists, music therapists, hypnotists and sex therapists. Black people are trained to accept these practices and are trained to eat what they are told to eat. Black people have become assimilationist and integrationist puppets.

White supremacist sciences and therapists are used to design food containers and packages, food jingles, food tastes, food commercials and subliminal persuasions and behavior controllers. The total effect of food marketing makes the Black consumer free to choose the wrong foods. The Black consumer is manipulated and addicted to foodstuffs.

As part of the marketing strategy, illness is blamed on germs, not on junk food. It is part of the terrorists' tactics to ridicule any junk food addicted person who stops eating their chemical garbage. The ridicule and insults can come from friends, family and strangers. The terrorists teach the junk food addict that getting sick, being sick, feeling sick is normal. Black people are made ignorant of food warfare.

Foods are loaded with drugs. In an indirect way, drugs are pushed through food. Food drugs have the chemicals that enslave the body in sickness and handicap the mind. It is difficult for the food junkie to understand or accept reality. Food terrorists make food addicting with chemicals such as, salt and sugar, then claim that Black people are freely choosing to eat the food that they want to eat. This is the same as addicting a person to alcohol or crack cocaine, then saying that because the addict keeps choosing to take the drug, they are exercising freedom of choice. The junk food addict is free to keep choosing junk food to eat because the terrorists are constantly creating the addiction. The terrorist will not turn off the addiction. Since the addiction is not turned off, they say the addicts' constant consumption of drugged foods means that they like being addicted.

221

The Food Chemical Companies say if people did not like junk foods they would not eat them. In other words, an alcoholic drinks alcohol because he likes alcohol, not because he is addicted to alcohol. The chemically controlled mind believes the food drug pushers' brainwashing and advertisements. The food-addicted parents addict their children to food drugs, salt and sugar. There is always a food drug fix available. The sugar addict always has a candy bar, liquid sugar (soda), sugary chewing gum or some other form of sweets available.

The food drug addict does not know that they are addicted. The terrorist says that if the addict (junk food consumer) is stupid enough to like the addictive foods, then they should have the right to keep selling them the junk.

A food drug addict is a living sacrifice to White Supremacy. They are physical proof that the advertisements are successful. The mind-and behavior-altering drugs (chemicals) in the foods clone the Black people. The white corporate own government agencies, food relief agencies, Food for the Hungry religious groups give and sell junk food to starving and poor Black people. The government agencies such as the Department of Agriculture, Foreign Agriculture Service, the Food and Drug Administration, the Red Cross and the United Nations give free demonstrations on how to prepare junk food and free samples in order to addict Black people.

If white society seems concerned about Black people's health, it is merely a method of deceit used to destroy Black people's health. White terrorists use food to control and keep Black people sick. Sickness drains Black people of energy. Sickness is a profitable business controlled and created by the corporate own Sick care industry. Sickness and White Supremacy are the only things democratically given to all Black people. Sovereign Human rights are not given to Black people. Only sickness, White Domination, White Supremacy and White Racism are given to Black people.

The terrorists make Black people believe that drug medicine, natural vitamins, minerals, amino acids, herbs or surgery or inoculations can protect the health of the body from diseases caused by junk foods. There is no miracle drug, herb or therapy that can make junk food addicted Black people healthy. Non- GMO organic foods are the only miracle medicine; medicine is natural foods. Non-GMO Organic food can be eaten raw or steamed and in the correct food combinations to maintain wellness.

Food terrorists use their belief in theory based science superstitions and myths to create horrible food concoctions. For example, White people's ritualistic eating of the grease or pus (essence) of the animal's corpse and the wearing of fur is believed to give the power of the murdered animal. Historically white people ritualistically rubbed animal grease on the body (grease bath) to protect them from diseases. Caucasians still use sheep grease (lanolin) to make their hair curly.

Historically, White people lived their lives without taking baths. They believed that eating or rubbing boar (pig) grease gave the strength of a pig and deer grease gave one the ability to run like a deer. Rabbit grease was believed to give fertility, grease from cooked corpses of Africans gave savage sexual ability, cat grease protects one from mice, etc. They used the animal's rotten grease to make candles. These candles were believed to release the power of the animal's spirit. The candles, when burnt, gave off a foul odor and black smoke that would fill the hut or cave.

White people believed that a breakfast of chicken fetus (eggs) and plant seeds (wheat, rice, corn, oats) used as cereals regenerated the body. They believed that white cow's milk purified the body. Their breakfast foods were put together out of ignorance, superstition and their famine ridden society and currently with fantasy theory based science. Black assimilation and integration multicultural people follow the White race's practices.

The White people used herbs on foods out of superstition. The ancient White people believed that the cold season could be changed to a hot (hot pepper, horse radish) or warm season inside the body by using irritant herbs (mustard pepper). Their herbs served as irritants to the delicate skin of their constipated digestive tract. They called these herbs "seasonings." Herbal irritants, such as mustard seed and black pepper are popular in food concoctions.

Many of the sauces poured on cooked animal flesh were derived from their ancient past. Historically, White people would use a Sauce made of strigil to season dead corpses. Strigil sauce's main ingredient was the pus from a dead whale's intestine. It was similar to A-1 sauce. They liked rotten fish oil in sauces such as Worcester Shire Sauce.

White people and assimilation and integration Black people like to eat the buttocks (behind, ass) or thighs of dead cattle, chickens, turkeys or pigs. They believed that muscle flesh of animals helps to make muscles in their bodies. Added to this, they believed that the hair from pigs (boar's hair) used to make hair brushes could give strength to their hair.

Ancient White people conduct spiritual rituals with animals. For example, the head of an animal (goat, pig) was believed to possess intelligence and represent a gate to a higher evil or heaven. Often, they would put an apple or fruit on dead flesh to gain the ability to give spiritual rebirth. Consequently, they would eat a pig's head with an apple in the mouth or a goat or sheep's head with fruit in the mouth. In order to gain the birth of new strength and muscles, they would put fruit such as pineapple slices on a pig's ass (ham) and then eat it.

They ate food because of superstitions and ignorance and never associated with nutrition, cleanliness or health. Consequently, they did not wash their own bodies, vegetables or the corpse of the animals that they ate. Their idea of cleaning an animal was to drain the blood from the carcass. They would eat dead animals' genitals, semen, ovaries, or cooked Black peoples people's sex organs in order to feel sexually aroused. The food terrorists still have insane attachments to foods that are deeply embedded in their subconscious minds based on ignorance. The terrorists are predatory in their approach to food and exploit Black people with food.

Predatory animals and the predatory White race captures and kill animals. Predatory terrorists capture the land and food supply, then kill the Black people with a junk food diet. Ironically, the White people are the same with farming. They capture the plants with cultivation farming, then process the vegetables which kills the nutrients, then they embalm the dead plants with chemicals (preservatives) and then they eat them. White Supremacists captured Black people and Africa's land, then they preserved the African culture by imitating it, and then they destroyed the Black people by "Seasonin," inferioriorizing and victimizing the Black race. They then kill Black people with drugged foods. Terrorists have the same behavior towards Black people, land and God as they have within themselves. They do not trust their own bodies and are in fear that their health will fall ill to disease at any moment. They mistrust their natural bodies. They mistrust God. They mistrust the nature and totally mistrust Black people. White people have Cave Trauma and self-hatred.

The food terrorists use the same predatory behavior as they did during invasions of Africa, during slavery and colonialism. During slavery, all foods, clothing, discipline and religion came from the slave master. After slavery, Black people became wage slaves or sharecroppers. Wage slaves earn only enough money to survive and always stay in debt. Sharecroppers bought food, supplies and clothing on credit. They paid their debts and rent by giving a large share of their crops to the slave master. They bought all of their goods from the overpriced company store (former slave master's store).

White people use their corrupt predatory capitalist system. Capitalism is a Caucasian money ritual whereby they steal (sell-overpriced goods) and labor from the consumer. They steal by selling cheap goods, at high prices. They then put high interest rates on credit (loans). Caucasian money rituals and ceremonies are called finance, marketing, economics and business. These money rituals and ceremonies use deceit, stealing, lies, sex, exploitation, homosexuality, cheap labor, drugs, spiritual perversion, immorality and dysfunctional families. Fidel Castro said "(White) Capitalism has no moral and ethical values, everything is for sale. It is impossible to educate people in such a (White) environment: people become selfish and sometimes turn into bandits".

Black people that attempt to participate in white people's money ceremonies or rituals must follow the unwritten and unspoken rules of dishonesty, mistrust, deception and ungodliness. White people's money transactions are exclusive and not inclusive of Black people—White only. Black people are aliens in white people's money transactions. Black people are a negative drive for white people and are systematically rejected and punished by White people for participating. For example, assimilated and integrated Black people that accumulate wealth or earn high salaries cannot openly support Black riots, Black revolutions or Black militant groups. If they do show any support, they will be killed, jailed, have their character assassinated or in some way be punished. Black people's money in white societies can only be invested or spent on approved white concerns.

White people view money as stored labor and a way to control people. All profit (stolen money) is considered good. Profit is merely used as a form of White Supremacy.

The new form of slave masters is the oligarchy's multinational corporation. Multinational corporations own the wage slave, the factories, banks, credit cards, prisons, colleges, religions, militaries, governments, media, hospitals, clothing manufactures, farms, pharmaceutical cartels and food stores. They own Black people's taste buds. Black people eat only what the multinational companies tell them to eat. Addicted taste buds only eat what the multinational companies tell them to eat. Junk food Black people become educated so they can work for the new slave master-multinational corporations.

The Black people are addicted to the slave plantation's GMO soul food garbage diet of fried rice, fried okra, fried chicken, greasy overcooked green vegetables seasoned with a pig's ass (ham) or bacon (pork bellies), chitterlings (pig guts), pig hoofs (pigs feet), salt (sodium chloride poison), vinegar (acidic acid poison), deadly food combinations such as milk, grease, vinegar (a drug), salt (a drug), sugar (a drug), chicken fetus, toxic night shade plants (peppers), onions, celery and overcooked demineralized GMO potatoes with nutrient-less Iceberg lettuce called potato salad. This soul food diet, causes disease and death.

The food terrorist armies used many tactics. They burned food crops homes, raped (men, women and children) and lynched Black people to make them abandon their farmlands. After the Civil War (northern colonies invasion of the southern colonies), a military field order gave land and mules to Black people. President Andrew Jackson declared that no general in the military had the right to by pass the governments legal process, the order was not a government approved and it was illegal. Congress ordered the people to move off the land. The Black people refused to move and armed themselves with guns to protect the land. White people said the land was stolen property. The government declared an unofficial 'Negro War" and sent the United States Army in to attack the Black people. The army attacked, murdered, raped, lynched, terrorized, burnt food crops and homes. Then they moved the people off the land at gun point.

The Black people that were not murdered during the Civil War were land less had to become sharecroppers. After the war, white soldiers were given land and the black soldiers were given hats or bicycles. Black people bought land that was illegally stolen by whites for what was claimed to be tax frauds. Black people became landless peasants who had a choice of starving to death as wage slaves or moving to northern ghettoes. Black people became refugees, exploitable, landless peasant wage slave laborers. This same food terrorist tactic was repeated over and over in Africa or anywhere that the white people wanted to steal land and steal labor (wage slavery).

The Food terrorist created food starvation as a means to make Black landless refugees. It has never been a case of Black people starving because of lack of farmland or lack of food or overpopulation. It has always been a case of white Food terrorists causing starvation to disguise their control of land and food. Food terrorist thugs such as the United States Department of Agriculture, Foreign Agricultural Services, Department of Commerce and the Agency of International Development, use wheat to destroy African farmers. They use Public Law 480 to switch Black people and Africans' livestock to an acidic, wheat-centered diet.

White people's rituals (laws and agreements) with each other, government control agencies, judicial systems, alliances and consumer protection agencies amount to the insane controlling the insane. The oligarchy's weather modification agencies are out of control. Weather modification is the process of changing the weather with concentrated heat radiation or chemicals or metals (aluminum). Chemicals are sprayed into clouds to force them to retain more water, which results in rain. However, making rain in one area causes a violent interruption of the natural weather cycles. This results in the negative rebound effects of droughts, hurricanes, forest fires, insect attacks on food crops and people and crop destruction.

Weather modification companies' reactions to bad weather is another chemically change of the weather which causes another negative rebound in the weather. They use the weather or climate change to destroy each others' crops in order to create food shortages which result in increased profits. The weather modification companies have weather wars among themselves. The National Science Foundation has stated that billions of dollars and an uncertain number of deaths are caused each year by weather modification.

These companies are controlled by the out-of-control corporate owned government. This means the insane are controlling the insane.

Food terrorists use weather climate change and food as a weapon. These weapons create diseases and death in the name of "money" or "profit." Profit and paper money (currency) are white peoples' way of worshipping White Supremacy. White peoples paper money (U.S. dollar, British pound, etc.) are their corporate owned governments paper credit cards and represent money stolen from their citizens. White people's terrorist use of food, climate and weather indicts them, and history verifies this indictment.

Historically, European civilization exploited Africans with food The Portuguese (name means stomach people) invaded Africa, burnt homes, raped men, women and children and destroyed crops in order to force Africans to work on peanut, rice, coffee, cotton and other quick cash crop plantations. This tactic of "rape, pillage and burn" was used in many African countries. The United Nations Environment Program and the International Crop Research Institute for Semi-Arid Tropics stated that the damaged land, crops and food supply are lost forever. Terrorist destruction of farms and farmer's forces Africans to be wheat dependent. The combination this disease-causing diet and the disease-causing chemical pollutants called fertilizer, pesticides and medicine destroys the so-called immune system. Food has been the most reliable weapon the white peoples corporate owned oligarchy has used to a control Black peoples. Black people become addicted to GMO junk food and emotionally, mentally and physically controlled by addiction and diseases until death.

The food terrorist use Black people's denial of disease to addict them to GMO junk food, drugs, sex, White religions and White cultural captivity. Food addiction indicates a failure to accept self. Failure to accept self is denial. Black people fail to accept their racial and cultural superiority. Black people are obligated to their ancestor's demand for a revolution for freedom (i.e. race war). Denial is used to hide pain. The emotional pain of being defeated by white people, enslaved and colonized has never been confronted or resolved.

Denial disease relies upon the continuous inability to face true reality. True reality is substituted with a false reality. Denial allows its victims to victimize self by accepting White reality as Black people's reality. Denial is a disease forced upon Black people by White people. The White people's psychotic reality denies their physical, emotional, mental, and cultural inferiority by creating a fantasy craziness called White Supremacy. They cannot and will not accept their inferiority and criminal deeds against Black people. If Whites accepted their crimes against Black people, then self-punishment or suicide would be the only logical action for Whites to take. Denial is the basis for the slave and slave master relationship. It is a failure of a people's group personality (culture) to allow their diet and self to be continuously enslaved by primitive Whites. Black people have failed to accept that White people are insane with moments of sanity. Denial of the mental illness of the white race supports denial of white people's Cave Trauma. They ignore and dismiss Black people's slavery trauma. Denial is needed to hide from reality. Black people deny junk food addiction and addiction to White people. Addiction is the failure to accept reality.

Black people free of the emotionally crippling impact of slavery/colonialism realizes that white people's junk foods are an extension of white people's insanity. Their worldview is based on ignorance, superstitions, and a mistrust of nature. Denial is a silent weapon used to destroy the Black people's ability to heal themselves from the pain of slavery or colonialism. Black people in denial use drugs, alcohol, sex, social media, violence upon each other and food to satisfy the sensual taste buds and the hurt of slavery. Food not only becomes a form of pleasure, and is used to soothe and pacify the ugly pain of denial.

Food terrorists must maintain the Black peoples' denial disease in order to maintain White Supremacy. They use nutritional Uncle Toms Black scientist or fictitious nutritional Uncle Toms such as Uncle Ben (rice) and Aunt Jemima (pancake), LeBron James, Oprah, etc. in order to keep Black people addicted to junk food, denial and fear. These nutritional Uncle Toms are victims of the food terrorist.

Fear combined with denial are the psychological devices used to sell food. Food terrorists believe that the more "rich food" you eat, the more health you will attain. Health is associated with quantity of food, not the natural quality of non-GMO organic food. Poor quality processed junk foods, dairy products and cooked chemicalized animal flesh cause nutritional starvation. These foods cause the body to rot. The muscles get hard, the bones get soft and the teeth rot and fall out. The feet, armpits and body stink with foul fumes caused by constipation or pollution of foods. Junk foods wrinkles the skin, the eyes and ears. Circulation decreases and the physical degeneration caused by drugged foods is called old age.

The "rich foods" are greasy, oily and heavily seasoned with herbal irritants. The "rich foods" also contain high amounts of acidic MSG, cooked meats and various cooked concoctions with stupid combinations of sugar and starch, or starch and protein. They are worshipped as "good food." People are made to believe that if you miss one of these rich meals, or miss any meal, you will lose energy and evil bacteria or virus will attack your body, causing a disease. They eat in fear these attacking germs.

White people have a compulsive eating disease, which is based on a history of cave life, famines and starvation from the Ice Age era (10,000 years). Post Ice Age era (5,000 years) and Cold era (2,000 years). During the Cold Age, white people started inhaling the fumes of their own bowel movements (manure) and sleeping with dogs, goats or pigs in order to use the foul odors as a sort of antibiotic evil spirit.

They would drink, have bowel movements and bathe in the same polluted water that they used to cook food. Cleanliness was not related to health, but related to myths, superstitions and fears of nature and the belief that nature or an evil spirit was always attacking them. White people's pagan rituals of fighting evil germs with antibacterial creams, lotions, soaps, mouthwash, toothpaste, deodorants, douches and cleansers is unscientific and creates antibiotic resistant and superbugs.

They kill germs with antibiotics, alcohol or bleach. They sterilize cow's milk (pasteurization), pots, surfaces, clothes, dishes and utensils. They forget that sterilization only lasts a few minutes before the germs return. Black people have adopted the White people's insane notion of killing evil germs and their sanitation medical rituals and ceremonies. Black people become twice as addict to white ignorance. Black people are attached to the white insanity by the white belief system and by their denial of the slavery trauma.

White people's fear and denial of reality makes their medical rituals and ceremonies seem logical. For example, they believe that taking a poison that is against life =anti-biological (antibiotic) is sensible. It is fear that supports denial and denial that supports denial, which is the foundation of the addiction to junk foods. The corporate elite oligarchy marketing tactics do not separate the rich and the poor, slave and slave master, technology and pollution, food and disease, peace and war, sex and love or good and evil. Their mind bonds and mixes ideas and behaviors together that are not related. Food is mixed with politics, wars, economic profit, chemicals, pollution, violence, etc.

Black people only see food as a connection to ancestors, God and nutrition. Food to White corporations is a weapon to control and terrorize. Black people's connection to food has to be a self-defense reaction to the food, the race war, White Supremacy and the disease industry as one in the same problem. White people do not and cannot separate tactics or actions outside their reality. Food terrorism has to be destroyed because it is part of and not separate from White Domination, Cave Trauma, White Supremacy and their juvenile civilization.

Food terrorism is part of a chain reaction of factors that react to each other and support each other. In this chain reaction, Black people are mentally and socially terrorized. The terrorist tactics keep Black people's mind crazy. For example, white people's money rituals of the institution of banking is alien to most Black peoples. People lend money to the bank which is called a deposit, then the bank gambles with the money. If the bank gambles and loses your loan money the government gives them more money(bailout) to gamble with and lose. This is not logical. It is the white people stealing money from poor Black people and calling it banking. Banks are not a building or business, but a social institution created by the white race to support their race exclusively. A bank is a coalition of white people who share the same rituals of thinking and behaving. Institutions require a ritual so they can trust and have reliance upon each other. Ex-slaves and colonized Black people are culturally homeless and their culture was shattered and is not intact to protect them so they are easy to "seasonin (brainwash)" and made to mistrust each other. The terrorists continue to maintain an atmosphere of mistrust or "seasonin."

During slavery Black people were made crazy by "seasonin". "Seasonin" was (is) a psychological conditioning process in which slaves were made to recite positive affirmations about the goodness of slavery and the White race and negative verses about the Black race (catechism) combined with performing the same menial task daily. The "seasonin" could last from a few weeks to months for chattel slaves. "Seasonin" slaves were made to mistrust other slaves and to feel that "niggers ain't no good and cursed by God." Modern "seasonin" occurs when Black people are trained by food commercials to sing positive music jingles and or recite positive slogans about harmful junk food.

The constant use of "seasonin" by Food terrorists is apparent in banks. Black people were made to mistrust each other. Because Black people mistrust each other they cannot as a group save money and lend money (interest free) to each other. They are "seasonin" to put money in the white slave master's bank. It is anti-Black to use White banks. White banks are White nationalist banks because they support White businesses that terrorize Blacks. White nationalists share the common disease of White Supremacy. Ironically, during post-chattel slavery Black people had savings clubs in which each member would contribute part of his pay each month. Each member would get a loan of $1,000 or more every six months. These savings clubs became part of burial societies and churches and they no longer exist. However, the contemporary "seasonin" process of the terrorist still exists.

White Supremacy terrorists must continue to make Black people insane (crazy). An insane Black person is an alien to their own culture. Cultural suicide occurs when Black people pay money for disease and death causing junk foods. A terrorized Black person sees food terrorism as separate and divided from White Racism, politics, jail, special education and disease. When a Black person lives in White culture and Black culture they are divided and conquered. A conquered mind is an alien and assimilated and integrated in White culture is confused, crazy and mentally terrorized mind.

White Supremacist teaches the craziness that Black people in white cultural captivity and controlled society have freedom of choice. Freedom of choice implies that you have "free will." Black people have the freedom to follow White rituals and ceremonies but no control over them. Life, Liberty and the pursuit of happiness can only be realized if you have a group that can protect you and attack your enemies. "Free will" requires that a group has ownership and control over resources and the military power to protect the group. Therefore, Black people fantasize that they can seek justice in the judiciary system by following white legal rituals and ceremonies. However, White people as a group control the judiciary system. Therefore, justice can be denied an alien ("seasonin" African). Similarly, Black people are free to choose different types of junk foods, but lack the power to ensure that it is not GMO or contains toxic poisons.

It is a terrorist tactic to maintain Black "seasonin." Black people "seasonin" themselves by various subtle means. For example, the Ebonics (Ebony =Black phonics) languages of Africans are labeled as Black English Negro Dialect, Gullah or bad English. Ebonics is the language that Africans speak. It may use English words, but it has distinctly African conceptualizations, word order, rhythms and consonant clusters at the end of words (i.e. "I be goin."). The Caucasians speak a Latin and German derived language (60% German words) which they call English. They do not label English as a bad Latin, German Dialect, bad German, or White German. English is labeled as a language. Mislabeled and negative connotations applied to Ebonics helps to make the Black people culturally alienated, confused and terrorized.

Properties and stores in the ghetto are owned by White people or their puppet racial groups (Asians, Arabs, Koreans). However, terrorists blame the creation of the ghetto poverty on Black people. Black people rent the ghetto, they do not own it. The White terrorists are in the ghetto business, poverty business, junk food business and the disease industry because it is economically and psychologically profitable. Profit is anything that supports White Supremacy. The only way for white people to make a profit from Black people is to keep them "seasonin" crazy (socially engineered) and terrorized.

A pregnant teenager is a tool of the terrorist. Teenage pregnancy is labeled as hypersexual, immoral and a symptom of a dysfunctional Black race. These increases stressors in the Black community. Stress, hypertension, violence, fear and denial cause an increase in marijuana alcohol, drug and junk food consumption. Historically, the white population in America was started by teenage pregnancy; slavery was maintained by teenage pregnancy, single unwed mothers, produced Black violent children and cheap child labor. During slavery, White men (pedophile) were raping Black girls and boys and the white (pedophile) women's rape of Black boys and girls produced mullato children that was free labor.

All Black people that are married by White people's rituals, ceremonies and religions are "unwed" and have bastard children. Teenage pregnancy is not the problem. It is the social conditions created and maintained by Supremacist terrorists that are the problem.

White cultural captivity social terrorism cascades and perpetuates food terrorism. For example, Black people that suffer from White racism, "seasonin", stress, hypertension, fear, denial and violence, eat more junk food. They are easily made addicted to the chemicals in GMO junk food and drugs. These chemicals not only alter the thinking, but also cause retarded genital growth, infertility and sexual identity problems. This adds to the slavery traumatized Black people being afraid of other Black people. This slavery traumatized "seasonin," causing Black people to identify with White culture.

Assimilated and integrated Black people call themselves Americans (Whites). "American" is a mislabel that denotes slavery, murder, rape, stealing and White nationalism. White people invaded Turtle Island. White people renamed the island America and themselves Americans. Black people cannot be Americans because they never voluntarily gave up their African citizenship. The mislabeled American assumes that Black people paid for their transportation to America as slaves and voluntarily gave up their sovereign human rights or African citizenship. Assimilated and integrated Black people celebrate White American holidays, eat American junk foods and contribute to the tension of terrorism.

Black people are miseducated in white schools and colleges become aliens to African Maat culture. They graduate and are respected (academic success) and suspected (became white). White institutions support the myths, superstitions, and lies of White Supremacy. Black college graduates and executives in White corporations are respected and suspected. They believe and fantasize that the European culture's idea of academics is the only type of academics of value. Black people in these white curriculum, white and black schools are majoring in White Studies. White Studies alienates the mind of Black people from African culture. Black aliens believe that health means the absence of obvious diseases. They go to optometrists who wear eyeglasses and dentists who have no teeth. They are trained to be blind to contradictions about health practitioners.

Black cultural aliens believe in the sex contraction that homosexuals can have sexual intercourse. Only a man and a woman can have sexual intercourse. Homosexuals merely masturbate each other. Black aliens believe that sexual intercourse means the same as love. They refer to having sexual intercourse as "making love or sleeping together ". These assimilation and integrated Black people have difficulty adapting holistically to African culture. Their attempts to adapt cause stress, confusion and terrorism to other Black people. Terrorists destroy holistic Maat sex and cause problems in the Black race. They are cloned with junk foods, junk medicine, junk religions and junk sex.

Aliens use the language they are "seasonin" with by Caucasian media (movies, computer programs, television, books and textbooks). Their language is based on the movie rating categories of Parental Guidance (PG 13) and Restricted (R). Consequently, they believe adult language means the use of curse words, profanity and obscenity. Black people's adult words are "I respect God in you." "I honor your presence," etc. Often, cloned Black people use the words "boyfriend and girlfriend" to indicate a sexual relationship. In African culture, a sexual relationship is based upon a mating with God and families (marriage). They refer to each other as a "mate." Caucasian language concepts maintain "seasonin" resulting in a Black mind too crazy to stop having junk sex and too crazy to stop being crazy.

The Black aliens who victimize African history, ancestors and the raw food diet are "seasonin." These Black aliens believe that their great ancient culture became weak, had serious social problems, religious conflicts, too much humanity, tribalism and egotism, which caused Black civilization to self-destruct. It is within the natural cycle that all creation (people, plants, cultures, planets and religions) adjust, readjust and change. The White exploitation of Black people in their changing process is a crime. White people are guilty of committing crimes against Africans in the process of change. The White Supremacy, crazy White people, have committed the crime and then blamed the victim. In other words, a woman who is raped is blamed for being raped =victimizing the victim. White terrorism is a disease trait of White syphilization (civilization). Black people that have intimate relationships or sexual intercourse with white people and have culturally mixed-up mullato children that help to maintain social White assimilation and integration of the Black race.

African Ecology and Caucasian Pollution

The world's first ecologists in recorded history were Africans of the Nile Valley. Ecology is man's relationship to the environment (plants, earth and animals). Humans must bond to their mother and father (the seen) and the spirit (the unseen) before they can relate to the environment (the seen created by the unseen). Black people learned Maat, harmony and human relationship, which is called spirituality. Therefore, African ecology is merely an extension of the relationship between their mother and father (seen) and Mother and Father God (unseen). Africans did not pollute or destroy the harmony of nature because to do so is a form of self-destruction.

Pollution of the earth (Ta) is historically an act of White civilization. In the White cosmology (worldview), the planet earth exists to serve their needs. It is not a give-and-take relationship. It is not a spiritual relationship.

Therefore, they treat Mother Earth as a slave. Caucasians rape the land of resources, mutilate (clone) and pollute the air, water, soil, sound (noise pollution), vision (artificial and perverted natural light reflected from buildings, glass, cars, concrete, asphalt, etc.), clone and exterminate plants, insects, animals and people. The earth, outer space and Blacks have become polluted garbage dumps of White technology. African civilization demonstrated the correct holistic behavior relationship to have between Ta (earth), in Ake-Bu-Lan (Africa), in Khui Land (the ancient state of Egypt), and in the nation of Khemet (black soil valley areas of the Nile).

The Hyksos (Caucasians from the Oxus Valley area), and other Europeans who invaded or traded with Africans were called vile, primitive and wretched people. White people had a limited vocabulary, did not bathe, were flea-infested, practiced group sex, raped, stole, murdered, were bed wetter's, drank pus to cure disease, had no religions, were disorganized liars, urinated in the streets, were superstitious and ignorant, believed the earth was flat and were constantly diseased. Their behavior among themselves and negative treatment of the land caused Africans to pity them and want to help them become civilized and ecology minded.

The African worldview (cosmology) sees each of us as custodians or servants of the land. The land is a living spiritual gift from God. Loving the environment and earth is Erapi-hati-a (hereditary) for Africans. Black people's bodies are the Pher (house) that ecologically resides on Ta. Black people give to Ta and Ta gives to Black people. This is the homeostasis (balance) that African culture has taught human beings (hue=black, man =thinking). The Ta (earth) is viewed as a spaceship (mothership) that carries Black people on a journey by day and by night through the heavens so that they can rise in God's presence. Africans who believed their spirit would resurrect in the West were called Osirians. They were believed to have gone west to be born anew in the Sun God's (Ra) presence. They were called Westerners. The White people's ecology is not a harmonious relationship with earth. They take all that they can from the earth and give back pollution and destruction. This is contrary to the ecological wisdom of the human body.

Junk food is processed and against the ecological wisdom of the body. For example, vitamins, minerals, fibers and proteins are milled or chemically taken out of whole wheat, brown rice and sugar cane, leaving a pasty, concentrate processed substance (synthetic manure). Basically, the food factories have machines that are similar to the liver, pancreas, stomach and intestine. These machines digest the food (process) and the end result of processing a food is a bowel movement. Technically, a processed food is synthetic manure. Eating processed (machine digested) food is against the body's wisdom, circadian rhythm and ecology. The normal ecology of the body follows a solar and lunar cycle, melanin rhythm and allows each organ to use the food's nutrients. The end product of whole food digestion is manure. Processed junk food starts off in the stomach as manure. This is contrary to the body's natural ecology. A junk food diet causes disease and death.

Black people claim the spiritual nature of life and foods by eating non-GMO organic foods. The spiritual rights of food as a spirit is ignored by White theory based nutrition, science and medicine.

White theory based science reflects white peoples' world-view and behavior. For example, any human (or vegetable) right that is not claimed by violence is not respected. The white people do not respect the vegetables, spiritual rights. They apply the same human ritual and ceremony behaviors called laws to all aspects of life.

Ignorance of white people's rituals (laws) of human behavior is no excuse for accidentally violating white people's rituals (laws). They demand that everyone know their rituals or be punished.

The White corporate elite oligarchy company's relationships to people, science, the body, nutrition, and food is a series of rituals and ceremonies which they call "law" or a "Fact." The White fantasy (theory) science rituals (experiments) are used to determine what is real and what is unreal. When a White scientist can perform the same chemical trick or physical ritual twice, then it is considered a fact. In other words, since God has not made the same person exactly twice (duplicated perfectly), then God is not real. In nature, even identical twins are not exactly the same. White science rituals are not directly related to nature, spirituality and God. They are related to their rituals. African science is directly related to the ecology of nature and God. Therefore, Ancient Black people did not pollute or disrespect the ecology of the earth or the human body.

The human body is an ecologically perfect system. For example, the liver takes waste from by-products of digestion and turns them into bile salts, which are used as digestive enzymes that break down food. The lungs breathe in air, and exhale carbon dioxide. The lungs use the carbon dioxide to regulate breathing in and breathing out (negative drive). The large intestine (colon) recycles electrolytes and water in food by extracting the minerals and water from digested foods. Minerals are recycled and used to make hair and finger and toe nails. The body's ability to recycle nutrients and melanin is hampered and destroyed by synthetic junk foods, polluted water and air, eating animal flesh, dairy products, alcohol, cooked cannabinol or nicotine drugs, White sugar, salt (sodium chloride), oils, bleached flour and vaccine drugs.

Vaccine drugs are pollutants that poison the ecology of the body. Pollutants, poison and waste stored in the body cause diseases. Taking vaccine drugs are a superstitious ritual performed by White theory based medicine in health treatment ceremonies called medical care. Vaccine (inoculations) drugs are based on the ignorant belief that the human body will not react, so-called immunity. The body always reacts to stimulants, food, drugs, rain, the sun, sound, touch, taste, odors, spirituality, electromagnetic forces and the environment. A body that does not react to disease either positively or negatively is not immune, but dead.

The body is never immune to life. Bodily cleansing or so-called dis-ease reaction is a life function. A living human cannot be immune to living or bodily reactions. In any case, vaccine drugs are made of the diseased cells of animals and humans. Vaccine drugs use a concoction of pus and unsterilized human or animal blood, Hela cells (short form of a Black lady's name, Henrietta Lacks, uterine cancer cells), added to diseased kidney cells from the Green Monkey, cells from the pig's stomach called trypsin and toxic poisons. This polluted concoction is injected into the veins of Black babies and adults with a hypodermic needle and called medicine.

All vaccine drugs are chemical garbage that destroys health. This includes the "pus soups" called polio, diphtheria, measles, mumps, rubella, small pox, malaria, tetanus and Influenza vaccines. White junk food companies put polluted drugs into the body to protect the body's natural ecology. This is in contrast to African centered medical scientist that extend their relationship with nature by using non-GMO organic food as medicine. Oddly enough, the ancient African's garbage dumps were spiritualized with plants and treated like living spiritual organisms.

The ancient cities of Africa had city dumps that did not pollute or destroy the ecology. These city dumps were surrounded by plants. Plants served to use the rich compost of the garbage dump, protected garbage from insect overpopulation, keep the soil in balance, maintain moisture, stop soil erosion and provide food, herbs and beauty. The garbage dumps contained plants such as henbane, apricot, flax, acacia, marigold, olive, myrtle, chrysanthemum, plum, fleabane, basil, and pomegranate.

Ancient African builders used medicinal herbs, fruits and vegetable plants in designing temples, cities, irrigation channels as well as garbage dumps. Ineni under King Tuthmosis I (1528-1510 BC) was an herbalist who designed gardens and garbage dumps. Sennufu the mayor of Thebes during the rule of Amenophis II (1425 BC) was in charge of the medicinal herbs and vegetables around the city dumps and cemeteries. There were many medicinal herb stores (flower shops) in the Egyptian Empire. They supplied medicinal herbs for private and public dumps, gardens, clothing, food storage, ornaments, wearing apparel and offerings. The herbalist Nekht during the rule Amenophis III (1375 BC) was in charge of the official medicinal herbs and ceremonial usage of herbs for the city.

Ancient Africans, in order to prevent the wasteful accumulation of paper packaging, used herbs for packing, storage of food and the protection of food, clothing and household items. Herbal packaging was used to protect cloth and foods that were to be transported by ships, horses, camels or wagons from insect damage. There were herbs pictured in the Theban Tombs of the 18th dynasty. Herbs gave a pleasant scent to stored items and respected a spiritual energy. Natural, herbal packaging could be brewed as teas or used as poultices in medical care. This is in direct contrast to the White corporations' wastefulness and pollution.

Ecology of the body and Ta (earth) are one. Living with spirituality means respecting the body and eating natural foods and morality for the body is not consuming anything that pollutes the body. This belief is built in the African family, diet, medicine and Maat lifestyle (culture). The African Maat lifestyle uses animals and plants in the written language, arts, cyclic laws, astrological science, architecture and fabric designs as a way to emphasize a spiritual ecology with nature.

In every area of African society, a reverence and respect for the environment is evident. For example, the Egyptian kingdoms we named after plants, insects and animals such as Bull Cult, the Bee King (Lower Delta Kingdom) and Papyrus (reed) King (Middle Kingdom). In African ecology, the family technology was used. The Ancient African people viewed Ta as Mother and Father Earth. Disrespect for the environment was considered disrespect of the privilege to obey God's will. Any destruction of Ta was destruction of God's spirit reflected by your Mother Father (parents and family). Therefore, any destruction of Ta also destroys your "hue (Black) man (living)" being.

Ecology keeps the holistic balance of a person. This human ecology is reflected in the person's relationship with their family, culture, diet and God. The practice of human ecology is learned by a harmonious interaction with other races and nature. Consequently, environmental ecology merely mirrors humanistic ecology. The smallest unit of ecology is the family. There must be harmonious, unconditional love between one race and another race or there cannot be ecology with the environment. It is a human imperative that ecology be preserved.

The world has become a garbage planet because of the pollution of white corporate own oligarchy companies and China and Japan's corporate oligarchy companies. The white race's inability to protect and save themselves from disease and infertility reflects an error in human ecology and a mental illness. For example, the United Nations census of world population indicates that white people are at zero population growth. Black people in Haiti will double their population in 30 years, while White people in Italy may double (probability mathematical guess) their population by the year 3000. They plan to curb their decrease in population by constantly promoting sex in all types of advertisements such as toothpaste, automobiles, deodorants, toilet paper, soap, chewing gum and hair product commercials. They use movies, news reports, sports, religions, weight loss, magazines and music as a sexual stimulating tactic to increase their population.

White people's continued abuse of nature and Black people dooms them to be unhealthy. It must be remembered that they had a population decline of between 8th and 1/100th of the world population before they started the race wars with Black people and the Natives on Turtle Island (America). It was after the invasions of Africa that they had an increase to 1/6th of the world population. The current decrease in population is viewed by them as another cycle of the decrease then increase then decrease population pattern. In the past, their decreases in population was caused by pollution of the water, the absence of hygiene, famines, diseases and war. Their destructive human ecology causes the new types of destruction to the environment. It is totally insane to ask the White people to practice ecology without military enforcement.

The White oligarchies new types of businesses use genetics to clone vegetables, microbes and people. These freak species of vegetables, animals and microbes do not fit into the natural ecology. Nature does not have a method of control to keep these freaks (clones) in balance with the environment. This results in a new type of pollution heaped onto the current pollution. A freak ecology is required to balance these freak "life forms."

The White businesses that create these clones do so to maximize profits. Cloned microbes are used to accelerate food, animals and vegetable growth, give them a cosmetically healthy appearance and allow poor quality produce to live until sale time. Cloning companies use massive bioreactor tanks to grow genetically altered microbes such as E. coli, bacillus, thuringiensis, methylococcus, thiobacillus, bdellovibrio, etc. These microbes are used in copper mining, to make plastic, treat telephone poles, prevent frost on oranges, in therapeutic baths, public water, etc. They grow meat flesh with fermented clone fungus, make plastic rice and eggs with synthetic flavorings from clone animals. There is no agency policing, or military or legal power to make White people behave.

The ecology of planet earth is on a death course. Black children are being terrorized with cloned vegetables, artificial meat and synthetic dairy products, vaccines, drugs, environmental pollutants, and dysfunctional parents. The Black children are chemical freaks (hyperactive, learning disorders, etc.), controlled by freaks (junk foods, fairy tales, psychologist, etc.). Their holistic health degenerates with constant disease. This results in their being placed in Special Education classes (prison holding cells) leading them ultimately to be place in elderly concentration camps called nursing homes.

238

It is the moral duty or curse of Black people to save their children and save this planet from White Supremacy. There is no compromise with the curse. Either the Black people will give the planet ecological freedom or the White people will continue to imprison the ecology with pollution and biological freaks. Black people cannot leave the fate of the planet on Natural, Karmic, Devine, Prana Laws or a Prophet to correct the polluted, off-balanced ecology. It is the responsibility of all Black people to correct the Caucasian people's misbehavior because Black people are the living Natural, Karmic, Devine, Prana Laws and the living Prophets. Black people's duty is to make the earth healthy so that the children can be healthy. Without a healthy planet, there cannot be a healthy culture or healthy people.

A non-GMO organic natural food diet gives a healthy body, which allows people to have a holistically healthy spirit, family and culture. Health means to protect ourselves and protect our living quarters, called the earth. It is a matter of life or death. It is life of all living forms that is at stake. White people do not behave. It is Black people's Maat duty to make White people behave. White people must confront their Cave Trauma Disorder and White Domination psychosis.

A Diet Without Chemicalized Meat is Healthier

A recent study conducted by several medical doctors, show that Seventh-Day Adventist, for religious reasons do not eat meant have:

- ∞ 40% less coronary disease
- ∞ 400 % less death rate from respiratory diseases
- ∞ 100% lower mortality rate from all causes
- ∞ 1000% lower death rate from lung cancer
- ∞ 50% less dental caries among their children

The Homosexual Plague and Food

The Black Peoples Homosexual epidemic is a social engineered emotional and mental manipulation forced upon them by White Supremacy. Homosexuality is beyond an epidemic and has become a plague in Black communities. Homosexuality is normal for the nature of White people, but a disease by Black Maat standards. Homosexuality is not an accepted part Black culture. This plague is used to maintain male and female relationship problems and conflicts, divorces, single parents, populations, sexually confused children. Children raised by homosexuals cause sexual problems with heterosexual children. This makes them distort their perception of self. It destroys   Maat and replaces it with white societies sexual values. The white junk food business, movies, television shows, cartoons, games, commercials, actors, scientists and politicians promote and support it as politically correct sexual behavior. Every white television or movie or news reports, or school teachers must have a homosexual character or a homo sexual person known out of the closet homosexual in the cast. The white corporate oligarchy businesses are the main creator and promoter of the Homosexual Plague. They confuse and mix natures reality to promote homosexuality. Everything (social or material) in a capitalist society must produce capital. Consequently, homosexual behavior creates capital or it would not exist.

Sexuality is hormonally defined before being born in the third prenatal month the testosterone hormone level rises causing the baby to be a male. The testosterone hormone takes a default path causing the baby to stay a female. The decision on whether a person is male or female is made by nature before birth.

The sex organs in animals have a hormonal function. The ovaries and testicles secrete hormones. The mouth and buttocks and sphincter muscles of the rectum do secrete hormones. They cannot physiologically be identified as having a sex function. The mouth has teeth and enzymes which identifies its function of chewing food to eat. The sphincter muscles that controls the release of the rectum's manure identifies a man's behinds function of bowel movement manure control and not a sexual function. The mouth and sphincter muscle can be used for masturbation of another person's sex organ but not perform sexual intercourse. Sexual intercourse means the penis enters the course(shaft) of the vagina. Masturbation cannot physiologically be called sexual intercourse. Two people of the same sex can masturbate each other but not have sexual intercourse. Sexual intercourse has different rituals and ceremonies with each animal and insect. Some animals and insects dance, make sounds, do pretend fighting and change colors of a body part (some monkey's get red tails). Insects and animals do not copy the rituals and ceremonies of other insects and animals. There can be similarities in their sex rituals but they never copy others rituals. The homosexuals copy the sex rituals and ceremonies of the heterosexuals. In nature, the sex organs of different animals and insects are different. The homosexuals have the same sex organs as the heterosexuals. Sexual intercourse in nature can always cause the conception of a child. In human homosexuality, their sex cannot produce a child.

Sex and gender are different. Gender are the behaviors associate with males and females. For example, in this society females wear lipstick, high heels, eye make up and while sitting with a dress on females are not allowed to open their legs wide. This is some of the activities associated with the female gender. Copying the gender of a Lion does not make you a lion. Copying a male or female's gender does not change your sex organs. The homosexuals

240

copy the gender behavior of male or female heterosexuals. This does not mean a change of sex organs. Gender and sex are two different things. The advertisement industries use gender images, oral and physical sex movements, and sex organ images hidden in shadows, clouds, smoke, or color combinations, painting, foam, shapes and movements and shapes of food.

The junk food industry uses psychosexual packaging, sexual food shapes, hidden images of subliminal sexual intercourse with animals, same sex intercourse, pedophile sexual intercourse, suggestive images of masturbation and oral sex, erogenous body areas, and embedded sex curse words in advertisements. They socially abuse and condemn anyone or a social institution that will not support the homosexual agenda.

The entertainment media uses sexual symbolism such as shadows, tunnels, hairstyles, landscape, hills, clouds, water and sexually suggestive language to sell homosexuality. The synthetic chemicals and sex hormones in the foods stimulate the sex organs, emotions and mind. This causes stimulating, biochemical sexually addicting foods to be associated with stimulating sex. In other words, the Black people become chemically addicted to sex.

The chemicals, sex hormones, steroids, endocrine disruptors in junk foods can cause the corpus colostrum (middle brain) to malfunction and degenerate. The brain begins to distort and confuse normal messages and loses its ability to censor information. This denatures and perverts the biochemical ability to harmonize the Left-Brain (Male Principle) and Right Brain (Female Principle). This limits Black people's ability to bond harmoniously with the complimentary (opposite) sex, which can result in homosexual tendencies. In experiments, the biochemistry of vegetarian gorillas and monkeys was perverted when they were forced to eat junk food and meat. The perverted biochemistry combined with living in a type of European colonialism (science laboratory cage = ghetto) and social confinement, isolated from free moving animals in a free environment which makes them become culturally homeless within animal culture. This causes them to turn on each other sexually and physically. This contributed the break down and fragmentation of the animal culture. Homosexuality can contribute to the break down of sex as a social language. White peope do not connect sex to culture, spirituality and or see it as a holistic language. Each culture and race has a different sex ritual and ceremony. There is not one culture (white homosexuality) that fits all peoples. Each animal, insect and plant has a different sexual ritual and ceremony. White homosexuals violate natures social systems and force their idea of a multicultural homosexuality sexism on Black people.

White psychology, biochemistry and hormonal norms can cause physical diseases. This can result in emotional and mental diseases, which can lead to homosexual creation. For example, diseases of the lungs can cause denial and fear, disease of the pancreas indicate lack of control; heart indicate irregular lifestyle; circulatory, high blood pressure indicate mood swings; liver can indicate unstable personality, etc. Black people have become biochemically perverted. This combines with slavery or colonialism trauma causes Black people to become easy prey for the junk sex (homosexuality) and junk food industry. Black people are deliberately taught homosexuality is acceptable. This makes commercials to easily seduce heterosexuals into homosexuality.

The hidden (subliminal) and subconscious sex in the commercials is directed at the voluntary brain functions of the emotional mind and senses. The controlled thoughts of the voluntary brain's intellectual mind may say that there is not sex hidden in the commercials, but the uncontrollable involuntary brain's emotions and senses respond to the sex. The White culture miseducates, teaches memorization, and discovery of information and indoctrinates and trains the senses to respond to sex images involuntarily on a subconscious level. The food industry's use of sex hormones in foods, sexually stimulating colors, patterns, music, sex symbolism, psychological manipulation, masochism, sadism and shapes is subconsciously selling homosexuality imagines and feelings and thoughts to Black people.

The sex is suggestive as well as sensual, such as penis-shaped hot dogs, candy bars, fish and breadsticks; the use of circles to symbolize the vagina such as donuts, pizzas, cheerios, round candies, or grapes and cherries for testicles; whip cream (semen) on pies (vagina); pyramid shaped whip cream with cherry on top female breast symbolism, ice cream (semen) in a cone (vagina); melted cheese (semen) dripping from a menstruating tomato filled pizza (vagina); liquid caramel or chocolate (semen) dripping on or from a candy bar (penis); a woman's lips (vagina) sucking on a drinking straw (penis); two ice cubes (testicles) and a straw (penis) in a glass (vagina), soda (semen) pouring out the neck (penis) of a bottle or an explosion to symbolize a climax, the suds of soap, shampoo or detergent do not help with cleaning the suds are there to symbolized semen etc.

The leaf of lettuce on a hamburger (beef) sandwich symbolizes the fig leaf. The myth of the fig leaf that covered Adam and Eve's genitals. Lettuce is not put on a sandwich for nutritional reasons but for sexual stimulation. The Black scientist's book *Isis Papers* by Frances Cress Welsing and a Caucasian book *Subliminal Seduction* by Wilson Bryan Key can give information on this subject.

The ancient primitive heterosexual White civilizations included homosexuality as part of normal heterosexual life. White mind scientists (i.e. psychiatrist, psychologist) classify homosexuality as normal and overeating as a disease. Ancient European females and males had four simultaneous mates which were (and are) the (1) breeder - so-called spouse (2) prostitute (3) lover-same sex mate (4) and concubine (non=emotional attached girlfriend or boyfriend sex acquaintance). There are still remnants of these mating type relationships such as sex triangles and orgies that are part of soap opera dramas, movies, television shows, computer games, social media relationships, etc.

The ancient Greek and Roman heterosexual males and females would attend live pornographic sex plays and sexual stimulating same sex wrestling matches in the arenas and gymnasiums. White people measure each other's sexual ability by the movement and or shape of the buttocks and are constantly looking at each other's buttocks. White people emotionally find that the upper portion of the breast and cleavage resembles cleavage space that separates the two the buttocks. Therefore, the breasts are sexually exciting. White people suck on each other's tongues (French kissing) because the tongue is sexually associated with the clitoris (lesbians) and penis (gay men). Junk food commercials use emotionally stimulating and subliminal homosexual symbolism of the buttocks, breast and the mouth to mimicking oral sex to arouse Black people into eating junk foods.

Homosexual behaviors are deeply woven into the fabric of heterosexuality. White women with dresses sit with their legs closed or crossed because in the past homosexual men in skirts sat with closed legs so that they would not reveal the size of their penis to possible lovers. In fact, Caucasian women basically dress themselves like men so that they can be sexually appealing to White men. Consequently, they wear G-string panties and bikini underwear and bathing suits because they were worn by homosexual men in ancient times. White women wear the ear, vaginal, nose, and navel rings as a form of sexual bondage. They shave their arms, under arms, legs and vagina pubic hair to physical mimic young boys available for homosexual sex activity and wear wet lip looking lipstick to indicate that they have semen on their lips from doing oral sex. It is the White involuntary emotional mind that believes that the highest form of masculinity is male effeminate behavior. Therefore, the more male the female model's physical appearance small breast, no fatty round hips they resemble a young pre-puberty teenage boy ready to be homosexually raped, this makes the skinny female model appear sexy. The White woman is the most sexual attractive and feministic when she subconsciously resembles a pre-pubic boy. In other words, lesbianism is a high form of maleness which is a form of femininity. This is attractive to the White male. Therefore, white men enjoy watching lesbians having sex because it stimulates their homosexual eroticism. Masters and Johnson's sex research indicates that homosexual fantasies are sexually arousing for White heterosexual men. They constantly have female homosexuality in pornography movies.

For more information on White homosexuality a book such as *Love in Ancient Greece* by Robert Flaceliere can be helpful. Ancient homosexuals would kidnap young boys/girls during full moons and sodomize them as part of mating with them as a lover. This homosexual ritual was called a "honeymoon." Heterosexuals still use moonlight for homosexual sexual arousal. White people's ancient sexuality, rituals, customs, taboos, and ethics are based on rituals that call their social laws called "The Law of the Caves" which they erroneously call the "First Laws of Nature," "Human Nature," "Nature" or "The Laws of the Jungle." There were no jungles in Ice Age Europe just caves. The White peoples use the word "jungle" in reference to their society in order to inferiorize the 11% jungle on the continent of Africa. This use of jungles makes their civilization seem superior. White people get subliminal, perverted emotional sexual stimulation with an imaginary hyper sexed Black savage by using the word jungle. Imaginary and subliminal homosexual themes surround their heterosexuality behaviors.

The constant junk food commercialization subliminal homosexual images and sex words causes thoughts and behavior of homosexuality. Black people that eat junk food are economically supporting the homosexual social engineering programing of behaviors, emotions, and images. The Black people with signs and symptoms of "Homosexual Exposure" are those in constant social contact with a homosexual peer, friend, associate or relative with homosexual emotionalism and behaviors. Those exposed need treatments. Those with the homosexual behavior need detoxification.

It is mandatory for the Homosexual detoxification that homosexual victims stop eating sex hormone non-organic junk foods, attend an African Study Group, Female and Male Heterosexual Group, abstain from sexually stimulating homosexual movies, songs, books, videos, dancing and games, stop using sexual curse words, stop masturbation, abstain from sex for two to three months, stop all homosexual social activities , practice Maat, avoid all non-sexual intimate personal and social relationships with homosexuals, take a stress formula supplement, use herbs to physically cleanse the reproductive systems, use a female or male herbal formulas, be in contact with a detoxed homosexual mentor and or psychotherapist and take supplements to reduce craving for sex such as Glutamine, Vanadyl Sulfate, Glycine, Taurine, SAMe supplements and chickweed herb (reduces craving), etc.

Those that practice Homosexuality are in all religions, sports, movies, television shows, politics, entertainment fields, social life and children's classrooms. The Homosexuals have developed political and economic power, which allows them to force their homosexuality upon Black people. Black people's resistance to sexual emotional manipulation is weak. The weakness that makes a Black person easily to engage in homosexuality is directly and indirectly caused by reduced emotional stamina, decreased emotional ability to protect themselves, and an inadequate emotional vocabulary. The dominate white culture has approved homosexuality and use their White Supremacy, Cave Trauma Disorder and the damage of Slavery Trauma to force it upon Black people. If a Black person does not and will not approve homosexuality then they are somehow label as homophobic or hate homosexuals for reasons that are sign and symptom of a mental illness or Black person is not politically correct or practicing a form of racism that is equal to sexism. Many Black people do not approve of White Supremacist, abortions or Crack addicts and or alcoholics socializing with them in social activities. They are not labeled abortionphobic, crackphobic or alcoholphobic. It is a matter of African centered culture. Black homosexuals are not free to make a sexuality choice. Freedom of choice requires being able to practice your culture at all times and in all situations and you must have a Black race that defends your rights and able to attack your enemies. Unfortunately, the Black race is in white cultural captivity and are only free to serve white people as entertainers, or in politics, the military, educational system, health field, government jobs, prison etc.

Black peoples use of homosexual behavior is based upon being in a state of cultural captivity in the dominate White civilization. Captivity comes in many forms such as social, mental and emotional. Cultural captivity is indicated whenever a Black person accepts as non-cultural or not racist the white educational systems. A Black is in mental captivity if they believe that White religions do not contain white culture or that the white terrorist USA is a peaceful country or the greatest country in the world, synthetic food and disease as natural, malnutrition, taxes, predatory loans, accepts Fascism as Patriotism, eating disorders, homosexuality, credit debt, predatory mortgages, leases, etc. White Racism makes the Black cultural consumer dependent upon White culture for education, foul (full) employment, culture, money, or drug medicine and homosexuality. Black people are addicted to white people's culture and addicted to white people's sexuality which includes homosexuality. And, like all addicts they have many alibies, justifications and reason to stay addicted. Blacks are a captive audience and vulnerable and easy to economically exploit. Black people are cultural consumers that are sexuality consumed by White cave culture. They are constant victims of white cultural control by White Domination, White Supremacy, and White Racism. The White culture spreads its sexual ideas and behaviors thru social media, textbooks, movies, television shows, art, music, cartoons, science fiction movies, sports, and commercials. Black people are miseducated sexually and do not know African sexuality, mating rituals and do not say a prayer before sexual intercourse. Most Black History celebrations do not claim or present African centered sexuality. They assume that white sexuality is their sexuality and white people's food is their types of food.

The pharmaceutical corporations processed drugs, chemicalized junk food, hybridized, GMO nutrition less junk foods cause the body to be in sick. These foods and drugs make the body, mind, emotions, and spirit weak and sick. A sick emotional (season) Black person is an alien of their culture and only follows the alien cultures social rituals and ceremonies and this includes an alien sexuality. Black people are biochemically, sexually and socially controlled by white cultural junkies. An addict constantly craves a white cultural fix and pays for a homosexual fix that never fixes their African centered natural need to be African and free. The White culture never restores the African centered culture's sexuality.

Black people do not pay African centered attention to their own sexual systems they rent white culture's homosexuality. White people own their culture's homosexuality can make it important in social value. They can exclude Black homosexuals whenever they choose. Because, Black peoples culture and sexuality is not taught or exposed to Black people. Black people rent White culture, the continent of Africa and all resources and goods while the White culture owns their sexuality and homosexuality. White homosexuality has a value created by White people. Every time a Black person uses white sexuality and homosexuality, it is paid for by molesting African sexuality and taking away their culture.

The white cultures sexuality is an emotional type of surrogate Black family. Historically, the Black culture controlled sexuality, spirituality, social order, education and protection. White cultures sexuality is another White supremacy corrupt institution. All white institutions support white culture and in no way support Black culture. Their institutions are White Nationalist design by whites for whites and always exclude Black Culture. If the Black homosexual sees white culture homosexuality as humane and inclusive of Blacks then that homosexual institution cannot be White Nationalist. Homosexuality is White Supremacy in another form. A Black person that sees white homosexuality as separate (divided) from white culture, White domination, and White Racism, then that homosexual has been divided and conquered by White Supremacy. It is the creation of racism, wars, police brutality, and murders, and economic debt (taxes, loans, etc.) that causes disease and addiction. Addiction to white culture and their rituals and ceremonies of homosexuality is in a state of emotional fantasy. When a Black person believes that their emotions and mental state is the same as a white homosexual or they believe they have the same rights or same prejudices as a white homosexual then they have been emotionally and culturally divided and conquered by White Supremacy.

White Sugar and Homosexuality

Concentrated sweeteners especially white sugar are the main addicting drug of the of the food corporate elite oligarchy. White sugar is a mixture of synthetic chemicals, bleach, acids, antibiotics, carbon dioxide and cooked sugar crystals. A combination of cheap, diseased scrap meat (TB, cancer, etc.). Contaminated blood albumin of pigs, cattle and chickens used in sugar to flush protein particles out of sugar beets/ sugar cane. This means all concentrated sweeteners such as white sugar is a pork sugar. The purpose of adding sugars to foods is to cause addiction to the foods.

Pork and other slaughter animal's albumin is used to make the sweetener aspartame used in NutraSweet, Splenda (roach killer chemicals plus pork sugar), Sweet and Low, Equal. Pork sweeteners such as white sugar and aspartame help to create an unstable personality with irritability and mood swings that result in dysfunctional behaviors and jail. Unstable personality can be easily manipulated into assimilating and integrating into White people's sexual behavior such as homosexuality. Aside from this, processed concentrated sweeteners like white sugar are dangerous.

The white sugar stimulating food commercials create and maintain eating disorder dis-eases. White sugar addiction causes uncontrolled impulse and behavioral disorders that result in biochemical perversion that causes behavioral perversion. Addiction to sweets is a vicious cycle of controlled eating of sweets then relapse into uncontrollable sugar eating. Relapse can be triggered by food commercials. Most people with a sweet tooth/sugar addiction know that they have it and if they do know, they never can stop eating sweets and or sporadically. People with a sweet tooth (sugar) eating disorders eat to relieve stress, tension, racism, depression, anger, worry, anxiety, attention deficits and hyperactivity, have eating binges, weight-loss diet binges, have sex hormone attacks, abusively use laxatives, colonics, chewing gum, hide food, constantly eat at movies, sports events, while watching television, riding in cars or planes or subways, busses or trains, constantly eating sweets or sweet junk food snacks, chewing gum, sucking on sugary breath mints, drinking sweet sodas, etc. They may have all these behaviors or a few and are in denial that they have a sugar eating disorder. The concentrated sweetener industry wants people to constantly eat sweets so that they can constantly earn profits. With each craving for sweet snacks and foods is attached the emotion of the need to give or receive love. The commercials of sweet foods keep the diet out of order and the sugar addiction out of order. Psychosexual stimulation, craving and addiction of Africans is aimed towards homosexuality.

African and Caucasian Sexual Beliefs

Caucasian	African
Surgery and chemicals can change your sex and redefine sexuality	Surgical and chemical sex organ mutilation cannot redefine sexual gender
A male / female that follows the sexual behavior of another gender becomes that gender	A monkey cannot follow the sexual practices of a lion and then call him / herself a lion
A woman's breast cleavage are sexually erotic because it resembles the cleavage of the buttocks	Buttocks are associated with bowel movements (Europeans associate the cleavage of the buttocks with the cleavage of the breast)
The behind (buttocks) are sexually erotic	The buttocks are associated with male homosexuality
Homosexuality is a lifestyle choice	European "Seasonin" creates African self, mother, father, relationship and/or Black race hatred
Homosexuality is psycho-social	Homosexuality can be caused by synthetic chemicals or radiation, which causes deterioration of corpus colostrum and/or damage to the smaller bundle of nerves in the hypothalamus resulting in homo-masturbators.
Sex drive	Reproductive drive
Genetic possibility for disease is normal /healthy	Genetic possibility for diseases is not normal. The genetic hybridization of disease is cloning people for disease industry
"Nature" is a non-cultural scientific term	The word "Nature" and "Science" are political and social terms of a culture. They are culturally based.
Evolution	Adaptation
Opposites Attract (man attracted to woman means one is opposite in sexuality)	Balance Attracts (man attracted to woman means both seek harmony / balance) They are complimentary sexes.
Homosexual	Homo-masturbators (Same sex masturbators) anti-sexuals (the mouth, teeth, tongue and lips are made for eating, the anus is made to pass out manure)
Same sex intercourse	Only a female and male can have sexual intercourse (the penis enters the course (pathway) of the vagina

248

African Sex Organ, Energy and Movement

Female Sex Organs
> Inside body (Earth element)
> Close together
> Move East to West (Fallopian Tubes)

Male Sex Organs
> Outside (Testicles) and Inside (Prostate) = Air Element
> Far apart
> Move South to North (Scrotum and Testicles) move up and down

Caucasian Homosexuality Recruitment Techniques

∞ Homosexuals must constantly recruit or become extinct as a group because they cannot reproduce.

∞ Promoting sex change surgery and hormones as normal. It is mutilation of the sex organs with a knife or synthetic sex hormones.

∞ Women dressing in ancient Greek homosexual clothes (i.e. bikini, G-string, high heels, pony tail (penis) and pigtail (penis) hair styles suggest that the tail is attached to buttocks

∞ Fashion industry controlled by homosexuals = "Cross Dressing" = "Homosexual Dressing" (Zipper in front of ladies' pants, bikini underwear for men - with no front flap, male boots for ladies, "unisex clothes, homosexual hair styles," etc.)

∞ Advertisements and commercials that focus on Buttocks (displaying cleavage of breast and symbols of the vagina, penis, and buttocks)

∞ Non-gender specific (cultural) dancing Homosexual

∞ Promoting and inferiorizing heterosexual activity as violent or unstable (domestic crimes, rape, divorces, single parents, adultery, etc.)

∞ Sexual symbolic use of guns (penis), ball games (testicles), symbolism of baskets, holes and pool pockets as hole of the vaginas, goal post is women's open legs for sex, the score of "0" (vagina) is destroyed by the number "1" (penis).

∞ Homosexual themes in elementary school story books (i.e., I *Have Two Mommies)*

∞ Sex words that have no gender that are applied to homosexuality -- "Go to bed" "Make love" "Sleep together"

∞ Homophobia defines people that reject homosexuality for physical, social or spiritual. The do not fear or hate homosexuals and do not accept the behavior as normal.

∞ Songs, movies, soap operas, books and sexual crime news reportage used to create hyper sex and homosexuality as an outlet

∞ Heterosexuals presented as having many relationship problems, while presenting harmony in homosexual relationships

∞ Non-gender = Unisex = One Sex = Homosexual deodorant, perfumes (cologne) tattoos, ear and body rings, clothes, hairstyles and slang words.

∞ Advertisements and commercials that focus on:
  ∞ Non-reproductive sexual behavior projected as normal (masturbation, pornography, phone sex, watching sex stimulates homosexual eroticism)

∞ Women being called by Lesbians names = "Guys," "Man"(sexual cross-over language)

∞ Homosexuality explained as a normal acceptable "Lifestyle Choice"

∞ Advertisements and commercials that focus on:
  ∞ Exercise equipment marketed with sex poses and homosexual symbols
  ∞ "Double Your Pleasure," advertisements that show fun between same sex - homosexual theme
  ∞ Homosexuals being idolized on TV shows, Talk Shows, professional athletes, movies, etc.
  ∞ Drag Queen (Female) dressing by Black male actors = homosexual subliminals

∞ Job applications and tests for jobs are deliberately designed to cause homosexual ideation to score higher (i.e., The Brain Watchers, Martin L. Gross)

∞ Religious shows used to raise emotions and misdirect emotions by making homosexuality as normal spirituality

∞ Homosexuality pictured as a happy, normal life = GAY

∞ Advertisements and commercials that focus on:
- Beer with white head of foam (semen)
- Sexually shaped foods and candy
- Penis-shaped candy bars with nuts, named after men (i.e., Clark bar, Babe Ruth)
- Lip movements suggesting oral sex
- Hot dogs (penis) placed in between buns (buttocks)

Homosexual Addiction

TREATMENT
∞ Must bond to African Maat-defined heterosexuality (culture)
∞ Must have basic needs of spirituality, emotions, family, shelter foods, freedom, health, and met
∞ Must provide personality and sexual adjustment
∞ Counseling must be at arm's length and not allow homosexual flirting, erotic gestures, jokes, and body movements.
∞ Abstinence from all homosexual related activities, intimate non-sexual friends, and homosexual and heterosexual intercourse

Homosexual Addiction

Steps in Treatment

1. Bond to Maat, African culture, and natural foods

2. Confront issues of sexual abuse of rape, incest, etc.

3. Identify activities, feelings, and thoughts that trigger homosexual feelings and sex activities

4. Confront emotional and spiritual issues concerning sperm abortion, rape, sex abuse, child abortion (murder), infertility, fibroids, and prostate disease

5. Heal relationship with self, family, friends, culture, etc.

6. Design methods to change negatives behaviors and emotions to positives

7. Evaluate achievements (rewards, punishment, etc.)

8. Follow treatment schedule, goals, relapse therapy, etc.

9. Stay in constant contact with mentor (advisor) detox homosexual, heterosexual, support or study group, female/male group, psychotherapist, etc.

Withdrawal Crisis

∞ Craving Addictor
(Social, Emotional, Biochemical Triggers)

∞ Depression
(Death of a behavior, Lifestyle, Friendship, etc.)

251

∞ Denial of Addiction/Disease
(Alternative lifestyle, Genetic, don't like opposite sex because of negative sexual experience, etc.)

∞ Stressor can cause Relapse (Death, unemployment, divorce, food addictions, masturbation, money problems, Alcohol, Drugs, White Supremacy)

Withdrawal Steps

Anxiety
Fear
(Won't get better, Challenge of heterosexual life, Rejection, etc.)
Anger

Self-Hatred		Race Hatred

Analyze Self ← → Analyze Addition

Analyze Self	Analyze Addition
↓	↓
Bond to Culture (Reclaim African Life)	Co-Dependency (Reclaim European Sex Life)
↓	↓
African Centered	European Centered Alien Sexuality
↓	↓
Life	Death

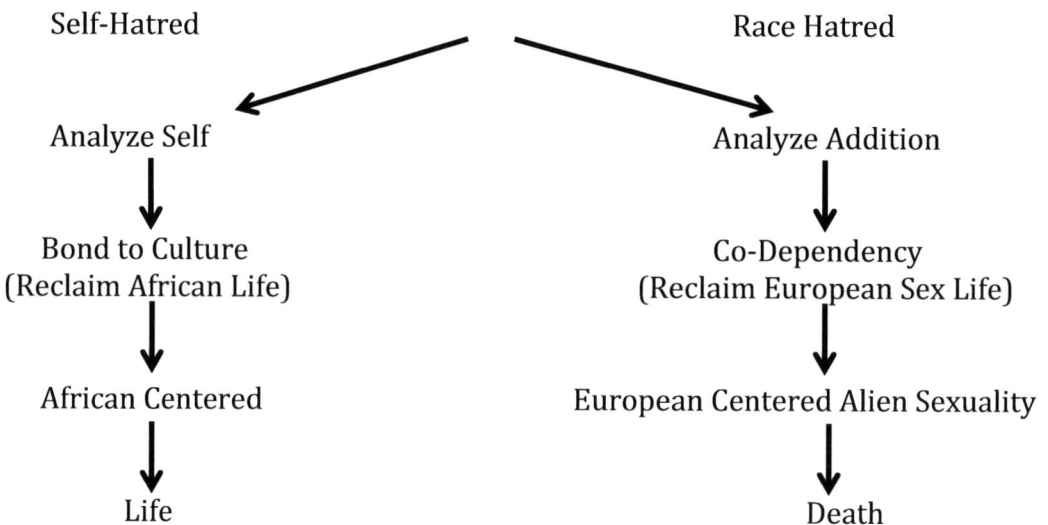

Homosexual Treatment / Detoxification

Diet
●No junk foods, alcohol, drugs, cooked cannabinol (marijuana)

Supplement
●Beta Carotene

●DHEA

●Phenylalanine

●Pumpkin Seed Oil Capsules

- Evening Primrose Oil Capsules
- GABA
- Glutamine
- Manganese
- Melatonin
- Chromium

- Histidine Glycine
- Selenium
- Serotonin
- Tyrosine
- Vanadium
- Vitamins A, C, E, B6

Psycho Social Treatment

∞ Abstinence from heterosexual and/or homosexual intercourse

∞ Abstinence from sexual-related dancing, movies, songs, etc.

∞ Participation in African spirituality group, women's group, men's group, cultural group, study group, support group

∞ Mentor (Sponsor): talk with daily. Mentor must have empathy and/or have been detox from homosexuality

∞ Positive emotional support from family and/or peers

∞ Abstinence from socializing and/or activities with active homosexuals

∞ Meditation, Egyptian Yoga

∞ Abstinence from sexual-related "words" and clothes

Herbs

Bilberry
Catnip
Chamomile
Chaste Tree Berry
Chickweed
Echinacea
Elder

False Unicorn
Feverfew
Gingko
Golden Seal
Gotu Kola
Ibogaine
Kudzu

Milk Thistle
Pau D'Arco
Sarsaparilla
Saw Palmetto
St. John's Wort

Juice or Foods

Alfalfa
Beet
Burdock
Celery

Cherry
Currant
Kelp
Lemon

Papaya
Pineapple

Factors

- ∞ In recorded history is a practice of European and Asian civilization and White cultural captivity.
- ∞ Is directly and indirectly (sublime) a part of European heterosexual activities
- ∞ Social conditions (engineering) creates homosexuality
    - o (schoolbooks, movies, television, clothes, organizations, etc.)
- ∞ Is a sign and symptom of European causes
    - o Slavery Trauma
    - o Cultural Stress
    - o Population Control (Genocide)
    - o Dysfunctional Genders, Relationships and Families
- ∞ Is part of Africans trying to be accepted by Whites and form of self-hatred and hatred of Africa co-dependency psychosis, assimilation, integration
- ∞ Homosexuality is a disease for Africans but normal for Europeans

Science and Addiction

White people's chemistry is the theory based science of studying the activity of chemicals called elements. Elements are non-living things (do not have carbon) and are not alive such as oxygen, calcium and hydrogen. They are the building blocks for organic carbonated living things and so-called organic chemistry (have carbon). Elements such as carbon, hydrogen, sulfur and phosphorus form atoms, which join together to form molecules. The elements sodium combines with Oxygen form Potassium. The element Potassium and Hydrogen combine to form Calcium. Each element is a universe within itself that has a type of family structure. The way a culture sees an African family kinship group and sees the world and the family is reflected in his culture's science of chemistry. The White theory scientist, in order to understand chemicals, first destroys the elemental family with heat or another substance. White scientist do not study elements in their natural relationship to other elements or elements in their environment. Instead they study their culture and then study their culture as living and nonliving substances in an artificial fantasy environment called a laboratory.

The theory based White scientist can only gain knowledge by destruction of life. The more destruction the White civilization causes and produces the more "scientific" and wealthy they become. White people's theory (belief, fiction) based science is a "science fiction" science. White scientists act out their cave cultural superstitious rituals, ceremonies in a laboratory by exploiting chemicals. No scientist can divorce himself from his culture's worldview (cosmology). They cannot become "objective." This is a human impossibility. White people label this destructive biochemical alterations, rituals and ceremonies as science. They act out their culture in labs.

In the food industry, White scientist use chemistry to destroy the natural nutrients of food by processing foods into biochemically-altered food "stuffs." Food "stuffs" (drugs) are sold by fast-"food" chains, sugar refineries, dairy, meat, fish, soda, snack and flour mill industries. The destruction of food creates diseases. Diseases create wealth for the Disease Industry (i.e. hospitals, pharmaceuticals, doctors, laboratories, etc.). The "food" disease industries cannot be separated anymore than can technology from pollution. In the White civilization, you cannot have one without the other. Everything white people do has a side effect, with their construction comes a form of destruction.

In order to change the food industry or any part of white society, the cave culture and White Supremacy foundation has to be changed. White rituals, ceremonies, theories and myths would have to be changed. Black people are hurt by white people's rituals and ceremonies and addicted to white people's rituals, ceremonies, theories and myths. White people's rituals are erroneously called science, law, economics, nutrition and culture. Caucasians culturally based thoughts and behaviors are hazardous to Black people.

Alimentary canal food processing plant

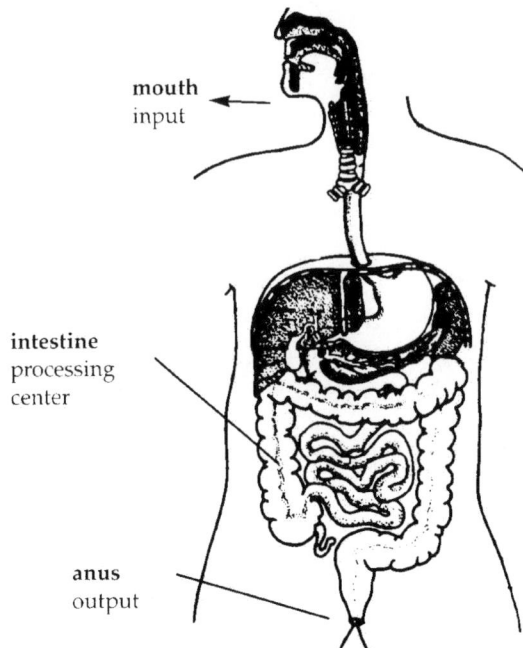

Processed food is synthetic manure type of dirt. The machines and synthetic chemicals in the food-processing factory imitate the Liver (makes a type of lye), pancreas (alkaline food), digestive enzymes (break apart), stomach, intestine, colon (takes out water) and rectum. These machines chemically and mechanically chew and digest (process) the food, which means they break apart the bonding between the vitamins, gases, minerals, water, fiber, proteins and oils. The end result of your body digesting (processing) processed is feces, manure, a bowel movement or scat (also named given to a type of jazz singing). A totally processed food by definition is a bowel movement. The processed hole in the villus (hair) inside the intestine and then into the blood to the Liver. The whole food such as an apple has to be broken down into very small particles. The small particles of eaten food has to be able to pass through a hole in the intestine's villus. The villus is a type of hair with a hole in the center similar to a drinking straw. There are many processed foods such as Bleach White flour, White rice, white sugar, concentrated sweeteners, salt (sodium chloride), oil and white grits are a processed bowel movement of a factory. These are waste by products of a factories digestion-a foodstuff, food contraband, starvation food, junk food etc.

Alimentary canal food processing plant

mouth _____
input

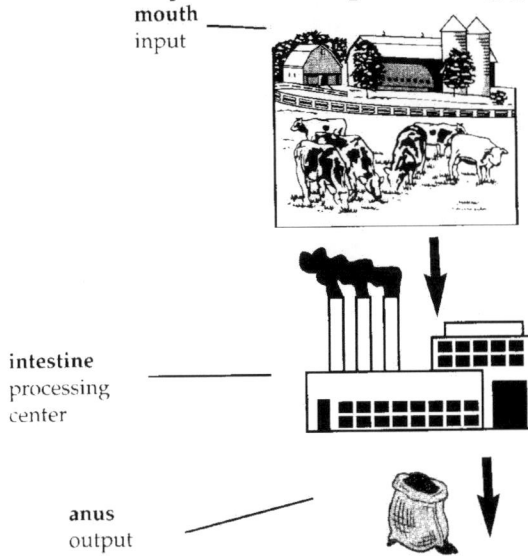

intestine _____
processing
center

anus _____
output

Caucasians suffer from Supremacy Psychosis, Cave Trauma, diseases and famine, violence prone to violence, consumed with self-hatred, invaders and food illiterate. For ages, they have turned natural organic foods into synthetic chemicals, GMO foods, and chemically altering the soil to alter foods. They use chemicals in warfare to invade countries and to control people. They used the alcohol chemical on the Native "Americans," opium on the Chinese and alcohol, cooked marijuana oil drug, heroin, Ritalin (hyperactive drug) and cocaine on Black peoples. White people have been (and are) addicted to synthetic chemicals such as white sugar, cooked nicotine, cooked caffeine, sodium chloride (table salt), energy stimulating drinks (types of caffeine), sex stimulants, cocaine, vinegar, oil, opium, muscle building steroids, valium, amphetamines, etc. They are addicted to the taste of burnt sugar in molasses and Bar-B-Q burnt wood oil smoke in meats. They are addicted to rotten food such cheese, yogurt, buttermilk, beef jerky, rancid oil salad dressing and sauces, hardtack (dried fish), beer (fermented-rotten barley), wine (fermented-rotten grapes) as well as the rotten cooked blood and pus of juicy steaks, chicken, pork, etc. Historically, White people ate many foods based upon them smelling like urine and/or feces (manure). For example, cucumbers were eaten because they smell like semen, roasted animals smell like rotten decomposing human bodies, asafetida smells like farts, cabbage smells like salted rotten fish, some cheeses and onions smell like human feces, tobacco resembled the smell of stale urine, vinegar is similar to human sweat or an unclean vagina (sexually erotic to White people), fish are similar to vaginal yeast infection smell, etc. The more food is corrupted, made into a synthetic rotten processed eatable junk food, loaded with toxic chemicals and hormones, burnt or smoked the more they like it.

The more the Black people are destroyed or processed (social engineered) and assimilated or integrated into White culture the more the White people like them. Black people have become synthetic, clone, drugged, and fermented (rotten Black people= culturally home less). Poor Black people are forced to buy cheap sugary junk foods because organic non-GMO foods are too expensive. Black people have become culturally homeless and biochemically and emotionally altered slaves serving White slave masters or searching for White masters to serve. Socially engineered Black people worship White people's **superstition myth based theory** science, biology, chemistry, economics theories, rituals (laws), and sugary junk food diet etc.

Synthetic chemicalized, sugars cause mental, emotional, and physical changes in sperm, eggs, children, and babies. Black babies have undeveloped immune systems while the adult elderly have deteriorated immune systems. Concentrated sweeteners are twice as harmful and addicting to the children and elderly Black people. Biochemically altered newborn babies are born with diseased emotions and mentality and bodies because of their parents were cesspools of synthetic chemical sugars. Many Black babies are born as sugar addicts, and are severely emotionally, mentally, and biochemically altered.

Black people are addicted to toxic concentrated sweeteners because of the biochemical trauma of Cesarean section (C-section/birthing interrupts). The C-section interrupt the birth bonding process, alters the biochemical personality, cause emotional problems, allergies, learning problems, asthma, self-control deficiencies and suffer hyper-sex. Processed sugars lack over 90% of the natural occurring vitamins, minerals, proteins and fibers. They are especially low in a B vitamin called thiamine. Thiamine, along with the B complex (family), is needed to control moods, violence, aggression, etc.

Junk food has synthetic toxic coal tar dyes such as red and yellow food coloring. Food coloring and synthetic sugars irritate the brain and causes allergic reactions. Nitrate give meat a fresh red blood color (including fish). Nitrates cause mental illness, hyperactivity and violent moods. The synthetic sugars added to foods are addicting. Synthetic sugar causes a craving for synthetic sugars in the food. For example, an alcoholic craves alcohol. The Eating Disorder and constant craving for the concentrated sweeteners (sugar), hormones, salt, nitrates, carbon, MSG and coal tar food dyes causes food addiction. A child in a state of sugar craving will be illogical in thought, emotion, have mood swings, attention deficit, mild senility, irritated, and have behavioral problems. The child constantly goes through sugar withdrawal and needs a synthetic sugar fix.

Biochemically altered and hyperactive children are usually raised by biochemically altered and hyperactive parents who live for the next synthetic sugary food fix. They are continuously stimulated from sugar, in withdrawal, or irritated because they are between sugar fixes. They and their children have sugar binges (Mac attacks). They have sporadic and constant headaches, pain, stress, constipation, energy loss, sugar cravings, weight increase and decrease, fatigue, birth control, sleep disorders, rashes, indigestion, colds, etc.

Irradiation of food is dangerous. Irradiation is the use of toxic radiation chemicals to preserve or kill worms and bacteria in foods. Radiation causes disease such as cancer. Radiation-sprayed foods store low-level radiation. Irradiation destroys electrically positive charged protein amino acids such as arginine and lysine. Lysine is used to help stop infections and arginine is used in reproduction of cells. Radiation stops the cell's ability to live, protect itself and reproduce new cells. Radiation, synthetic chemicals, hormones, pesticides, herbicides synthetic coloring, and preservatives and processed sugars in foods are destructive to health. Synthetic sugars turn into alcohol and are tasty forms of embalming fluids used on dead bodies (corpses). Preserved (embalmed) Black people move from chattel slavery to chemically controlled slaves.

Processed sugars biochemically altered Black people are seasoned socially engineered cloned GMO slaves. They have outsourced their intelligence to white people. They sing or rap sugary junk food jingles that praise the tasty goodness of poisonous chemicals such as carbonated sodas. Carbon Dioxide in sodas are a contradiction because the lungs exhale toxic carbon dioxide waste produced by breathing in oxygen and the digestion of foods. Then Black people go to the store and buy sugary carbon dioxide because Black people are train to drink the sugary carbon dioxide waste that their lungs are trying to get rid of. Their minds, emotions and behaviors are "seasoned" by commercials to practice the direct opposite of health, which is disease. The slaves were "seasoned" to like the White people and are addicted to white people. White people are the instruments of social, emotional, and sexual tools that destroy Black women, children, men, African culture, and the continent of Africa.

A "seasoned" biochemically altered Black person has thoughts and emotions that take a chemical side chain loop reaction response to Maat ideas spoken by other Black people. The synthetic sugars in the body and brain cause reception of stimuli to be misdirected, distort information they receive, misinterpreted, or block information. For example, the sound of music may cause sex stimulation, sex may cause violence, violence may trigger a euphoric high, a high may trigger homosexuality, and the sight of the elderly may trigger hate.

African culture may trigger fear, fear may trigger denial of slavery, learning may trigger self-hate, etc. The nerves are saturated with sugary synthetic chemicals and hormones in sweet food. This causes Black people to react to artificiality and not to reality. Black people to mimic white people's sugar addiction, mental illnesses, emotions, thinking and behavior. In other words, they act unnaturally, unreal and crazy in normal social situations.

Sugar addicts are walking time bombs of diseases and mental confusion. Black people have illogical, emotional, spiritual, mental and or disease outbursts from the release of stored sugar in their fat cells when stressed. Even water can be biochemically altered. Public drinking water is basically chemically deodorized, ammonia treated, bleached and fluoridated toilet water with micro fibers, prescription insulin and illegal drugs chemicals from urine in it. Fluoride stimulates passive and docile behavior. Fluoride and processed sugar also destroy teeth and irritates nerves. Chemicals in antiperspirant deodorants stop the glands from working normally (i.e. pineal, uterus, prostate, adrenals, eyes, etc.).

Any chemical such as processed sugars stops, slows down, or builds waste constipates the brain. Black people get negative chemical stimulation from the toxic radiation that turn into chemicals that are produced by microwaves, cellular phones, low frequency radio stations, lasers, computers, television screens, etc. *No "benefit" of Caucasian "science" comes without destruction (side effect).* The "benefit" and "destruction" of biochemical alteration by Caucasian "civilization" cannot be separated. For example, a "seasoned" Black person who learns to obey white people's rituals (rules) simultaneously learns to disobey Black peoples Maat rules. A "seasoned" Black person is taught and supervised by Whites is simultaneously being taught not to be supervised by Blacks. It is built into white rituals and ceremonies. You cannot have one without the other. However, there is an alternative.

Unprocessed sugars, organic non-GMO foods should be the diet of Black people. Natural foods are central to Black people's freedom. Black people must be able to image and talk about eating natural foods. Black people image by thinking in pictures. A whole picture image gives mental, emotional, spiritual and cultural meaning to social movements, ideas, events, food, herbs, culture, and history. Black peoples written language is a whole picture image language, which includes a spiritual symbol, action symbol and phonic (sound) symbol. The foods that ancient Black people ate were organic whole foods and their whole picture language described the organic whole food. The Black people should be able to image the preparation of natural organic whole foods. These foods must be imaged with delight.

The Black family such as babies, pregnant women, the sick or the elderly must be able to eat organic non-GMO sugars in natural foods. The traditional ancient Black family did not eat processed sugars that could harm a baby, sugary alcohol drinks, eat salt (sodium chloride), vinegar, cooked grease trans oils, concentrated sweeteners, white sugar, rotten food, cooked animal blood, cooked pus and flesh. The ability to image organic non-GMO foods in a natural cultural social environment was destroyed by the White institution of slavery and colonialism. Slavery started Black people eating processed sugar. Slavery perverted the appetites and television shows, computer games and movies created the images that sugary junk food is good.

Black people that eat organic non-GMO foods free of synthetics will no longer be chemical sugar addicted slaves that serve the White slave masters oligarchy owned food corporations, and disease(sick) industry hospitals and drug companies. Black people on a natural organic non-GMO food diet without processed sugars will bring an end to the nutritional destruction of the Black race.

Weight, Over Waste (Overweight) and Lies

The white peoples worldwide-distributed normal body weight chart, is the standard weight chart that was formulated in 1959 by insurance companies. This chart ignores the physical differences in races, this is in direct contradiction to the facts. For example, White people have more muscle mass (big calves, big thighs with flat buttocks muscles) while Black people tend to have less muscle mass and more skin surface (due to longer arms and legs). This means Black people have a greater ability to cool themselves in hot weather. White people have more ammonia, sulfur, and salt in their biochemistry, have the least amount of skin pores, the most bodily hair, a larger muscle mass and lack the ability to be cool in hot weather.

An overweight person can have excess water retention (edema). On a processed food diet they can have the weight of 7 to 15 pounds of feces impacted in the digestive tract. An obese person has excess bodily fat. Therefore, a person can be overweight and not have obesity.

The corporate own insurance companies set the normal weight tables at a low weight per height ratio. This causes many people to be declared over weight, an overweight person's insurance rate is higher. It was to the insurance companies economic advantage to falsify weight tables.

The normal weight table was reformulated in 1990 to reflect the true weight for height of Caucasians. However, the vast majority of white health practitioners and drug companies still use the 1959 tables. This causes them to classify more people as ill to increase the dosage and strength of drugs prescribed to a person.

Comparison between the 1959 and 1990 tables
Weight Chart

Height	Women-Men			
	(25 and older)		(19-34)	(35 and up)
	Women	Men		
5'0"	103-115		97-128	108-138
5'1"	106-118	111-122	101-132	111-143
5'2"	109-122	114-126	104-137	115-148
5'3"	112-126	117-129	107-141	118-152
5'4"	116-131	120-132	111-146	122-157
5'5"	120-135	123-136	114-150	126-162
5'6"	124-139	127-140	118-155	130-167
5'7"	128-143	131-145	121-160	134-172
5'8"	132-147	135-149	125-164	138-178
5'9"	136-151	139-153	129-169	142-183
5'10"	140-155	143-158	132-174	146-188
5'11"	143-158	147-163	136-179	151-194
6'0"	147-162	151-168	140-184	155-199
6'1"	152-167	155-173	144-189	159-205
6'2"	156-171	160-178	148-195	164-210
6'3"	160-176	165-183	152-200	168-216

Nutritional Approach

∞ Eat raw organic non-GMO food such as fruits, vegetables unprocessed grains, beans.

∞ Food should be eaten FRESH and RAW.

∞ Eat in a calm unhurried state of emotions and mind

∞ Dark green leafy vegetables and the juice of dark green leaves or fruits should add 1 glass of spring water per liter before drinking

∞ No dairy products. No fried food.

∞ No animals. No fish. No fowl. Dead animal cells produce dead moods and thought cells.

∞ Do not take synthetic drugs of any kind. No prescribed, over the counter or street drugs.

∞ Drugs destroy the immune system.

∞ Herbal extracts and teas work better and faster than synthetic pills and capsules.

Blood Cleansers
∞ Burdock
∞ Dandelion Root
∞ Elecampane (lung congestion and blood)
∞ Garlic (for white blood cells)
∞ Green vegetables
∞ Milk Thistle (protect liver and blood)
∞ Pleurisy (lung congestion and blood)
∞ Red Clover
∞ Spirulina
∞ Wheat grass juice (for red blood cells)
∞ Wormwood (parasites and worms)

Immune System Builders
∞ Exercise - the best immune system builder
∞ Garlic (antibiotic, parasites)
∞ Vitamin C (-25,000-60,000mg (300/2hrs.) (infection)
∞ Echinacea (infection)
∞ Grape Seed Extract (infection)
∞ Pine Bark Extract (colds, infection)
∞ Maca, Yohimbe (stimulate energy to the sex organs, female should use it with Damiana)
∞ Goldenseal Extract (good for all types diseases)
∞ Vitamin E -up to 800 I.U./day (blood thinner)
∞ Ginseng (energy)
∞ Lecithin - for the nerves
∞ Lysine 1000mg (infection, herpes)
∞ Foti (energy)
∞ Ginger (digestion, edema)
∞ Glutathione (removes cellular waste)
∞ Creatine (build healthy tissue)
∞ Vegetarian Glucosamine (helps repair cells, tissue)

Skin
∞ MSM tablets and lotion (anti-inflammatory, alkalines)
∞ Lysine crème
∞ Zinc crème (used by sex organs)

Yeast Infection
- ∞ Pau D Arco and Thyme

Sleep
- ∞ Valerian
- ∞ Catnip
- ∞ Chamomile
- ∞ Kava
- ∞ Passion Flower
- ∞ Hops
- ∞ 5 HTP
- ∞ Melatonin

Digestive Enzyme Tablets
- ∞ Improves metabolism of supplements, herbs and food.

Medicine Food

White Folks Thinking

White people tend to process words, memorize ideas, and discover ideas. They do not think. Thinking is the ability to create thought with a thought = improvise.

Black people think and White people copy = memorize thoughts. Black people have been taught an unreal fantasy idea of how the emotions and the mind functions. White people assume the mind is based upon Oedipus myth and the Left and Right Hemisphere Theory(superstition). White people's fantasy mind function from the real function, Black people must follow the Maat principle, which clearly states that we must separate the real from the unreal.

Sigmund (Sickman) Freud helped to establish the unreal fantasy idea of the Caucasian mind. He used a Greek children's fairy tale to explain the mind called the Oedipus Complex. He decided that each character in a fairytale story represented a fragment of the mind (i.e. Oedipus, Conscious, Subconscious, Ego, Id, Superego, etc.). This is similar to watching an animated children's cartoon or movie and saying the cartoon characters represent the true and pure psychological aspects of the mind.

A Greek or Roman myth is a story in which the characters have Latin or Greek names. If the characters in the myth (story) had English names the myth would be called a children's fairy tale or folk tale. The mind does not function like a fairy tale. The Greek Oedipus fairy tale does not explain the mind.

The White people's idea of their mind and how their mind functions is a fantasy and totally unreal. An idea or scientific fact based on a fantasy is a fantasy. If you use a lie to explain a lie then your explanation is a lie. A real idea of the white mind and how it functions can be obtained by a historical examination of their past cave civilization behavior, thinking, emotions, family structure and the way the cave people treated each other. History more than anything reveals the real mind of the white people, their psychological personality.

Psychopathic Racial Personalities, Narcissistic Avaricious Disorder, Post Traumatic Cave Disorder, and White Supremacy Psychosis were used to murdered and exterminated natives in every country they have invaded. White people are constantly violent and stay in a constant state of war with others. They constantly exploit and steal others natural resources and human resources with violence. They are in denial that they are violent and have a superstitious nature. Their superstitions are the number 13 is unlucky, Friday the 13 is an unlucky day, and the superstitious Halloween Holiday of worshipping the dead and evil.

The problem with White psychology is it treats emotional problems as a mental problem. It is defect logic. Emotions have a different neuronet pathway from a mental synaptic pathway. In other words, White people use a street map of New York (mental problem) to find the solution to traveling in Chicago (emotional problem).

If I were to tell you that the Black peoples mind is based functions the same way as the characters in Cinderella or Goldilocks and Three Bears you would clearly see the absurdity of White fairy tale psychology. White people's minds function based on a fairy tale and myth is in itself crazy. It is from this fairy tale myth theory based psychological construct (foundation) of craziness (mental illness) that the White people explains their cave civilization and their collective mental illness (craziness). White people's mental illnesses are in itself craziness based upon theories of craziness which maintains a level of craziness. The absurdity of this situation is that Black peoples use White people's fairy tale psychology to understand the mentality and emotionality of the Black mind. Black people use White psychology to find the solution to Black problems and emotional and mental problems. This means that any solution Black people derive for overthrowing White Supremacy, Oppression, Colonialism, White Domination and White Racism will fail. Build into any solution that uses White fairy tale psychology will be craziness of the unreal (fairy tale). A real problem (White Domination) cannot be solved with an unreal psychological solution (fairy tale craziness).

265

Chapter Five

Chemical Madness

"At some point – like right away – we are going to have to deal with the destructive effects of fast food, TV, integration and village breaksdown…"

Kiarri T.H. Cheatwood

Chemical Madness

The poisonous chemicalized GMO Junk Food Diet Increase with a Life span decrease and Disease Increase

Average Life Expectancies at Birth

The maps show countries where the average life expectancy at birth is within the age limits stated below. The graph shows the percentage of the total world population born in countries belonging to the different groups.

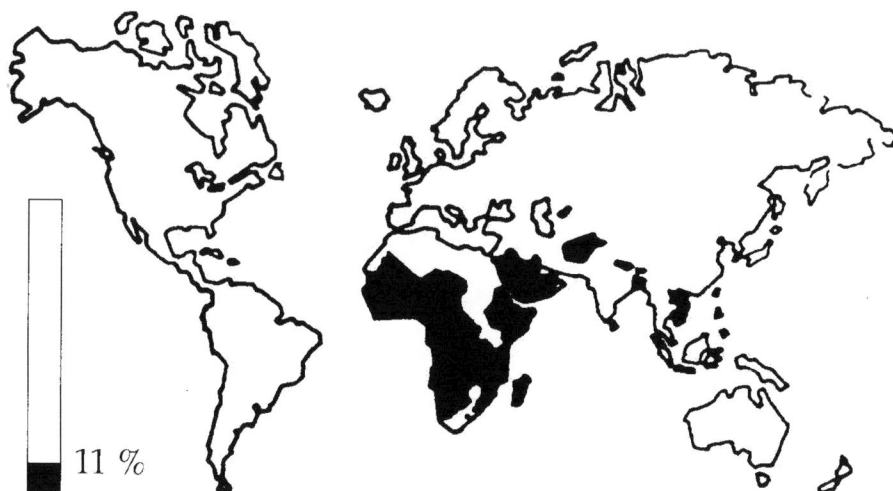

11 %

38-46 years

Developing countries in Africa and Southeast Asia have the lowest average life expectancy figures. This is related to the nutrient poor diets, synthetic chemicalized junk food and White corporate elite oligarchy control of their natural resource and political control in Africa.

White people's non-college graduates have the highest death rate and addiction to drugs as compared to other White age groups. In other words, White people in the USA have emotional traumas, prescription drug use, dysfunctional families and White Supremacy addiction leading to early deaths. This means that a White education and the economic exploiting of the poor by the white oligarchy has the side effect of death.

List of some African countries in the 30 to 40 years Life Expectancy Group

Angola

Botswana

Cameroon, Gabon

Chad

Coast, Upper Volta

Congo, Zaire

Equatorial Guinea

Ghana

Leone, Liberia, Ivory

Madagascar

Malawi

Mali, Guinea, Sierra

Mauritania

Mozambique

Namibia,

Niger

Nigeria

Senegal

Somalia, Ethiopia

Togo

Zambia

Zimbabwe

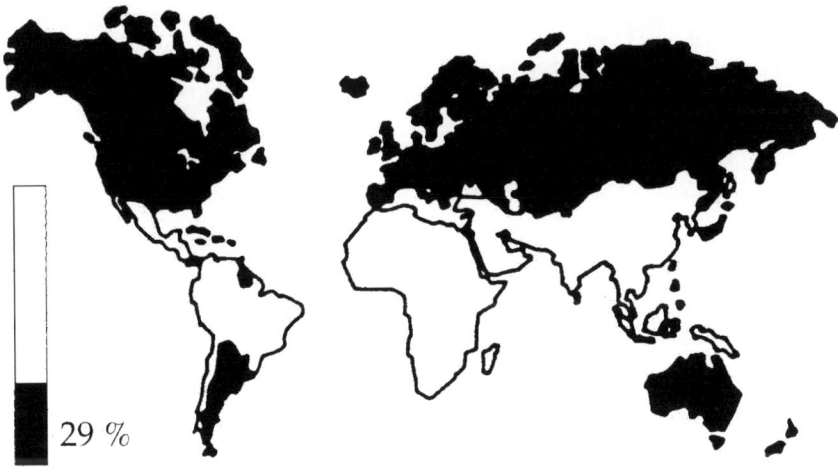

29 %

66-74 years

North America and European countries are in this group. Denmark, Iceland, Norway, and the Netherlands all have the highest figure of 74 years. This verifies the that White corporate own industries (carbon emissions, pollution, oil spills radiation, etc.) and chemicalized GMO junk food companies are deliberately killing Black people.

The EPA estimates that Chemicalized Indoor Air is 1,000 Times Worse than Chemicalized Outdoor Air

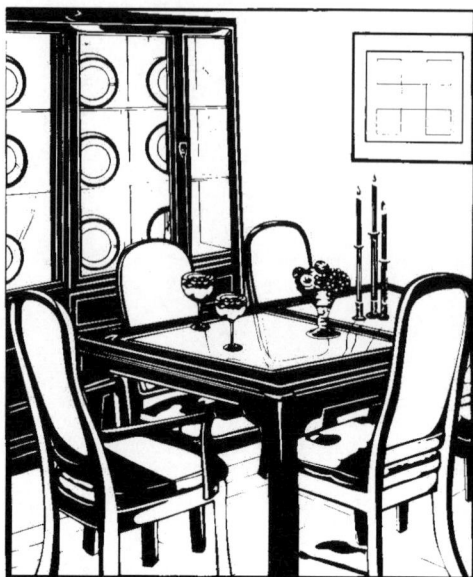

Some of the Possible Effects of Indoor Air Pollution are...

- ∞ Bronchial Constriction
- ∞ Cancer
- ∞ Depression
- ∞ Dizziness
- ∞ Drowsiness
- ∞ Eye, Skin and Nasal Irritation
- ∞ Fatigue
- ∞ Headaches
- ∞ Memory Loss
- ∞ Pulmonary Irritation
- ∞ Gynecological Problems
- ∞ Respiratory Irritation
- ∞ Shortness of Breath
- ∞ Slow Poisoning

The EPA (environmental protection administration) Estimates That 20% of All Workers Will Get a Major Illness from Chemicalized Indoor Air Pollution

Common Contaminants in Your Building Are:

∞ Air Conditioners
∞ Air Fresheners
∞ Animal Dander
∞ Bacteria
∞ Benzene
∞ Carbon Monoxide
∞ Carbon Tetrachloride
∞ Dust
∞ Dust Mites
∞ Formaldehyde
∞ LED lights
∞ Mildew
∞ Mold
∞ Noxious Fumes
∞ Odors
∞ Paint
∞ Pollen
∞ Plastic
∞ Radiation toxins (computers, digital machines)
∞ Smoke
∞ Static Electricity
∞ Sulfur Dioxide
∞ Viruses

Contaminants can originate from:

∞ Adhesives
∞ Air Dust
∞ Appliances
∞ Cleaning Supplies
∞ Clothes Dryers
∞ Concrete
∞ Construction Materials

271

- ∞ Drapes
- ∞ Dry-Cleaned Clothing
- ∞ Electric cables
- ∞ Furnaces
- ∞ Gas Burners
- ∞ New Fabrics and Carpet
- ∞ LED lights
- ∞ Radiation from cell phones, computers
- ∞ Manure vapors from toilets
- ∞ Paint, Glues
- ∞ Particle Board
- ∞ Pets
- ∞ Plywood
- ∞ Wall Paper

Do You Live
In A Sick Home?

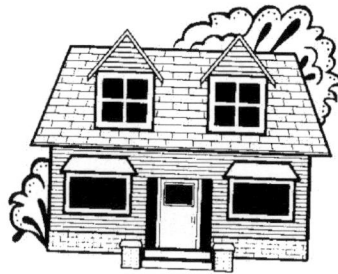

Do You Work
In A Sick Building?

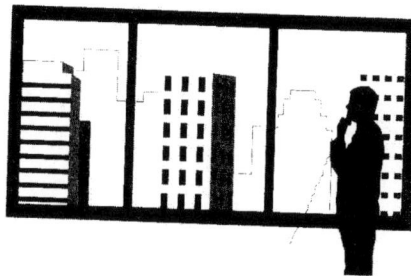

Do You Attend
A Sick School?

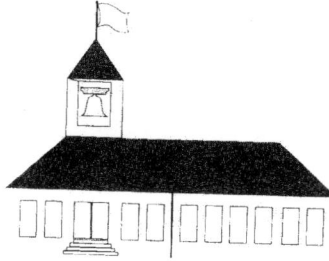

Noise Pollution

The sounds of noise are measured in decibels. Noise above 60 decibels is toxic, causes nerve damage, free radicals, tension, alter attention, and can cause mental fatigue. Research has shown that performance errors can occur within 10 minutes of exposure to 100 decibels. Sound must convert to a liquid (neurotransmitters) to travel in the blood to the brain. The ears are sensors that detect sound. The ears do not know what they are hearing. The brain interprets sounds you hear, taste, touch, smell and see. You hear, taste, touch, smell, see and feel pain with your brain. Loud sounds above 60 decibels are poisonous free radical toxins. Toxins (cocaine, alcohol, sugar, cooked cannabinol, salt (sodium chloride), etc.) are addictive. You can become addicted to loud sounds and not the loud music especially children. They only enjoy the chemical made from the loud sound and do not enjoy the music. The loud sound feeds their addiction. Their hearing decreases and they cannot hear normal levels of decibel sounds. Their internal ear gets damaged.

Some common noise levels (decibel)
Whisper 20 dB

The average home 40 dB

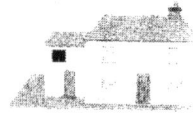

The average car 70 dB
(and some Black homes and schools)

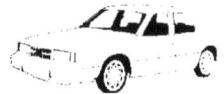

The average airliner cabin 85 dB
(Ghetto street noise)

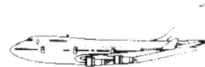

Subway Station 105 dB

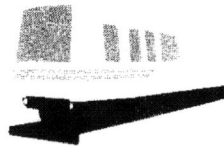

12 lb. cannon blast 300 dB

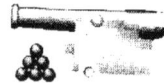

100 decibels are considered very noisy, while 140 is painful. Go up to 160 decibels and deafness occurs. Another 40 - to 200 decibels - can kill.

70 decibels Loud radio in an average house. A noisy restaurant. Ghetto automobile traffic. This type of noise makes it difficult to hear telephone conversations.

80 decibels Road construction site. This sounds twice as loud as 70 decibels.

274

90 decibels Loud shout. Busy city street. This sounds four times as loud as 70 decibels, is annoying and causes neurological damage after eight hours of continuous exposure.

100 decibels Subway station. Running printing press. Train horn 33 yards away. This noise is eight times as loud as 70 decibels.

110 decibels Sheet metal grinding. Loud music. This is 16 times as loud as 70 decibels and requires shouting to be heard.

130 decibels Pneumatic chipping and riveting, machines from the operator's position. This is 64 times as loud as 70 decibels. Shouts can't be heard. This noise level is considered intolerable.

Toxic noise sound levels can damage the ear over time.

Ritalin
(a type of crack-cocaine)

Stimulant Medication Side Effects

Common Initial Side Effects
- ∞ Abdominal pain
- ∞ Anorexia
- ∞ Easy crying
- ∞ Emotional
- ∞ Oversensitivity
- ∞ Headaches
- ∞ Irritability
- ∞ Weight Loss

Less Common Side Effects
- ∞ Anxiety
- ∞ Decreased social interest
- ∞ Depression *(rare)*
- ∞ Dysphoria or exaggerated feelings of depression and unrest without apparent cause *(especially at higher doses)*
- ∞ Hypersensitivity rash, conjunctivitis or hives
- ∞ Impaired cognitive test performance *(especially at higher doses).*
- ∞ Insomnia
- ∞ Less than expected weight gain
- ∞ Nervous habits *(such as picking at skin, hair, etc.)*
- ∞ Rebound attention deficit hyperactivity disorder *(ADHD)*
- ∞ Rebound over activity and irritability *(as dose wears off)*
- ∞ Withdrawal effects

Rare but Potentially Serious Side Effects
- ∞ Depression
- ∞ Growth retardation
- ∞ Hypertension
- ∞ Motor tics
- ∞ Psychosis with hallucinations
- ∞ Tachycardia (fast heart beat)
- ∞ Tourette's disorder (uncontrollable movements, talking, thinking, emotions)
- ∞ Stereotyped activities or compulsions

Side Effects Reported with Cylert (Pemoline) *Only*

- ∞ Chemical hepatitis (elevated liver enzymes, jaundice, epigastric pains).
- ∞ Choreiform movements (nervous condition marked by involuntary muscular twitching)
- ∞ Dyskinesias (defect in voluntary movements)
- ∞ Lip licking or biting
- ∞ Night terrors

Behavior Symptoms of Hyperactivity or Attention Deficit Disorder

Aggressive Behavior (Male principle expression of disease)	Passive Behavior (Female principle expression of disease)
Aggressiveness	Accident prone
Angry outbursts	Anxious
Bully	Daydreams
Clumsiness	Depressed moods
Compulsive aggression	Distractibility
Eats lots of sugar and drinks a lot of caffeine	Eating problems
	Emotional instability
Inability to concentrate	Fearful
Inability to make and keep friends	Hyperventilates
Junk-food eater	Insecurity
Lying	Lying
Not good in sports	Mood swings
Poor handwriting, drawing, and reading skills	Poor math calculations
	Poor muscle coordination
Poor muscle coordination	Poor reading skills
Poor sleep habits	Poorly developed musculo-skeletal system
Quarrelsomeness	
Resentment of punishments	Reasoning difficulty
Restlessness	Show off, constant emotional activities
Self-mutilation	
Show off, constant physical activities	Skin problems such as rash or hives
Stealing	Sleep problems
Temper tantrums	Slow reader
Unable to complete projects	Stays close to mother
Unaware of danger	Temper tantrums
	Withdrawn

Psychiatric Terms/Meanings

Psychological terms are political and social tools used to manipulate and control Blacks. They define Blacks as dysfunctional. This makes Blacks beneficial for Caucasian society.

- ∞ **Aggressive Tantrum** - aimless, thrashing, flailing limbs, wiggles legs
- ∞ **Attention Deficit** - easily distracted, loses things, fails to finish task, doesn't listen
- ∞ **Dementia** - forgetful, memory problems
- ∞ **Developmental Arithmetic Disorder** - difficulty understanding and solving mathematical problems
- ∞ **Drapetomania** - a mental illness which causes a slave to think about running away from the plantation or attempts to escape from freedom
- ∞ **Dysaesthesia Aethiopica** - a mental illness which causes a slave to be disrespectful or disobedient to Slave Master
- ∞ **Dyslexia** - fails literacy test, misspells words, cannot read, puts letters backwards
- ∞ **Hereditary Violent Genetic Disease** - protesting, acting militant or confronting White Supremacy or expressing doubt about White authorities, at risk social conditions (ghetto, poor education) which genetically makes you inferior
- ∞ **Hyperactivity** - impulsive, constantly moving, excess talking, impatient, makes excessive mistakes, excessive running and/or climbing
- ∞ **Hypo activity** - withdrawn, passive, plays alone, talks very little, seems lost
- ∞ **Orthorexia Nervosa**-tends to be obsessive about eating health food, can be concern about proper food combinations.
- ∞ **Oppositional Defiance Disorder** - acting independent, having self-identity
- ∞ **Pain Disorder** - having headaches, backaches
- ∞ **Passive Tantrum** - frown, cries, grimaces, beats on objects/furniture, throws and/or breaks objects
- ∞ **Persecution Complex** - getting into confrontations with authorities, getting into fights

The above terms are political and social and are used to manipulate and control Black Folks in order to make them dysfunctional and an economical benefit to White Supremacy's oligarchy.

Chemically Induced Teen Suicide

Blacks in the U.S.A. are #1 in the world in Black teen suicide.

The below Vitamin deficiency causes suicide and behavioral problems in school:

1. Low Vitamin B intake causes mental and emotional imbalances in teen.

2. Teens chemicalized GMO junk food diets are deficient in vitamin B content.

3. They addictively consume concentrated sweeteners, sodas, junk foods, and alcohol, which biochemically reduce already critically low levels of Vitamin B in the body, dehydrate the cells and cause nutritional starvation.

4. The signs of vitamin B deficiency are characterized by ***delusions, disorientation, mood swings, and depression.*** These symptoms are consistent with early **Beri Beri,** a Thiamine, and Vitamin B deficiency disease.

5. The major symptoms of B Vitamin deficiency are anxiety, fear, depression, hostility, rage, vagueness, forgetfulness, instability, craving for sweets, mental confusion, vague fear, mindless sex, irritability, and a **constant feeling that something dreadful is about to happen.**

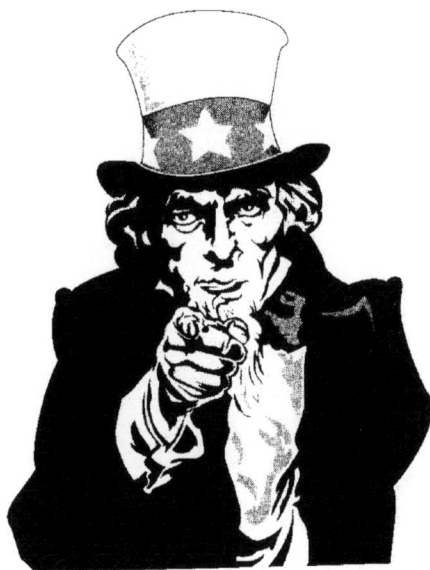

Black Children and Adults
I WANT YOU IN PRISON-You My Nigger

Black people's nutritional deficient, consumption of chemicalized junk foods, chemicalized water, pesticides, herbicides, synthetic fertilizers, and legal and illegal drugs put them at a higher risk for crimes and prison. Court is where the negative behaviors caused by Post Traumatic Slavery Disorders, White Supremacy, and mal-nourishment from junk food goes on trial. The junk food industry is found innocent while the Black people are found guilty and sent to jail. The oligarchy's corporate controlled food Industry creates the social and nutritional condition of Genocide. Genocide occurs when you create the condition that destroys a people. In the white courts, dysfunctional behavioral responses caused by the junk food diet are innocent and the negative behavior that is a result of malnourishment is turned into a misdemeanor or felony crime.

Fast food stores and restaurants use addictive synthetic chemicals, meat glue, sex hormones that stimulate hypersex and sublime sex connotations in their advertisements. Their commercials create and stimulate self-hatred in Black folks by using the minstrel clown character (negative image of the Blacks) Ronald McDonald.

White Supremacy commercials, television reality shows, computer games, court shows with judges, shows with Black characters that do not or cannot be African-centered and Maat-Centered. This subconsciously culturally castrates Black people. The advertisements emotionally and psychologically help Black consumers to hate themselves. The stimulation of self-hatred causes the need to medicate the self-hatred with sugary foods and junk foods. This means it causes Black people to buy more and more junk foods that increases fast food's sales and profits.

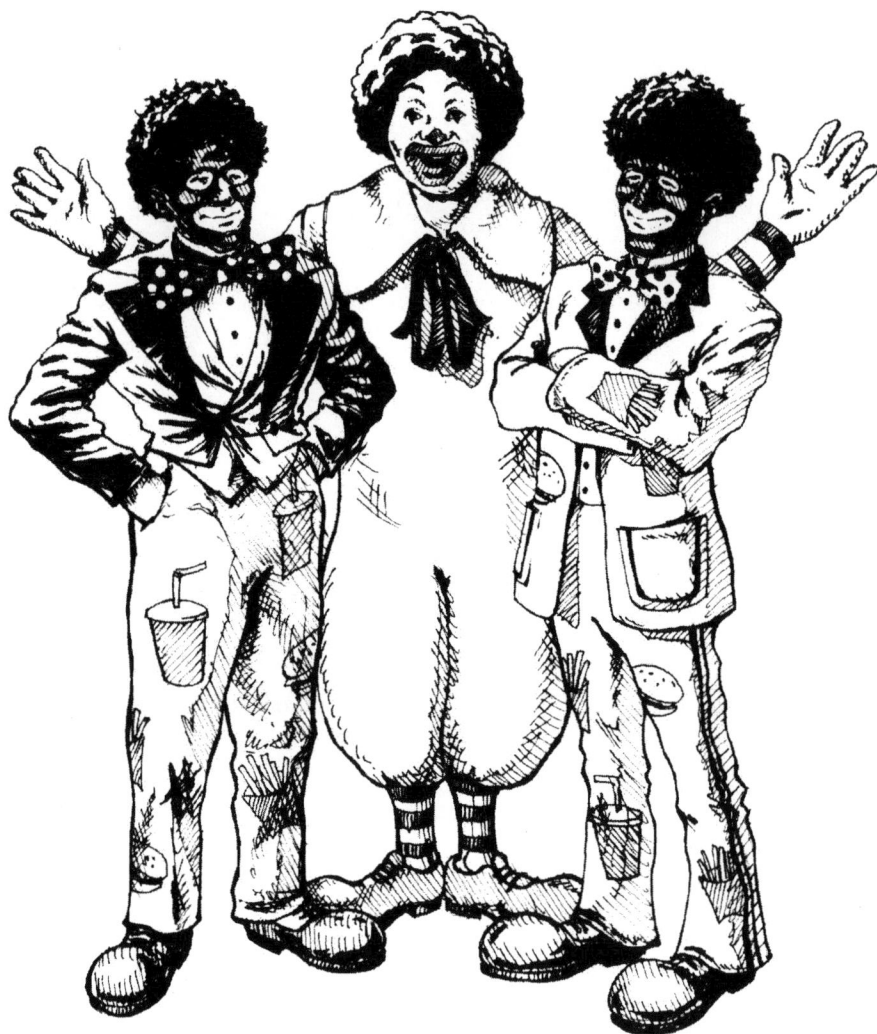

```
DATE:                    INMATE EARNING STATEMENT      PAGE:
INMATE PAYROLL               PAY DATE: 12/31/97         USER ID: annler

INST:    FACT:     GROUP:            CREW:

Name                                 Grade:
Reg-Num:

                      Amount    Hours
Standard Pay       $  44.05   191:30     Date Computed           01/05/98
Group Incentive Pay    0.00     0:00     Anniversary Date        12/01/97
Indiv. Incentive Pay   0.00     0:00     Longevity Months               1
Overtime Premium Pay   8.05    35:00     UNICOR Work Months             1
Holiday Pay            3.46    15:00     Accrued Vacation Hours    003:45
Administrative Pay     0.23     1:00     Prev Yrs Vacation Hours   000:00
Vacation Taken Pay     0.00     0:00     Unpaid Call-out Hours       0:00
Vacation Cashed Pay    0.00     0:00     Rework Hours                0:00
Lost Time Wage         0.00     0:00     Unpaid Off-std Hours        0:00
Premium Pay            0.00              Final Pay?                    NO
Longevity Pay          0.00
Gross Pay             55.79
Adjustments            0.00
                    --------  --------
Net Pay            $  55.79  242:30
```

Reproduced above is a copy of a UNICOR pay statement with the inmates's identity blacked out. This worker has a base pay of 23 cents per hour and received a total of $ 55.79 for 242.5 hours of work.

The Corporate Prison System
Prisoners for Profit

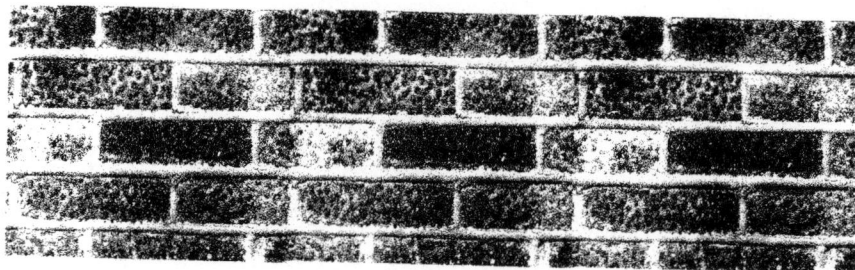

The private corporate oligarchy prison industry has tripled its profits in recent years. The USA has the most people in jail of any country (China, Russia, Egypt). It has the largest number of women in prison in the world. The prisons are private businesses and have to be guaranteed 90% full capacity as part of their contracts. They punish and warehouse prisoners and do not offer rehabilitation. Solitary confinement in prison is torture and illegal in many countries. It causes permanent emotional and mental damage. The prisons jail refugees, people seeking political asylum, families and children that have been charged with a crime or committed a crime. People are put in jail for thought crimes and put in jail without being charged with a crime. Very, very few prisoners are allowed DNA tests to prove innocence. The prisons are over crowed and building new facilities that will become over crowded which will increase profits for the private prison business.

Capacity on the rise

Actual and predicted capacity
of private prisons in the United States:

1996	77,584
1997	111,588
1998	142,799
1999	179,884
2000	223,002
2001	276,455

Slicing up the market
Two companies dominate the industry.
Percentage of the market share based
on U.S. contracts:

Corrections Corp of America	52.03 %
Wackenhut Corrections Corp	25.11 %
U.S. Corrections Corp	5.20 %
Management & Training Corp.	3.84 %
Cornell Corrections Inc:	3.37 %

Source: Private Adult
Correctional Facilities Census,
10th edition, prepared by the
Private Corrections Project
Center for Studies in
Criminology and Law,
University of Florida

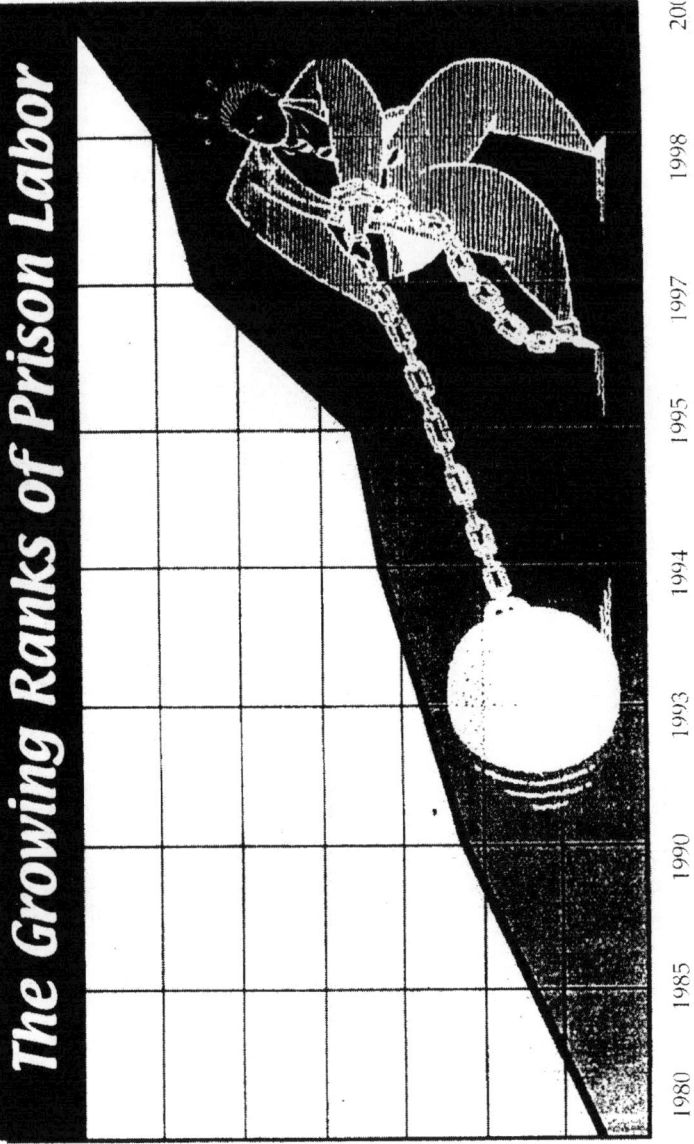

The Growing Ranks of Prison Labor

State and Federal Prisoners

2,000,000
1,750,000
1,500,000
1,250,000
1,000,000
750,000
500,000
250,000

1980 1985 1990 1993 1994 1995 1997 1998 2000

286

Chewing Gum
(Commercial Toothpaste has the same ingredients as)

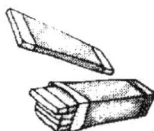

Ingredient	Harmful Effect
BHA (Butylated Hydroxyanisole)	Cancer
BHT (Butylated Hydroxy Toluene)	Cancer
Plasticizers	Solvent (Dissolves Skin), Digestive Problems
Aspartame	Nerve Damage, Cancer, Cysts, Tumors
Polysobutylene	Solvent, Skin Irritant, Suffocation
Polyterpene	Respiratory Failure (Death), Skin Irritant
Aluminum	Brain Damage, Clogs Glands
Propyl Gallate	Skin Irritant
Polyvinyl Acetate	Damages lungs and kidney, Tumors
Coal Tar	Cancer, Degenerative Diseases
Wood Tar	Cancer, Insanity
Petroleum Tar	Cancer, Degenerative Disease
Paraffin	Cancer, Degenerative Disease
Approved Non-food Dirt (Dead insects, Rat manure Filth)	Unknown
Unspecified Ingredients (Over 20 not listed)	Unknown
White Sugar	Kidney failure, Diabetes, Blindness, Addiction, Cancer
Dyes	Cancer

White Spots on Black Folks' Skin

The effect of junk foods, meat, drugs (legal and illegal), sunlight deficiency, synthetic chemicals, smoking marijuana, sleep deprivation, fluoridated water, herbicides, radiation, pesticides, GMOs. Steroids, and nutritional deficiencies causes

- ∞ Melanin Deficiency (Internal organs use external melanin)
- ∞ Cellular and food waste constipation
- ∞ Sunlight Deficiency (sunlight helps retain minerals, pH level, electrolytes, produce Melanin)
- ∞ Retention of waste in body due to salt addiction
- ∞ Radiation toxicity (i.e., computers, X ray, TV, appliances)
- ∞ Lymph gland congestion
- ∞ Excessive sex or sex stimulation
- ∞ Loud sounds (noise pollution)
- ∞ Toxic Liver damage
- ∞ Unable to metabolize food properly (digestion too fast, stomach skin thick, colitis, etc.).
- ∞ Body too acidic to use nutrients
- ∞ Fungus infections (Athletes foot, Yeast, Dandruff)
- ∞ Severe Vitamin C and D deficiency
- ∞ Potassium deficiency
- ∞ Decrease building of cells (Micronage)
- ∞ Vitamin A, B_{12} and/or Iron Anemia

Symptoms
∞ Deterioration of cartilage, cell glue, bones.
∞ High blood pressure, stress, cyst, tumors.
∞ Cracking, ridged and/or splitting fingernails.
∞ Waste in uterus, waste in prostate.
∞ Menstruation problems.
∞ Mood and thought problems.
∞ Urine alkaline and saliva alkaline.
∞ Micronage of cells.

Partial-birth Abortions

The murder of late term Unborn babies by sucking out brain (D&X). The Black mother is drugged and the murdered baby parts are sold.

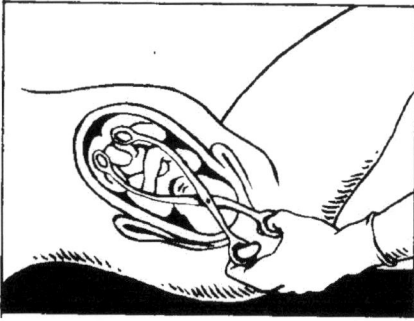

Guided by ultrasound, the abortionist grabs the baby's leg with forceps

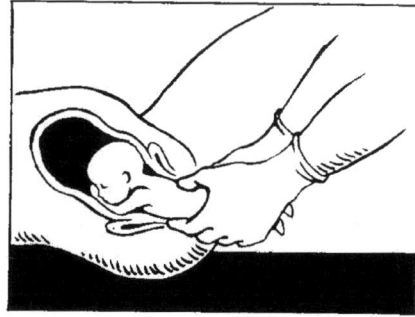

The abortionist delivers the baby's entire body, except for the head.

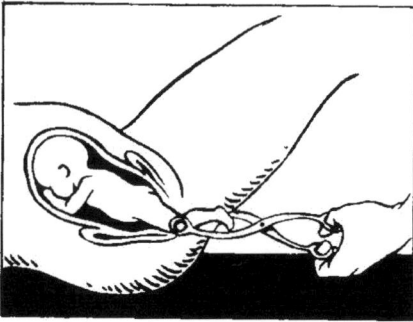

The baby's leg is pulled out into the birth canal.

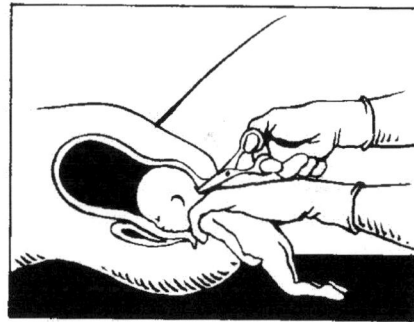

The abortionist jams scissors into the baby's skull. The scissors are opened to enlarge hole

"The abortionist punches a hole into the base of the child's skull with a scissor... They then spread the scissors to enlarge the opening. The abortionist removes the scissors and puts a suction catheter into this hole and vacuum sucks out the brain which murders the child. With the catheter still in place, he pulls the child out of the uterus of the mother. The abortion pill "morning after" murders the child and leaves the brain in the skull. If performed in a medical facility, the fetal tissue is sold to the organ donation corporate businesses. The tissue is used in foods to add flavor, used in cosmetics, and stem cell businesses.

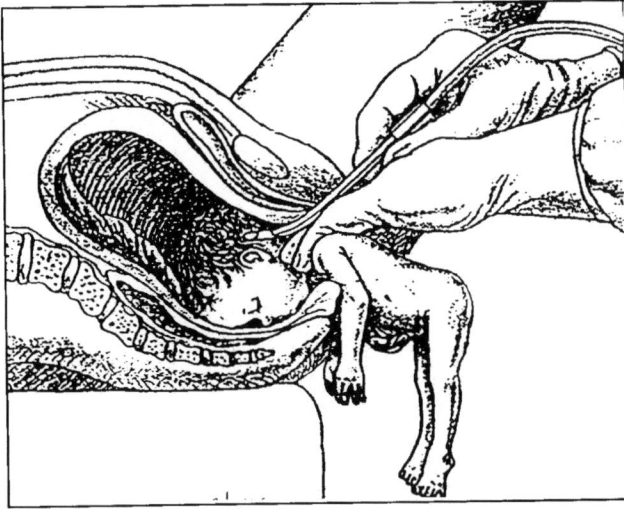

Murder tops the causes of death among infants

Parents on junk food, legal, and illegal drugs murder more infants. 10,370 injury-related infant deaths were reported between 1983 and 1991. After murder, which accounted for **23%** of the deaths, the leading causes were:

Suffocation **18%;**

Car accidents **15%;**

Fires **9%;**

Drowning **7%;**

Choking on food **7%;**

Chocking on objects **6%;**

Other intentional injuries **11%;** and

Injuries undetermined intent **4%**

Infants were more likely to die of injuries including murder, if their mothers were young, unmarried, had little education and their diets tended to be junk foods—nutrient deficient.

Vaccination (Chemical, pus and filth)

The chemical companies cannot be sued and are legally protected from law suits by the FDA. Vaccination is technically classified as a drug and poison. Vaccination drugs are made mandatory. There are states that accept Vaccination Exemption. The exemption must be requested in writing and sometimes require notarization, and/or written on a church's or lawyer's letterhead paper. The doctor should advise you of the side effects before giving the injections. The amount of diseases from vaccinations (i.e. mental illness, autism, paralysis, nerve damage) increases every year. The person with a flu vaccination spreads the disease to others for two months. They are shedding the disease. There is no scientific evidence that they work. Vaccinations are a ritual. They are based upon the Germ Theory, Contagious Disease Theory and the Immune Theory. Theories are beliefs that come from superstitions.

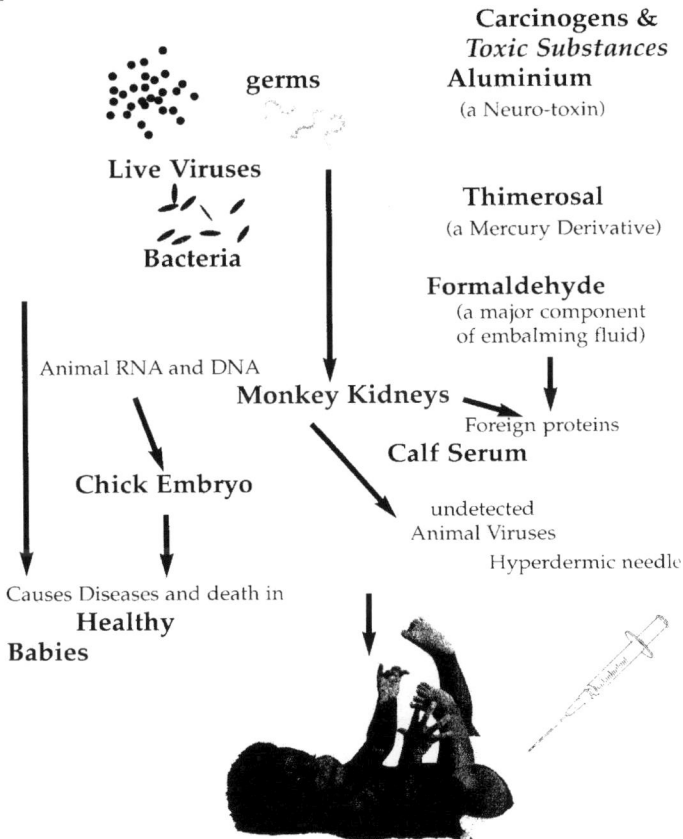

germs

Carcinogens &
Toxic Substances
Aluminium
(a Neuro-toxin)

Live Viruses

Bacteria

Thimerosal
(a Mercury Derivative)

Formaldehyde
(a major component
of embalming fluid)

Animal RNA and DNA

Monkey Kidneys

Foreign proteins

Calf Serum

Chick Embryo

undetected
Animal Viruses

Hyperdermic needle

Causes Diseases and death in
Healthy
Babies

AFFIDAVIT
DECLARATION OF VACCINATION EXEMPTION

"EXEMPTION FROM IMMUNIZATION", I hereby declare that I as guardian/parent/adult having responsibility for myself/child named herein _____withhold my consent and let it be known that said adult/minor is exempted from any and all vaccinations on the grounds that such is contrary to my personal beliefs.

IMMUNIZATIONS OF A PERSON SHALL NOT BE REQUIRED FOR EMPLOYMENT, ADMISSION TO A SCHOOL OR OTHER INSTITUTION...IF THE GUARDIAN, PARENT, OR ADULT WHO HAS ASSUMED RESPONSIBILITY FOR HIS OR HER CUSTODY AND CARE IN THE CASE OF A MINOR, THE PERSON MUST FILE WITH THE GOVERNMENT AUTHORITY, A LETTER OR AFFIDAVIT STATING THAT SUCH VACCINATION IS CONTRARY TO HIS/HER BELIEFS...

Any institution, school or medical authority which tries to enforce vaccination on children or anyone else is in violation of the laws of the United States, and may be subject to prosecution.

Amendment 14 of the United States Constitution:
"No state shall make or impose any law which shall abridge the privileges or immunities of the citizens of the United States, nor shall any state deprive any person of life, liberty, or property."

Amendment 4 of the United States Constitution:
"The right of the people to be secure in their persons shall not be violated."

INTERNATIONAL VACCINATION EXEMPTION
Exemption has been ratified and approved by the United Nations members under WORLD HEALTH ORGANIZATION International Sanitary Regulations Article 83, Chapter IV; "each individual has the right of vaccination exemption".

SUBSCRIBED AND AFFIRMED TO BEFORE ME ON THIS____DAY OF
_____, 19_____.

_____

SIGNATURE AND DATE

NOTARY PUBLIC
COMMISSION EXPIRES

(Your Address)
Date

Dear (School Nurse or whoever it has to go to):

RE: Religious Exemption from Immunization Requirements

Please be advised that I am hereby requesting a religious exemption for my (daughter/son). ____(name)_____. (Select and continue here with (A), (B) or (C).

(A:)   Our family follows the tenets and practices of a religion which strictly forbids....

(B:)   Our family are members of (or: **have recently joined a**) religion whose tenets and practices strictly forbid....

(C:)   Although my **(daughter/son)** previously received some immunizations, our family are now members of a religion whose tenets and practices strictly forbid immunizations of any type, including those injected, ingested or infused into the body.

Kindly enter this religious exemption into my **(daughter's/son's)** school records.

Thank you very much.

Sincerely,

(Your Name typed or printed)

Orange Chemical Liquid—Orange Juice

Commercial cooked (pasteurized) orange juice can have dangerous amounts of the following:

1. Water-extracted soluble orange solids
2. Dehydrated water-extracted soluble orange solids
3. Commuted (pulverized) oranges
4. Dehydrated commuted oranges
5. Dehydrated extract of comminuted oranges
6. Juicy orange pulp for manufacturing
7. Dehydrated juicy orange pulp for manufacturing
8. Noncarbonated flavored beverage
9. Concentrate for flavored beverage
10. Powered flavored beverage
11. Orange drinks and diluted orange drinks
12. Concentrates for orange drinks
13. Powered orange drinks
14. Orange-flavored drinks
15. Concentrates for orange flavored drinks
16. Powered orange-flavored drinks
17. Concentrated water-extracted orange juice
18. Orange blend
19. Orange juice drink
20. Orange drink
21. Concentrate for diluted orange juice beverages
22. Orange juice drink and blended orange juice drink
23. Concentrate for orange juice drink and for blended orange juice drink
24. Powered orange juice drink and powered blended orange juice drink
25. Concentrate for orange drink
    Concentrate for orange-flavored drink
26. Powered orange flavored drink
27. Cooking oranges creates white sugar
28. Tap public water, that is not purified or distilled
29. Orange colored coal tar dye (causes cancer)
30. Pasteurization (boiling) orange juice is too concentrated and should be mixed with equal amounts of water. If not it damages the pancreas.
31. Contains poisonous chemicals from fertilizers, pesticides, growth hormones and endocrine gland disruptors
32. Bleach
33. Safety for women, children, elderly or women that expect to become pregnant is doubtful

Condom—Rubber Coffins (Latex and Chemical poisons)

∞ Condoms cannot prevent emotional pain.

∞ Condom failure rate for pregnancy prevention is 13-31%[1].

∞ Condom Research: Latex condoms may have voids (holes) approximately 5 microns in size that occur naturally during the manufacturing process.[2]

∞ The powder in condoms cause cyst and tumors.

∞ The spermicide causes cancer.

∞ The condoms fail to prevent nearly 1 in every 3 HIV infections.[3]

∞ Sexually transmitted viruses and bacteria can pass through the voids (holes) in a latex condom.[4]

∞ The latex condoms cause Chlamydia, Pelvic inflammatory dis-ease — PID and cancer of the female reproductive system, anus and mouth.

∞ Voids (holes) occur in Sterile and Latex free condoms

∞ While having sex the friction heat expands the holes

∞ Cancerous chemicals in the latex gets into the vagina, anus and/or mouth

∞ Coal tar dyes and flavorings are cancerous

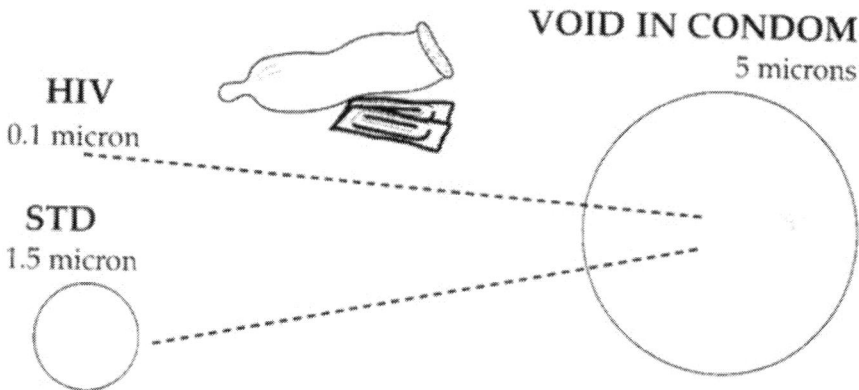

VOID IN CONDOM
5 microns

HIV
0.1 micron

STD
1.5 micron

[1] Family Planning Perspectives, V. 24, 1992.
[2] Roland, C. M., Rubber Chemistry & Technology, June 1992.
[3] Weller, Susan, Ph.D., University of Texas, June 1993.
[4] Carey, R. F., et al, Sexually Transmitted Diseases, July/August, 1992.
[5] Manual of Clinical Microbiology, 4th edition.

Disease by Blood Type

Black people are higher in Type A and B with a normal level of Type O and have a moderate RH—(negative) level, very rare RH+ (positive) and RHO.

The synthetic, chemicalized and GMO junk food diet causes specific diseases amongst blood types. Blood type cannot dictate a diet.

TYPE A				
Supplements	Exercise	Positives	Risk	Personality
Vitamin B, B_{12}, C, E, Folic Acid	Moderate	Digestive system highly responsive, long and high fermentative bacteria	Heart disease, Cancer, Anemia, Diabetes, Liver and Gall Bladder Disease	Humanitarian, Organized, Harmonious, Intelligent, Spiritual
TYPE B				
Magnesium, Zinc, Lecithin, Echinacea, Gotu Kola	Moderate	Digestive system highly responsive, long and high fermentative bacteria	Lupus, Diabetes, Fatigue, Multiple Sclerosis, Stress, Digestive	Adaptable, Empathetic, Aggressive, Sensitive
TYPE O				
Vitamin B, K Calcium	Intense	Digestive system highly responsive, long and high fermentative bacteria	Arthritis, Endometriosis, Ulcers, Allergy, Hypothyroid	Determined, Constructive, Leader Type, Communicator
TYPE AB				
Vitamin C, K, Manganese, Potassium	Challenging	Digestive system highly responsive, long and high fermentative bacteria	Prone to Anemia, Cancer, Heart Disease	Spiritual, Diplomatic, Charismatic, Emotional

Insulting Black People

The word nigger origin is Niger from the Niger River. Slaves captured around the area of the river were called Nigers. Unfortunately, white people mispronounced the word and called those captured slaves Niggers, white people decided that calling black slaves by the African word Niger may cause them to identify with their country of Africa. This might cause them to know they were once free and were not born to serve whites. Therefore, white people decided to make the African word Niger into a derogatory, negative, insulting, slur, for Black people. The irony of this white word control is if Black people decided to make white people from England into a insulting word by calling these white people Engers, no white people would pay attention to the word Engers. They would still call themselves English, and not Engers. In any case, the word nigger can be used as a noun, verb, or adjective. Many peoples have variations of the word nigger and use it to insult Black people. Here are a few examples of nigger used around the world.

Language, Country, or People	Insulting Slur Word Meaning
Arabic	Abeed (slave), Mishwa (grilled Black skin), Fahim (charcoal), unevolved earth into humans- Nigger
American Indians	Muckadoo, Mud People have not been created into humans = Niggers
British	Es-obe (Apes) = low form of human = nigger
Brazil	Crioulo (nigger)
Cuba (whites)	Niche (nigger)
China	Hakui (burnt skin nigger) Hagwet, Hay quay (black ghost) not real people (Nigger)
Chad (Whites)	Niger (nigger) River people
Canada	Cppmadian, Nigloo (nigger)
Dutch	Nig-Nog, Niknok (nigger)
Finnish	Neekeri, Nekru (nigger)
German	Schwarz (Black)
Hawaiian, Polynesians	Boffer (nigger), Papolo (dark purple skin)
Israel	Kushi (Cush black country), Shvatsa, Shvarlz (black)
Italians	Melon (watermelon) Johnny (rider)

	Moolingnon, Melanzena (dark purple, eggplant) a plant, not human = nigger
Irish Americans	Nagur (nigger)
Japan	Doujin (dirt person) Kurombo (black)
Jews	Shbatsa (yieldish form of nigger)
Kenya (whites)	Mau Mau (violent nigger) Gikuyu for rebels, Jambo (black sambo[niger])
Korea	Yont'an Sarem (black coal)
Mexicans (white, a minority of Blacks)	Miyate (niggers)
Portugeses	Baracoons (jail the niggers)
Panama	Chombo
Poland	Czamuch (nigger)
Persia	Meshky (Farsi language for nigger)
Phillipinos	Belvga (nigger) Egot (nigger)
Russia	Shahtor (black coal nigger)
Rhodesia	Munt (person is black, nigger)
South Africa (whites)	Platneus (flat nose). Caffre (nigger)
South America (whites)	Congolip (big lip nigger)
Russia	Chenozhopyl (black ass)
Thailand	Tycoon (Thailand coon = nigger)
White West Africans	Buckra, Boogie (devil spirit)
White Hispanics	Mayate, Mono (monkey) (nigger)
White Zimbabwe	Floppy (big Floppy Lip, nigger)
Vietnam	Mi Dang (black American, nigger)

Blame the Bacteria or Blame the Virus

The body constantly maintains a fluctuating biochemical balance of bacteria, virus, fungus, yeast, hormones, amino acids, genes, fats, and enzymes ratios. For each disease, there is bacteria that are high and some low, virus that are high and some low which can be identified by microscopes. Every time there is a negative or positive change in the emotions or state of mind or pH, the bacteria and virus ratio will change. However, this type of biochemical change is subtle while the change in bacteria and virus ratio is more obvious.

The drug companies use bacteria and virus to blame for diseases because it is easy to test and validate. There are over 1,000 different species of bacteria that live in the body at all times. The bacteria out number human cells 10 to 1. Virus (bacteriophages) outnumber bacteria 10 to 1. There is an estimate of over 100 trillion bacteria and quadrillion virus. Therefore, the disease (pharmaceutical) industry can always find an unknown, or specific bacteria, or virus to blame for a disease. Producing a drug, research or vaccination drug for each and every bacteria or virus is an unlimited and an unlimited source of income potential. This is the main reason they operate their business on beliefs instead of facts. They use the Germ Theory (belief=fiction) which supports their Contagious Disease Theory (belief=fiction) that helps their Vaccination Theory (belief). They use "science fiction (belief)" as science. Anyone that points to the errors of their beliefs is ridiculed, label in some way insane, or unscientific and blamed for trying to spread disease. Either they blame a bacteria or virus or they blame the person or research that disproves them as false and unscientific.

Skin Tight

Black peoples fashion of wearing tightly fitting so-called sexy clothing is killing them. The wearing of tight fitting clothes causes compression of blood vessels. The compression narrows the blood vessel which reduces the flow of blood, nutrients and cellular waste. This causes cells, tissues, nerves and bones to have starvation resulting in disease. The squeeze of the blood vessels similar to a tourniquet which reduces blood to the nerves, and muscles. Some of the symptoms are:

- Back pain- nerve damage from nerve compression
- Constipation/Abdominal Pain- decrease movement of food, slows down digestion, squeezes organs to close together.
- Headaches/Blurred Vision- decreases blood circulation to the brain caused by tight collars, button down shirts, neck ties
- Heart burn/Acid Reflux- squeezes organs against liver, stomach, pancreas, which impacts the flow of alkaline digestive enzymes
- Fainting- decrease blood flow to lungs. The lungs to do not fully expand causing decrease oxygen to brain and cells
- Tingling Thigh Syndrome- squeezes nerves causing nerve damage
- Yeast Infection- decreases oxygen to sex organs increases heat and moisture to sex organs which increase yeast/fungus growth

Safe Foods become Bad Foods

The fast foods are killing Black people. When some foods are cooked then re-heated the nitrates in then change to Nitrites. High levels of nitrites can be cancer causing in foods such as:

∞ Beets
∞ Celery
∞ Chicken
∞ Eggs
∞ Mushrooms
∞ Potatoes
∞ Spinach

These cancerous foods are sold by the fast food and pizza restaurants.

Oily Mess

An isolated element from a plant is a concentrate and drug. Opium isolated from poppy seed, cocaine from cocoa leaves and oils from plants are drugs. Many olive oil products are diluted with cheap sunflower, cottonseed and canola oils. The can be up to 90% cheap oils with 10% olive oil. The cheap diluted oil is sold at the price of 100% olive oil. The diluted oil is perfumed with poisonous chemicals that make it smell like olives and poisonous green dye coloring to make it look like olive green (University of California Study). Below is a few olive oils that are not 100% olive oil:

- ∞ Antica Badia
- ∞ Bertolli
- ∞ Carapelli
- ∞ Colavita
- ∞ Felippo Berio
- ∞ Mazola
- ∞ Mezzetta
- ∞ Pompeian
- ∞ Safeway
- ∞ Sasso
- ∞ Star
- ∞ Whole foods

Women and Sexual Disease

In the Black community girls should be made aware of sexual problems such as the below:

Problem	Symptom
Pubic Hair	Hair follicles can get inflamed caused by shaving, depilatories, sweating, Treat with warm compress
Bumps in and around vagina and labia	Swollen Bartolin gland, clogged pores, and channels
Vulvodynia	Very painful labia, and/or vagina
Dry Vagina	Caused by birth control pill/patches, allergy, stress, extra absorbent tampons, stress
Bulge near Vagina	Caused by varicose veins
Vagina Bubbles	HPV, herpes bump
Vaginismus	Muscles in vagina constrict and close the shaft blocking penis penetration
Itchiness	Fungus/yeast, diabetes, antibiotics
Itch and Burning Sensation	Gonorrhea, syphilis, chlamydia
Burning sensation and constant urination	Sexually transmitted disease
Bleed after sex	Infection, vaginal lesions (sores), dryness, cancer
Vaginal pain, painful sex, fever and secretions	Chlamydia, gonorrhea, frequent urination, with vomiting
Odor with secretions can burn	Vaginosis

Always Drunk

The addiction of White people to stay intoxicated with alcohol (i.e. mildly drunk, partially drunk, totally drunk) is normal in their culture. Alcohol intoxication, mild or severe, causes a mild temporary state of mental illness. It is a mental illness because it causes the inability to stay focused, thoughts wander, mood swings, emotional imbalances, etc. White people enjoy making themselves temporarily crazy. This is called being drunk and feeling good. They socially accept making themselves mentally ill and mildly drunk. Consequently, they consume alcohol in many forms (beer, wine, whiskey). They need to be crazy (mentally ill) for social activities.

- While watching sports (football, basketball, soccer, boxing, etc.)
- Social events (parties, night clubs, pubs etc.)
- On airplanes
- On dates
- At meetings
- Visiting each other
- Fighting wars
- Engaging in sex
- After exercising
- Negotiating contracts
- While driving cars
- Using equipment that requires full attention
- While taking prescription and non-prescription drugs
- When interacting with children
- When supervising others
- While watching television
- During pregnancy
- Holidays, weddings, funerals, birthdays
- Given to their children and pets
- Before bedtime
- After work
- To relax

Most of the time Black people talking to whites that are in between drinks, mildly drunk episodes (craziness). Many times a Black person is a social obstacle blocking the alcoholics drunk. Therefore, Black people are treated as a social obstacle in a white person's life. Alcohol is a chemical poison that destroys nerves, brain cells, tissue, bones, liver, organs, and lives. It is emotionally and physically addicting. Alcohol consumption should require a medical prescription for its use. The problem for communication with the majority of white people is at all times they are:

- ✓ Mildly drunk (mildly crazy = mentally ill)

- ✓ In mild alcohol withdrawal and slightly irritated
- ✓ Their alcohol craving causes them to want another drink
- ✓ Already in a mild alcohol withdrawal state
- ✓ In between their drunken state (pauses in craziness)
- ✓ In between hang overs (side effects of mental illness)

Their decision and behaviors are alcohol stimulated mental illness or alcohol depressed mental illness. They never consider themselves as a society of mentally ill drunks. Being mildly drunk (crazy), or in mild alcohol craziness withdrawal is Politically Correct Alcoholism (PCA). They would never consider a brain surgeon taking a few drinks before operating on their brain. And, yet White people take a few alcoholic drinks, or are in a mild withdrawal while they operate on Black people lives, intelligence, emotions, and make decisions to hire, fire, or pass laws, dismiss laws, or imprison Black people. Essentially, Black people's lives are in the hands of White people on prescription and non-prescription drug addicts and white alcoholics craziness. The constant consumption of alcohol is the normal life. White people do not consider consistent or daily drug test or alcohol test before White people in society are allowed to be with or around Black people. Black people are surrounded by alcohol crazy White people. You will not see an alcohol test given to White people leaving a soccer, basketball, baseball, hockey or restaurant. They have safe levels of drunkenness for automobile drivers.

Chemical Malt Liquor and Beer

Methanol
wood alcohol, poison, mental illness, cancer, liver, kidney and sex organ damage

Ethanol
narcotic, starch alcohol, poison, narcotic, explosive, liver, kidney and sex organ damage

Butanol
poison, narcotic, explosive, cancer, petroleum, alcohol, liver, kidney and sex organ damage

Isobutanol
poison, natural gas, alcohol, eye, lung, skin, liver, kidney and sex organ damage

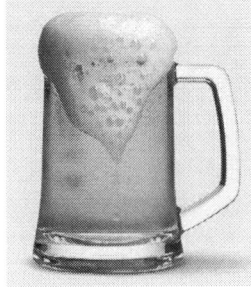

White Sugar
nitroglycerin, diabetes, blindness, gangrene, addiction

Acetaldehyde
poison, paralysis, nerve, brain, lung, skin, digestion and sex organ damage

Histamine
shock, swelling, skin rash, headache, low blood pressure, digestive problems

Phenol
carbolic acid, poison, convulsions, cancer, circulatory collapse, paralysis, coma, numbness, burns, digestive problems, skin rash

Propanol
poison, narcotic, toxic gas, disinfectant, cancer

Isopentanol
alcohol, poison, irritates eyes, lungs, liver, kidney and sex organs

Cobalt
metal, digestive problems

Lead
poison, nerve and brain damage, digestive problems

Iron
poison, skin disease, coma, hypotension, restlessness

Carbon Dioxide
high blood pressure, mental confusion, lung disease, digestive problems

Public Drinking Water
Used to make beer, is not purified or distilled and contains lead, ammonia, iodine, fluoride, aluminum, chloroform, atrazine, benzene, chlorine, arsenic, copper, nitrate/nitrite, rust, insulin, prescription drugs, illegal drugs, plastic, microfibers

GMO Barley
Herbicides, hormone disrupters

Viagra (Citrate Salt of Sildenafil):

Synthetic nitric oxide increases and disturbs blood inflow to brain, glands, eyes, lungs, heart, liver, kidney, and prostate. The effect of over exercise, exercise in the evening and late at night, inadequate sleep, legal and illegal drugs, steroids, sex hormones, GMOs, herbicides, radiation, cell phones, computers, sex addiction, emotional abuse, junk foods decrease nitrites. Over exercise causes the loss of nitrites to stay in a stress biochemical state. Consequently, there are not nitrites available for erection or orgasm.

Nitric (Nitrous Oxide)
(Laughing gas, causes psychotic Illusions)

Chemical Problems
Viagra cause abnormal increase in Nitric oxide
High concentration is narcotic
Burns and irritates skin
Decreases oxygen
Explodes cells
Used in explosives and fertilizers Nitric (Nitrous) Oxide
Side Effects[6]
Headaches
Infections
Urinary tract infections
Peptic ulcers
Arthritis
Chest pain
Mood swings
Frequent urination
Incontinence
Multiple myeloma
Blood Cancer (Leukemia)
Hypotension
Diabetic problems
Hypertension
Weakens immunity
Lung and nasal congestion
Blurred vision
Dizziness
Back pain
Heart problems
Depression

Thirst
Increases breast size
Colds and influenza
Sickle cell
Flushing
Nerve problems
Bleeding disorder

[6] Pfizer info sheet

The Untold Caucasian History
(Dirt, Fart, Feces, Fun and Sex)

The European relationship to health is reflected in their relationship to the soil (Mother Earth), which they call dirt. The soil nourishes the plants that we eat. A healthy relationship with dirt (soil) indicates a healthy relationship with your body. Many factors helped to create a negative, hostile and, in many ways, distorted relationship between the White people and dirt.

The Cave civilization, Ice Age and Cold Age that followed created nutrient-poor soil. The many mudslides, floods, thunder storms and subsequent forest fires caused erosion and stripped the land of valuable topsoil. This caused good dirt (topsoil) needed for food crops and animal feed plants to feed animals to be scarce. This inadvertently caused the loss of adequate food supplies, food shortages, famines, and starvation. The ancient European cave population consisted of gangs, thieves, roaming bandits, cannibal gangs, wild dogs which ate humans, people attacking each other, diseases, violence, water shortage, rape, looting, filthy and unlighted dark homes and cities, dead bodies, manure hills, and people who stayed dirty in fear of water.

The dirt (soil) without top soil was unable to provide adequate food. There were many cave taboos about cleanliness, myths and superstitions about dirt. The cave dwelling language refers to dirt in many ways, such as dirty shame, filthy rich, dirty dancing, dirty lie, dirty words, dirty dog, dirty nigger, dirt poor, dirty sex, etc. The cave civilization belief was that the white race evolved from dirt and that humans are made from dust (dirt). In reality, humans are approximately 80% water, which means they may have been made from water and not dirt. Cave people developed the belief that dirt is money, such as, yellow dirt (gold) or transparent crystallized dirt (diamonds). In their cave past it was believed that dirty children were healthy. Cave Women's dirty faces with cosmetics clay dirt was believed to block out the germs and the evil sun. If the cave woman was unwashed and had a foul body odor and a foul smelling, hair or musky smell it was considered sexy.

The ancient White writer, Jean-Paul Sartre (1905-1980), wrote in *Huis Clos* that hell is full of dirty people. Dirty people were believed to contaminate society and needed to be murdered. When cave people murdered each other (genocide) they refer to it as "racial cleansing." This is an expression for getting rid of dirt (genetically inferior, dirty people).

The original reason why the Khazars and White Moslems did not eat pigs had nothing to do with the bacteriology or worm infestation of the pigs. The Khazars worshipped the pig and thought the pig was sacred to their God. They did not eat pigs to honor their God similar to east Indians and cows. If cleanliness of the animal was the reason not to eat pigs, then cats would be eaten as food instead of cattle and fish (they swim in their own feces and urine). Pigs in the wild are clean animals and will constantly bathe. However, in captivity and raised indoors in animal farms. They do not have access to pools of water so they bathe in their own manure. On the early explorations (invasions) of Africa and the Americas, the Caucasian sailors would eat the dogs, then the cats, then the rats and pigs, then eat their leather boots, shoes, hats, ropes along with eating insects. White sailors, soldiers, and peasant populations normally ate bone meal cooked in fat and insects and the food found in a dead animal's intestines and stomach along with the animal's feces.

The ancient white cave civilization behaviors indicate a mixed and confused relationship between dirt, food, sex, medicine, health and disease. In primitive cave rituals, feces (manure) is symbolic of gifts, death, money, babies, the penis, art, spirits, sex, poison, foreigners, disorder, gold, the vagina, golden eggs, candy, food, etc. In books such as *The Ontogenesis in the Interest of Money* by Sandor Ferenczi (1914), *Studies in Psychology of Sex* by Havelock Ellis (1906) and *Character and Anal Eroticism* by Sigmund Freud (1908) It was reported that anal sexual ideas of White people began in childhood. They made weird feces myths because babies played with their own feces in the diaper. It is believed that White babies play with mud, sand, pebbles, hair, buttons, fingers, lips and coins because it is associated with feces. The coins (money)were a part of the subconscious belief that feces were an extension of the sex organs. Therefore, buying sex from prostitutes is an emotionally erotic extension of feces. In the White subconscious mind the need for domination of natural and human resource provides are economic control (power) over others. This is part of Cave Trauma Disorder, Narcissistic Avaricious Disorder and Psycho Pathological Disorder. These disorders are an extension of their sexuality and sex is an extension of feces and urine.

Historically, Ancient White people used human feces in religious ceremonies. Ancient Greeks rubbed feces on their bodies to atone sin. Urine and feces were used during funeral ceremonies and rituals. Joshua used feces in the Bible's Zechariah 3:3-4. Books such as *Scatalogic Rites of All Nations* by John G. Bourke (1891) customs with feces is indicate this.

A German harvest festival game, involved farm laborers covering each other with feces and then throwing each other on a hill of feces. A harvest game in Netherlands and New Zealand allowed farm workers to run and catch each other, then bury the caught person in dirt up to his waist and then defecate in front of and on the caught victim's face.

Historically Caucasian criminals in the act of a crime would have a bowel movement on the floor at the crime scene. This was considered a spiritual way to prevent the criminal from being caught. If caught the English prisoners were given bread and drinking water with chicken feces in it.

The "Feast of the Fools" which dates to the Roman Saturnalia Festival used feces in the worship ceremony. The naked participants would eat sausages (sexual, erotic penis symbol) at the church altar, paint their bodies, cross dress, and throw feces on each other.

The White historical figures involved in feces-related behaviors are plentiful. Robert Boyle (1627-1691) physicist/chemist recommended human feces be used as an eyewash. King James I (1566-1625) of England, Scotland and Ireland constantly had bowel movements on himself rather than stopping his social or sexual activities such as hunting. He was a homosexual and authorized the famous King James Version of the Bible. Martin Luther (1483-1546) said he got his spiritual inspiration while having a bowel movement. Luther believed that Satan had an anus face and farted on him. Richard III (1452-1485) of England while having a bowel movement decided to murder his nephew Terril. It seems that ancient White people believed that feces had some psychic ability. Psychologist Carl Jung (1875-1961) was obsessed with the idea that God sat on a toilet in heaven, and had a big bowel movement, which fell down to earth and broke the cathedral roof. This, he said, was God's way of telling him that his thoughts had no boundaries. Elizabeth Charlotte (1652-1722) in the court of Louis XIV in a letter to her Aunt Hanover (1694) said that during the day ladies constantly had bowel movements on themselves and would wait until evening to clean off the day load of feces. Francois Voltaire (1694-1778) while dying in bed ate his own bowel movement as a cure for his disease. Sigmund Freud (1856-1939) had erotic, sexual associations about his feces and his penis. He had constant constipation probably due to his diet and got sexual arousal from hard feces stuck in his anus.

The Caucasian nutrient poor soil (dirt) produces nutrient poor vegetables, which cause physical, mental, and emotional diseases. This causes mixed emotions about life, themselves, others, and dirt. Added to this they have disease-causing behaviors with feces. Their methods for wiping feces from their anus after bowel movements caused diseases.

Ancient Romans kept a bucket of salt water with a sponge attached to a stick soaking in it. The sponge-on-a-stick was used to wipe off the feces after they had a bowel movement. Seneca's Epistle No. 70 told of the sponge-on-a-stick ass wipers being used to choke people to death and to commit suicide. One of the members of the crowd that surrounded the Bible's Jesus at the crucifixion, poked a sponge-on-a-stick in his face (John 19:29), Matthew 27:48 and Mark 16:36). The poor could not afford this sponge on a stick luxury, so they used their bare left hand to wipe their behinds and the right hand for eating and shaking another's hand. The African slaves in America's slave colonies used their hands, grass, leaves, old rags, and soil to wipe themselves. White people thought the Black people that wipe themselves after a bowel movement had a primitive superstitious need for cleanliness. In the Middle Ages, some ass-wiper sticks were curved. This modern curved stick would confuse the wipers and often times they would mistakenly grab the wrong end of the stick. This has given rise to the expression "I got the short end of the stick (was wronged)," "I got the wrong end of the stick"," "this is a stick up" (to take advantage of, to clean out someone's money,) "stick it to him," etc. Before the sponge on a stick people such as Louis XIV used prostitutes, servants, and flea-infested wool or lace to wipe their behinds. Medieval monks used cloth, rags and/or pottery shards (dirt). In France, rich folks used grass and grew lawns for ass wiper use. Aristophanes wrote that the wealthy used onion leeks leaves. In Europe and America people use newspapers, letters and magazines as toilet paper. In 1907 crepe paper was invented to be used as toilet paper. In 1910 catalogue paper was popular as an ass wiper paper. This caused the Mail Order Catalogue Company to switch to glossy, clay coated paper to stop folks from ordering catalogues to use the paper in them for ass wiper toilet paper. Most White people and African slaves used leaves and corn cobs as wipers. White people's relationship to their body functions is surrounded by superstitions, disease producing behaviors and social practices of a dubious nature.

The hands, dirt and grass remained as staple ass wipers. Diarrhea and constipation could cause scarce ass wiper items. Enemas were a remedy for the constipating diet. *The Essence Gospel of Peace* (3 A.D. Aramaic document) says that constipation was very common and enemas were the solution. In Germany, Dr. Johann Kampf (15 AD) said that enemas could cure all diseases as well as constipation. In 1932 French scientists found that ringing a bell while giving cats an enema caused them to have a bowel movement any time a bell rang. They hoped to use the bell ringing techniques for constipation and sell anti-constipation bells. Enemas can become just as addicting as a laxative. The colon muscles get weak from laxatives and excessive enemas. An enema, colon cleanser, laxative formula, colonic irradiation and laxative stool softener addicts can stay constipated for a week or more if they do have an enema "fix."

Constipation causes flatulence-stomach gas-farts. Farts are a combination of nitrogen, oxygen, carbon dioxide, hydrogen and methane and hydrogen sulfide (rotten egg smell). Farts have served a social function amongst White people. Many fairy tales and stories include character farts. There were many fart performers in literature such as the Greek Aristophane's story *The Clouds.* Farts were edited out of the English version of Chaucer's original *Canterbury Tales.* Joseph Pujol of France, born June 1, 1857 in Marseille, was called Le Petomaine (The Fartist). He gave fart performances in 1892 at the Moulin Rouge (Red Mill). He was one of the very famous fart performers who amused packed houses of white people.

311

In Britain, up until the 1800's landholders had to appear before the feudal kings and had to perform a pagan ritual that included jumping up and farting in mid-air. It is part of cave civilization beliefs that bodily functions such as farts and excrement's (feces, urine) are symbols of life. Cave people believe that farts could be used as sacrifices to appease the spirit beasts. They believed good and bad spirits pass from one object into another object called sympathetic powers or magic. Emperor Claudius (41-54 AD) of Rome considered passing a law to allow farting at dinner. In France in the 1400's prostitutes who had to cross a bridge to sell sex had to fart while on the bridge as payment for using the bridge. Crates, (323-324) a stoic philosopher, had a farting contest with the philosopher Metrocles. Adolf Hitler (1889-1945) constantly farted. He took small amounts of belladonna and strychnine in unsuccessful attempts to stop farting.

The Bible mentions the god of human feces Baal Peor. Human as well as farts and feces sacrifices were made to Baal Peor (Psalms 106:28, Deuteronomy 29:16, Numbers 5). The African slaves were fearful of superstitious cave behavior of the uncivilized Dutch and other Whites because they did not bathe, were cannibals, drunkards, violent, homosexual, had a grunt sounding language, had bad breath, were illiterate, foul smelling, flea and lice infested, ate feces and constantly farted. White people were a diseased, animalistic, superstitious organized mob that had feces and urine in their underwear, had heterosexual and homosexual activities and masturbated in public, licked and spit on dinner tables and were usually unbathed.

White people's custom of eating human feces and drinking urine appears in the October 1880 "The Lancet" and the Bible's Isaiah 36:16, Proverbs 5:15, Kings 18:31 and in John W. Armstrong's *The Water of Life* and Dr. C. P. Mithal's *Urine Therapy*. White people urinating while having sexual intercourse is considered erotic *Urodynarnics, Principles, Practice and Application* by Mundy Stephenson and Wein, 1984. The Romans used urine as a mouthwash. White women in the city of Versailles urinated during church service. They would pass a urine bucket around to each other as a pagan spiritual ritual. In Scotland and France, after a White woman gave birth, her breasts were wiped with a man's urine. Stale urine was used as a cleanser called "Chamber Lye." Urine was used as a skin softener, shampoo and conditioner. Women used dog urine as an all-purpose beauty lotion.

An ancient European custom was to have married couples urinate on their wedding rings to spiritually protect the marriage from evil. The people who attended weddings were sprinkled with the bride's urine. In England and Ireland, the guest would drink the bride's urine. Ancient doctors such as Hippocrates, Paracelsus and Galen recommended urine as medicine. They

312

had a sympathy belief that urine's medical properties could be transferred to another person. They felt the same about other excrements(feces).

The Roman Empire had public buildings designated for the wealthy to vomit in. It was part of the sympathy belief that the wealthy's vomit smell can carry the spirit of wealth. The poor would smell the rich vomit to transfer the wealthy ability from the rich to themselves. Later in White history vomiting became associated with witchcraft and spiritual possession by demons. Therefore, vomiting became disgusting along with other bodily functions.

The scientist, religious men and medical practitioners told people not to bath. Feces foul odor were associated with healthy animals. St. Benedict who founded the Benedictine, monastic order, told people to stay dirty and to very seldom bathe. The early White Christians did not take baths, marry, drink spirits (wine) or eat flesh. They practiced a life of misery in order to enter heaven.

Hospitals in England and France were staffed with fleas and lice infested friars and other unbathed, dirty, foul smelling, constipated, farting, rotten teeth, had fleas, lice, germs, and bad breath people. The staff never changed underwear or outer clothing. A bath was considered a medicine and was not to be taken for cleanliness or pleasure. Dr. Russel wrote the book *A Dissertation Concerning the Use of Sea Water in Diseases of the Glands* (1754). He strongly advised against baths for cleanliness.

Queen Elizabeth (ruled 1558) only took one bath a month. White people generally, urinated, had bowel movements, drank and bathed in the same water. This was reported in *New Bath Guide* by Christopher Anstay (1766.) In stories such as *Gulliver's Travels* by Jonathan Swift bathing was reported as not customary. Gulliver and the people, called Yahoos, stayed dirty and did not take baths and were considered foul, smelly, stupid, and violent. They had feces and urine in their underwear and were wild. Today, if White people are having a wild fun time they will often holler "Yahoo." White people's hatred for baths is reflected in phrases such as "you are in a stew," "I am in a stew," etc. "Stew" is the old English word for bath. They kept themselves dirty and foul smelling and did not want to bathe. They would negatively refer to stew. Their health was poor and standards for health reflect it.

White people that lived in old Europe were infested with fleas. The custom of wearing fur coats comes from the abundance of fleas and lice. Fur was worn so that the fleas would get trapped in it instead of getting on the person. This did not work, but fur coats were believed to give relief from the insects. The medieval homes and early ghetto (village homes of Europe) were filled with rats, fleas, human, dog and rat feces, manure, urine, etc.

Fleas and lice were common in beds. Caucasians looked for miracle cures for their living conditions. When the cures did not work, they resorted to wearing amulets. They had three types of lice: pediculus capitis (head lice), pediculus curoris (body lice) and phthirus pubis (crab lice). Fevers caused by being bitten by lice were treated with opium. The padding for shoulders in today's White clothing started as a way to trap fleas and lice and to keep warm. The padding usually acquired a foul odor and flea colonies as revealed in *Pleasant and delightful Dialogues* by Minsheu. Bedbugs were infested in the homes and often fell from the ceilings into the beds. *[The Bed Bugs* British Museum (Natural History) Econ Series No. 5 1949]. Bedrooms had foul funky odors, feces and urine fumes, fleas and lice. This added another dimension to the already pervert bedroom sexuality.

The early White people had group sex orgies. Fathers and mothers had sex with their children and animals. Their society had heterosexual and homosexual random rapes, orgy rapes and gang rapes. White people's cannibalism adds another dimension to the social atmosphere as the sick, elderly, young strangers were hunted and killed and eaten for food or used for sex orgy feast festivities. King James (known for the King James Version of the Bible) was hyperactive, an alcoholic, constantly drooled at the mouth, was a homosexual and never bathed except for washing his fingertips before eating. He would get involved in homosexual activities in public and during mealtimes (letters and speeches of Oliver Cromwell Carlye). Danish King Christian IV visited England in 1606 got involved in heterosexual and homosexual orgies during feasts (reported by Sir John Harington). White people would get sexually excited from eating and licking feces. This was a type of coprophilia erotic love of filth *(Psychopathic Sexualis by* Krafft-Ebing). In Elizabethan England sex partners would get sexually excited by exchanging "love apples." A "love apple" is a peeled apple rubbed with the foul odors of underarm sweat or the stench of an unwashed vagina. "Love apples" were carried around by sex partners and sniffed as an aphrodisiac. Students giving apples to a teacher is a leftover fragment of this sex ritual. In a letter written by Napoleon he requested that his wife Josephine should not take a bath for two weeks so that they could have erotic sex. James Joyce (1822-1941) in a letter to his wife Nora wrote that he got aroused from her farting in his face, the sight of feces stains in her underwear and seeing her feces come out her anus. The combinations of filth and odors were a delight to the White cave civilization. The bacteria on the skin produces a musky odor (androstenol), goat like smell (isovaleric acid) and stale urine fumes (androstenone). Funky odors are sexually arousing for ancient and modern contemporary white people (i.e. musk perfume).

The body's odors are related to the body's sweat, sex organs, urine and feces. Feces is emotionally connected to "dirt" with its pagan rituals and sexual connotations. This is mixed into the subconscious mind of the white cave culture people. White people currently use many of their pagan rituals and ceremonies and social cultural behaviors and thoughts of their cave ancestors. Many pagan rituals are used in Greek fraternities, sororities, secret societies, Masonic orders, religious initiations, social gatherings, and sexual activities. Lynching of Black people is a form of sexual arousal. They would have slaves do pornographic shows.

Chapter Six

Once Upon a Time

"Our people must learn to make the analysis of what is good and healthy"

Del Jones
(The War Correspondent)

Tattoo Danger

The tattoo ink is put below the top layer of skin and used for permanent make-up cosmetics. It is estimated that 40% of adults in their 20s have tattoos as well as 10% of the children. There are at least 50 million Americans with tattoos. There are at least 20% of the teenagers with them. And, it is a fad amongst professional athletes (80%).

The tattoo can cause cancer, allergies, thyroid problems, increase skin aging, tumors, sperm defects, scarring, infections, photo toxins, react to MRI (Magnetic Resonance Imaging) and increase the absorption of radiation from cell phones, computers, and microwaves.

The tattoo industry is not regulated by the FDA. The manufactures of inks and pigments legally do not have to list the ingredients in the dyes. They use industrial grade chemicals in the dyes. These are the same ones used for printers and automobile paints. The dyes have to be kept smooth and without lumps therefore they use solutions such as denatured alcohol which can burn skin and causes cancer, benzopyrene causes cancer, and phenol causes cancer. They also use the toxic poison dibutyl phthalate, a plastic, titanium causes cancer, anti-freeze (glycol), and embalming fluid formaldehyde. These ingredients are put in the skin and absorbed in the blood and circulate in the body and brain.

The inks are made from ground up powder metals such as lead, copper, iron, aluminum, titanium, etc.

Ink Color Ingredients

White
- ∞ White Lead
  - o Cause eye and lung problems, nerve damage, reproductive problems
- ∞ Barium Sulfate
  - o Used to make paint, glass, rubber, forms poisons compounds
- ∞ Zinc Oxide
  - o Eye problems, digestion, skin, hair, kidney problems
- ∞ Iron
  - o Digestion problems, skin disease, reproductive problems

Black
- ∞ Soot/Carbon
  - o Causes lung problems, heart disease

Blue
- ∞ Copper
  - o Lung, brain kidney damage and liver problems
- ∞ Aluminum
  - o Liver and brain problems
- ∞ Silicate
  - o Demineralizes bones
- ∞ Pthalo cyanine
  - o Heart, liver, kidney, skin, and lung problems, used in furniture, skin aging, cancer, and toys

Brown
- ∞ Iron Oxide mixed with unpurified dirt (clay)

Green
- ∞ Chromium Oxide
  - o Allergy, inflammation, itching, skin sores, lung problems
- ∞ Malachite
  - o Kidney disease, toxin
- ∞ Iron
- ∞ Lead

Orange
- ∞ Disazodiarylide
  - o Lung and liver problems
- ∞ Cadmium Seleno Sulfide
  - o Kidney, lung, and bone problems

Yellow
- ∞ Cadmium Yellow
  - o Liver, lung and kidney problems, dizziness, headaches, chills

Violet
- ∞ Manganese Ammonium
  - o Swelling of cells, sex organ problem
- ∞ Dioxazine/carbazole
  - o Lung and digestive problems, coal tar cause cancer

Red
- ∞ Mercury/cinnabar

318

- o   Nerve damage, loss of sense, poison
∞   Iron Rust
∞   Naptha
- o   Feminization of boys, headaches, nausea, anemia, lung and kidney problems, sperm defects, thyroid disease
∞   Cadmium

Electronic Cigarettes Disease
(Cooked tobacco and marijuana)

The vapors are inhaled in aerosol solutions have cooked nicotine oil and cannabinol oil, THC drug cartridges and other liquids and flavorings. They cause oral and lung cancer. The high level of toxic nano particles with very small sizes cause nerve damage, diabetes, asthma, heart disease, strokes, cause antibiotic resistance.

They contain:
∞   Formaldehyde – embalming fluid cancer
∞   Propylene glycol – anti-freeze, mouth and throat problems
∞   Glycerin – damages the pancreas
∞   Carbon Monoxide – poison
∞   3 to 4 times stronger drugs

Water pipes are not safer. They only mix water vapor with the drops of cooked cannabinol and nicotine oils. They can inhale 100% to 200% more smoke than a single smoked cigarette or E-cigarette. Sharing the water pipe increases catching (transmitting) herpes, hepatitis, tuberculosis, and viruses.

The strength of nicotine and cannabinol have been hybridized to be stronger. The toxic chemicals in GMO marijuana are very dangerous. You would have to smoke 4 tobacco cigarettes to equal the effect of 1 marijuana cigarette. The vapor (electronic, water pipe) content of poisons is 2 to 3 times higher.

Cooked nicotine oil and cannabinol oil are addicting and have increased the amount of teenagers and children below 13 years old to smoke.

About the Author

Llaila (La-ee-la) Afrika is a holistic health practitioner. He has been in the health profession for over 40 years. His background includes working as a social worker, psychotherapist, group facilitator, community organizer, nurse, and naturopath. Llaila has a doctorate in Naturopathy diploma and is a Certified Addictionologist, Certified Acupuncturist, Massage Therapist and a licensed Traditional Healer in Ghana, Togo, and Benin. He is essentially self-taught in holistic sciences. Llaila is an author, teacher, lecturer, practitioner, and historian.

Llaila lectures and teaches certification classes with his wife Dr. Melanie Stevenson. The classes are of a wide variety such as Holistic Nutritional Counselor, Anatomy and Physiology, Massage, Needle-less Acupuncture, Ethical Midwifery, Hypnosis, Holistic Nutrition, Holistic Sex and Relationship, Holistic Skin Care and Analysis, Touch Diagnosis, Holistic Diagnosis, etc.

Index

323

SUGGESTED READING

A Healthy Foods and Spiritual Nutrition Handbook   *Keith T. Wright*

A National History of the Senses	*Diane Ackerman*
African Holistic Health	*Llaila Afrika*
AIDS, Africa and Racism	*Richard Rosalin Chirimunta*
Basic Herbs for Health and Healing	*Rashan Abdul Hakim*
Black Spark White Fire	*Richard Poe*
Blueprint for Black Power	*Amos N. Wilson*
Caribbean Medicine	*C. Wolde Kyte*
Claim the Victory	*Keefa K. Lorraine*
Colon Hygiene	*John H. Kellogg*
Dick Gregory's Natural Diet for Folks Who Eat	*Dick Gregory*
End Product: The First Taboo	*Dan Sabbath*
Forever Young	*Dr. Paul Goss*
Guyanese Seed of Vegetables	*Yvonne John*
Deserts the Vegetarians and Food Lovers Paradise	*Yvonne John*
Heal Thyself Cookbook for Natural Living	*Diana Ciccone*
Heal Thyself for Health and Longevity	*Queen Afua*
Health Teachings of the Ageless Wisdom	*R.A. Staughn*
How to Eat to Live: Volume I and II	*Elijah* Muhammad
How to Select and Combine, Fruits, Vegetables and Tubers, Through their Color-Powers	*Doctor Ignatius*
Le Petomane	*Jean Nohain*
Let Us Now Praise Famous Men	*James Agee and Walker Evans*
Melanin—Protective Intoxicant Capabilities in the Black Human and Its Influence on Behavior	*Carole Barnes*
Melanin—The Chemical Key to Great Blackness	*Carol Barnes*
Memories, Dreams, Reflections	*Carl Jung*
Message in A Bottle	*Alfred "Coach" Powell*
Mother Nature	*Dick Gregory*

Nutrition, Herbal and Homeopathic Guide to Healing	*Ra Un Neter Amen 1*
On Farting	*Michael Kimball*
Optimizing Health Nutrition	*Ra Un Neter Amen I*
Pyramids of Power (Ancient African Centered Approach to Optimum Health)	*John T. Chissdl, M.D.*
The Invasion of the Body Snatchers	*Del Jones*
Textbook of Black-Related Diseases	*Richard Williams*
The Fantasy of Dirt	*Lawrence Kubie*
The Foul and the Fragrant	*Alain Corbin*
The Harlem Hospital Story	*Peter Bailey*
The Healers	*Ayi Kwesi Arrnah*
The Last Great Plague Upon Man, AIDS Related Murder Tools	*Georges C. Hatonn*
The Medical Question	*A.A. Erz*
The Ontogenesis of the Interest in Money	*Sandor Ferenczi*
The Rejuvenating Plants of Tropical Africa	*Albert A. Enti*
The Science and Romance of Selected Herbs Used in Medicine and Religious Ceremony	*Anthony Andoh*
The Standard Edition of The Complete Psychological Works of Sigmund Freud	*James Strachey*
The Straight Dope	*Cecil Adams*
The Sweet Scent of Decomposition "Forget Baudrillard"	*Bryan Turner*
The United Independent Compensatory Code/System/Concept: A Textbook/Workbook for Thought, Speech and/or Actions for Victims of Racism (White Supremacy)	*Neely Fuller, Jr.*
Through the Alimentary Canal with a Gun and a Camera	*George Chappell*
To Save the Blood of Black Babies	*Kiarri T. H. Cheatwood*
Scatologic Rites of All Nations	*John G. Bourke*

Printed in Great Britain
by Amazon